Clinical Research in Communicative Disorders

Clinical Research in Communicative Disorders

Principles and Strategies

M. N. Hegde

Department of
Communicative Disorders
California State University,
Fresno

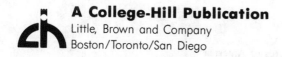

A College-Hill Publication
Little, Brown and Company
Boston/Toronto/San Diego

College-Hill Press
A Division of
Little, Brown and Company (Inc.)
34 Beacon Street
Boston, Massachusetts 02108

Library of Congress Cataloging in Publication Data
Main entry under title:

Hegde, M. N., 1941–
    Clinical research in communicative disorders.

    "A College-Hill publication."
    Bibliography: p. 431
    Includes indexes.
        1. Communicative disorders—Research—Technique.
    2. Research—Methodology. I. Title. [DNLM: 1. Communi-
    cative Disorders. 2. Research. 3. Research Design.
    WM 475 H453c]
    RC429.H43 1987   616.86′5′0072   87–3631

ISBN 0-316-35434-1

Printed in the United States of America

C O N T E N T S

Part One: Science and the Scientific Method

Chapter 1
Why Study Science and Research Methods? 2

The need to study scientific methods, 4 ■ The need to produce in-house knowledge, 6 ■ Why many clinicians do not do research, 8 ■ Problems associated with certain research practices, 9 ■ Problems associated with the education and training models, 13 ■ Evaluation of research, 16 ■ Study Guide, 18

Chapter 2
An Introduction To Research: The Formal and Formative Approaches 20

What is research?, 22 ■ Why scientists do research?, 23 ■ How is research done?, 31 ■ Serendipity in research, 37 ■ Concluding remarks, 40 ■ Study Guide, 41

Chapter 3
Science And Its Basic Concepts 43

Popular misconceptions about science, 44 ■ What is science?, 45 ■ Outcome of scientific activity, 50 ■ Variables and their types, 52 ■ Causality and functional analysis, 56 ■ Experiment and experimental control, 60 ■ Hypotheses in scientific research, 61 ■ Theories and scientific reasoning, 65 ■ Theories and scientific laws, 69 ■ Data and evidence, 70 ■ Study Guide, 72

Chapter 4
Types of Research 74

Ex post facto research, 75 ■ Normative research, 79 ■ Standard-group comparisons, 84 ■ Experimental research, 87 ■ Clinical and applied research, 93 ■ Sample surveys, 96 ■ Evaluation research, 98 ■ The relation between research types and questions, 99 ■ Study Guide, 101

**Part Two:
Clinical
Research
Designs**

**Chapter 5
Observation and Measurement   103**

Observation and measurement, 104 ■
Philosophies of measurement, 105 ■ Traditional
levels of measurement, 107 ■ Some measures of
communicative behaviors, 109 ■ Client-assisted
measurement, 117 ■ Indirect measures, 118 ■
Covert measurement, 119 ■ The observer in the
measurement process, 121 ■ Mechanical aids to
observation and measurement,124 ■ Reliability of
measurement, 126 ■ Study Guide, 129

**Chapter 6
Research Designs: An Introduction   134**

What are research designs?, 135 ■ The structure
and logic of experimental designs, 136 ■
Variability: some philosophical considerations, 137
■ Intrinsic Variability, 138 ■ Extrinsic Variability,
140 ■ Experimental designs: means of controlling
variability, 141 ■ Validity of experimental
operations, 143 ■ Internal validity, 144 ■
Generality (External Validity), 151 ■ Concluding
remarks, 159 ■ Study guide, 161

**Chapter 7
The Group Design Strategy   164**

Basic terminology and characteristics of group
designs, 165 ■ Preexperimental designs, 167 ■
True experimental designs, 171 ■ Designs to
evaluate multiple treatments, 179 ■ Factorial
designs, 181 ■ Quasi-experimental designs, 186
■ Time-series designs, 190 ■ Counterbalanced
within-subjects designs, 196 ■ Correlational
analysis design, 206 ■ Group designs in clinical
research, 207 ■ Chapter summary, 209 ■ Study
guide, 213

**Chapter 8
Single-Subject Designs   216**

Basic terminology and characteristics of single-
subject designs, 217 ■ Control mechanisms in
single-subject designs, 221 ■ Preexperimental
single-subject designs, 241 ■ The ABA design,
242 ■ The BAB design, 246 ■ The ABAB design,
247 ■ The multiple baseline designs, 250 ■ The

ABACA/ACABA design, 259 ■ The alternating
treatments design, 261 ■ Ineffective treatment in
multiple treatment evaluations, 265 ■ The
interactional design, 266 ■ The changing criterion
design, 270 ■ Designs to assess response
maintenance, 271 ■ Other single-subject designs,
273 ■ Single-subject designs in clinical research,
275 ■ Chapter summary, 276 ■ Study guide, 279

Chapter 9
Generality Through Replications 282

Direct replication, 283 ■ Systematic replication,
287 ■ Failed replications, 291 ■ Treatment
variables and treatment packages, 294 ■ Homo-
and heterogeneity of subjects: some
considerations, 296 ■ Study guide, 298

Chapter 10
Comparative Evaluation of Design
Strategies 300

Research questions and investigative strategies,
301 ■ Advantages and disadvantages of design
strategies, 310 ■ Problems common to design
strategies, 313 ■ Philosophic considerations in
evaluation, 315 ■ The investigator in the design
selection process, 315 ■ The final criterion:
soundness of data, 316 ■ Chapter summary, 317
■ Study guide, 321

Chapter 11
Designs Versus Paradigms in
Research 323

Limitations of exclusively methodological
approaches, 324 ■ Research methods and subject
matters, 324 ■ Philosophy as methodology, 326
■ Philosophy of subject matters, 327 ■
Philosophy of the science of speech and language,
329 ■ Philosophical ways of handling
methodological problems, 339 ■ The interplay
between philosophy and methodology, 342
■ Study guide, 343

Part Three: Doing, Reporting, and Evaluating Research

Chapter 12
How To Formulate Research Questions 346

Where are the research questions?, 347 ■ How to formulate research questions, 348 ■ Preparation of theses and dissertations, 359 ■ Study guide, 361

Chapter 13
How To Write Research Reports 363

Format of scientific reports, 364 ■ Writing without bias, 373 ■ Good writing: Some principles, 374 ■ Structural principles, 374 ■ Conceptual considerations, 384 ■ Writing style, 394 ■ Write and rewrite, 395 ■ Study guide, 396

Chapter 14
How To Evaluate Research Reports 399

Professionals as consumers of research, 400 ■ Understanding and evaluating research, 400 ■ Evaluation of research, 401 ■ Internal consistency evaluation, 402 ■ External relevance evaluation, 405 ■ Evaluation of research reports: an outline, 407 ■ Evaluation and appreciation of research, 411 ■ Study guide, 412

Chapter 15
Ethics Of Research 413

Honesty and integrity of scientists, 414 ■ Effects of science on society, 416 ■ The ethics of treatment evaluation, 417 ■ Protection of human subjects, 420 ■ Ethical issues relative to animal subjects, 427 ■ Dissemination of research findings, 428 ■ Study guide, 429

References 431
Appendix 437
Author Index 441
Subject Index 445

■ P R E F A C E

I am a student and an instructor of the philosophy and methodology of science and research. In my teaching, I have found it necessary to supplement information from a variety of sources. I knew that several of my colleagues who teach courses on science and research were doing the same to make their courses most relevant and useful to graduate students. To me, this meant that we did not have a comprehensive text book on science and research. This book is an effort to fulfill that need.

My own teaching experience, and discussions with many of my colleagues, suggested that such a book should address the following concerns. The first is the basic concepts of science and scientific methods. The book should point out the need to study science and research methods, and summarize the basic concepts of science and research. It should describe the true and lively process of research, not an idealized and frighteningly formalized process that typically discourages the beginning student from further study of science and research. The book should give an adequate description of the different kinds of research that are conducted in communicative disorders. A discussion of observation and measurement, which are the basic tools of science, would need to be provided.

The second concern is clinical research design. Most books on research designs tend to be statistically oriented, since the enormously prestigious analysis of variance is constantly confused with experimental design. The book should present the experimental designs, not methods of data analysis under the guise of designs of research. Furthermore, the book should address both group and single-subject designs. Generally speaking, most books that do offer information on research designs focus almost exclusively on group designs, while the clinically more relevant single-subject designs are not well represented. On the other hand, there are some books that focus exclusively on single-subject designs. There are not, however, many books that present adequate information on *both* the design strategies. Regardless of one's own methodological preference and practice, a critical user and producer of research must have a knowledge of group as well as single-subject design approaches. It was thought that a single source that offered descriptions and comparative evaluations of both the strategies would be useful to students and researchers alike.

A third concern is a discussion of some important philosophical issues that are an inexorable part of science and research. Research is based on philosophy as well as methodology. There is a tremendous lack of appreciation of the philosophical bases of research. Therefore, it was thought that the book should at least raise the issue of the philosophy of research, as a stimulus to further discussion.

The fourth concern is the practical aspect of doing, writing or reporting, and evaluating research. Students need suggestions on where to find and how to refine research questions, how to find current research trends, how to search the literature, and how to select designs that help answer those questions. They also need information on how to get started on theses and dissertations. Writing style and writing skills pose a major problem to instructors and students. It was thought that the book should offer basic information on principles of good writing. Furthermore, students should also know how to evaluate published research reports.

The fifth concern is the ethics of research. Science and research are ethical activities. From the beginning, science and research must be taught with due regard for the ethical principles that restrain research. A textbook on research should summarize ethical principles that govern research activities.

I have written this book with those five concerns as guiding principles. An overall concern was to make it especially relevant to clinical research in communicative disorders, and to write it in a less formal and, I would hope, more readable style that reflects the process of research more accurately than the style that typically formalizes research to an unnatural extent.

The fun I have had in writing this book is partly due to my fascination with science and its philosophy, and partly due to the encouragement and reinforcement I have received from my family, my students, Dr. Raymond Kent of the University of Wisconsin at Madison, and Dr. Sadanand Singh and his editorial staff at College-Hill Press.

My wife Prema and my son Manu have been a part of all of my writings. This book, which I began to write soon after completing *Treatment Procedures in Communicative Disorders*, would not have been finished without their full support. Using his computer, Manu has prepared all of the graphs printed in this book. Without his quick grasp of designs and data presentation techniques and his technical expertise in computer graphics, this book would not have been on schedule.

My students at both the undergraduate and graduate levels have been generous in their support and encouragement. They have always tolerated, and often appreciated, my unlimited passion to teach science and research anytime and anywhere. Many students in my graduate seminar on research methods have offered excellent comments on earlier versions of several chapters in this book.

I am grateful to Dr. Kent for his review of the manuscript. His constructive criticisms and suggestions have helped me improve the quality of this book, and his enthusiasm has meant a great deal to me. Any limitations of the book, however, are entirely my own responsibility.

Finally, I would like to express my appreciation to Dr. Singh and his outstanding editorial staff, especially Associate Editor Marie Linvill. Their constant support and courtesy have made it possible to keep writing and finish on schedule. ■

■ P A R T **O N E**

Science and the Scientific Method

■ CHAPTER 1

Why Study Science and Research Methods?

■ The need to study scientific methods, 4

■ The need to produce in-house knowledge, 6

■ Why many clinicians do not do research, 8

■ Problems associated with certain research practices, 9

■ Problems associated with the education and training models, 13

■ Evaluation of research, 16

■ Study guide, 18

C ommunicative disorders is both an academic discipline and a clinical profession. As an academic discipline, it seeks to study and understand normal as well as disordered communication. As a clinical profession, it is concerned with the methods of assessing and treating various disorders of hearing, speech, language, voice, and fluency. An academic discipline can research practical problems without applying the information it generates. A biochemist, for example, may research a new drug that can be used in treating a particular disease, but he or she may not actually treat patients with that disease. In communicative disorders, researchers of various disorders and treatment procedures may also apply that information in the treatment of disordered communication. In this sense, communicative disorders is simultaneously concerned with both scientific and professional matters.

During the historical course of the development of communicative disorders as a discipline, the professional aspects, rather than the scientific bases, received greater attention. This is understandable because the starting point of our discipline was a professional concern to understand and treat certain speech disorders, especially stuttering and articulation disorders. The profession had to start providing clinical services without the benefit of a lengthy history of controlled experimental research to back up clinical practice. Borrowing from various fields of basic study and applied research, the speech–language pathologist of the early days began to treat various disorders of communication. Equally understandable is the trend that dominated the next several decades, in which the emphasis was on expanding clinical services rather than conducting experimental research to produce a scientific basis for those clinical services.

One of the unfortunate historical lessons of many human service professions, including that of communicative disorders, is that clinical services can continue to be offered without a strong experimental data base. Such services may be supported by subjectively solidified clinical experience, uncontrolled observations, anecdotes widely circulated by "authorities" in the field, descriptive research, and speculative theories. Experimental research in which treatment techniques are systematically evaluated may be lacking. As a result, clinical services offered by a profession may not have a strong foundation of experimentally evaluated evidence. However, this may not deter a profession from offering services, partly because of practical exigencies and partly because something better is not available.

The problem with such a historical trend is that the situation does not change quickly when experimental research information begins to flow. The clinical practice of established clinicians may continue to be based on old and unverified bases. Often, it takes several years to affect clinical practice on a wider scale because the research information must be incorporated into the training of new clinicians.

THE NEED TO STUDY SCIENTIFIC METHODS

It is now widely recognized that the profession of communicative disorders needs to strengthen the scientific bases of its clinical practice. The need to put our clinical practice on experimental foundations is growing because of many legal, social, professional, and scientific reasons.

Legal and Social Considerations

The legal circumstances that are faced by the profession stem from various sources. One of the well-recognized sources of the influence of the federal government is the Education for all Handicapped Children Act. It went into effect in 1977 and introduced some significant changes in the delivery of special educational services, including those of communicative disorders. Some of the most significant requirements under the law are that the special educational services must be oriented to the individual and that the service programs must have specific procedures, objectives, and evaluative criteria. The law places considerable emphasis on *clinician accountability* in that the effects of treatment programs must be documented objectively so that they can be verified by independent observers. Such documentation requires that changes in client behaviors be measured systematically. As we shall see shortly, these and other requirements of the law are in harmony with the requirements of *scientific clinical practice.*

Other kinds of legal concerns necessitate a more objective and scientific clinical practice. There has been a slow but steady increase in third-party payment for clinical speech, language, and hearing services. Various government agencies and private insurance firms that pay for the services are demanding more and more systematic documentation of the need, the procedures, and the outcome of such services. Uniform and objective means of evaluating treatment effects are being encouraged by agencies that pay for services.

Many social concerns are also leading us in the direction of clinical practice based on scientific methods. The profession is taking several steps to increase the public awareness of speech and language problems and the services that are available to individuals with those problems. Consequently, an increasing number of individuals and families are seeking and paying for services in private clinics and hospitals. At the same time, many people who are seeking services are also inclined to question the effectiveness of those services. In case of speech, language, and hearing services, this trend is probably in its early stage, but it can be expected to increase. It is logical to expect that widespread social awareness of speech, language, and hearing problems, and higher demands for services, coupled with the higher costs of service delivery, will inevitably bring more thorough scrutiny of professional practices.

Professional and Scientific Considerations

Regardless of the legal and social requirements, there are professional reasons to develop a scientifically sound clinical discipline. Currently, there is much concern regarding our standing in the community of clinical professions and scientific disciplines. There is a growing concern that the profession of communicative disorders does not have high social visibility. Some persons believe that the profession is not well recognized by other established or recently developed professions, such as medicine or clinical psychology.

A profession can try to draw attention to itself by various means. It may seek better legal recognition and protection by more effective lobbying efforts. Extensive public relations and public awareness campaigns may be launched. Services may be more aggressively publicized by advertisements in local and national media. Since all professions have a business side, most of these efforts are necessary. The current thinking within the profession of communicative disorders is that the services can be marketed ethically and that there is a need to do so (Yoder, 1984). Such activities can yield relatively quick results. However, to build a lasting and more solid reputation, the profession, in addition to taking all those steps, must put its practice on a scientific footing. In the long run, no amount of public relations campaigning can compensate for questionable and subjectively evaluated clinical practice. In fact, generally beneficial public awareness can also expose the inherent and widespread weaknesses of a profession.

Better reputation and higher visibility are often associated with professions that are scientific and technological. A profession can be expected to make significant progress when practices are based upon methods of science and effects are evaluated in objective ways. The ideal to strive for is a solid scientific discipline and a clinical profession with a single identity. Currently, this looks like an ideal that is going to take some time to achieve, but we need to start working in that direction now. In recent years, many professionals and scientists have drawn attention to the need to strengthen the scientific bases of the profession of communicative disorders (Costello, 1979; Kent, 1983; Minifie, 1983; Moll, 1983; Ringel, 1972; Ringel, Trachtman, and Prutting, 1984; Zimmermann, 1984).

The typical argument supporting a more scientific orientation is made on the basis of the legal, social, and professional requirements described so far. Such requirements are compelling, and anything that makes us more scientific is welcome. However, a discipline or a profession need not be driven entirely by such requirements. In other words, one need not necessarily face legal, social, and professional image-oriented reasons and requirements to be more scientific. Although the statement may sound tautological, science itself is a good reason to be scientific. The logical beauty, methodologic elegance, and practical benefits of science antecede all of the legal, social, and professional pressures.

It is possible that had the profession heeded the call of science from its inception, most of the legal and social pressures would have become superfluous. Clinicians who by training and practice follow the methods of science do not need a push from Public Law 94-142 to write treatment targets in measurable terms. For such clinicians, the requirement that changes in client behaviors must be documented objectively will not come as news or as a legal nuisance. Their personal history of training and education will suffice for such purposes. Surely, social and legal demands can force clinicians to be systematic and objective in their clinical work, but those with a strong scientific background are inclined to be so regardless of such demands. The clinician who wishes to evaluate treatment effects under controlled conditions may not be driven by concerns regarding bad professional image. Such a clinician has better reasons, including science itself. In spite of not being overly concerned with bad image, scientifically competent clinicians probably help counteract its effects more effectively than those who are concerned but continue to offer questionable services.

These comments should not be construed as a negative evaluation of legal, social, and professional reasons to be more scientific. In fact, governments, social groups, and professional bodies have an obligation to protect the rights of people who seek (and thereby support) professional services. Societal and regulatory forces are necessary for smooth and socially beneficial operations of professions as well as sciences. Such regulatory forces have helped us move in the right direction. These comments are meant to underscore an additional and often neglected reason to be more systematic, responsible, and objective in clinical work: the philosophy and methodology of science, which are capable of providing unsurpassed safeguards for both the profession and the public. At the same time, science gives us an unlimited and exciting opportunity to make significant advances in all areas of professional endeavor.

THE NEED TO PRODUCE IN-HOUSE KNOWLEDGE

As noted before, all applied disciplines go through a period during which the scientific data base is still being formed while the need to practice the profession takes precedence. During this stage, the profession is dependent on other disciplines—both basic and applied—for a knowledge base. For certain kinds of information, the profession of speech–language pathology historically depended on some nonclinical disciplines such as linguistics, experimental psychology, and child psychology. It has also depended on clinical professions such as medicine, and basic sciences such as physiology and physics.

Speech–language pathology has been a borrower for a long time, perhaps too much of a borrower and too little of an innovator. It borrowed not only basic or applied information but also conceptual frameworks, theories, paradigms, models, and methods of investigation and data analysis. As a result, the slowly developing traditions of research have been extensively influenced by other disciplines that have offered methods and theories of varying degrees of validity, reliability, relevancy, and applicability.

Unless a discipline quickly begins to produce its own data base, it will continue to borrow theories and methods that may or may not be appropriate for studying its subject matter. The only way some professions can begin to generate their own data bases is to train their practitioners to do research. Some professions have the luxury of receiving a large and varied amount of custom-produced research information from outside their professions. Medicine, for example, has chemists, biochemists, physiologists, anatomists, biologists, geneticists, bioengineers, and a variety of technologists and technical product manufacturers, who do research and supply theoretical information as well as practical technology. Speech–language pathology, on the other hand, cannot depend on many different kinds of researchers geared toward supplying relevant basic and applied information. Much of the information and technology we borrow is not produced for us; its relevance to us is mostly incidental and, in some unfortunate cases, mistaken.

Specialists in communicative disorders must produce their own knowledge base and technology, but this does not mean that they should not borrow what is relevant and useful from other subject matters. Like other professionals, we will continue to borrow what is relevant and useful. Many fields of knowledge are interrelated, and therefore they benefit from each other's research. Nevertheless, what is urgently needed in our field is a systematic effort to increase the in-house knowledge base and technology. A discipline cannot always expect other subject matters to produce the basic scientific information necessary to understand its subject matter. A profession cannot always expect others to produce a relevant and effective technology. As stated by Kent (1983), "A profession that provides its own research base is much more in charge of its own destiny than a profession that doesn't" (p. 76). A similar opinion was expressed by Flower (1983), who stated that "if we must rely on others both to achieve the scientific and technological advances and then to apply those advances within our field, we cannot pretend to be a mature and autonomous profession" (p. 13).

The most significant problem with increasing the amount of in-house knowledge is the scarcity of research institutions and sustained research programs in communicative disorders. Many university programs in communicative disorders are not research oriented, and large institutions that specialize in research are few or nonexistent. Producing a systematic body of reliable and valid scientific information is a slow process even under the best possible conditions. Therefore, under the existing conditions, the accumulation of valid knowledge in communicative disorders will be a prolonged process. There seems to be no easy or quick solution to this problem. We must take several steps in order to increase the amount of research. Among others, we can seek more government and private research funds, increase the number of theses produced by master's degree candidates, accelerate research efforts at existing research and teaching institutions, and establish new programmatic research.

A different tactic, which can be used in addition to all others, is to recruit practitioners into the kind of research that does not detract from clinical activities. That is, the field can make an effort to increase on-line research by the practicing clinicians. Since the majority of persons in the field are clinicians, even a slight increase in the number of clinicians doing on-line research may have a considerable impact. This is the kind of in-house knowledge base that can have immediate and simultaneous clinical and theoretical significance.

WHY MANY CLINICIANS DO NOT DO RESEARCH

It is well known that a majority of clinicians do not do research. They are busy serving their clients, naturally. Even so, there are many other reasons (Costello, 1979; Costello, Punch, Schery, & Shriberg, 1984; Kent, 1983, 1985; Perkins, 1985; Ringel, Trachtman, & Prutting, 1984). Most clinicians do not have the needed extra time for research. Besides, when research is thought of as something unrelated to clinical service, the clinicians obviously cannot do research. Besides, the scheduling of their clients may be best suited for clinical work but bad for research. When clients are seen twice weekly for a few minutes each time, it may not be possible to collect certain kinds of data.

Settings in which clinicians serve their clients may not place an emphasis on research. Many public schools and hospitals do not require research from clinicians and may not even encourage it. From a practical standpoint, however, a considerable amount of research, both good and bad, is done when research is required or valued in a given setting. It may also be noted that bad research can be done even when someone "wanted" to do research while it was not required to achieve promotions or pay raises. In many settings research is often done over and above one's regular duties. When it is not required for professional advancement, the administration is not likely to support research to any great extent.

It is also possible that clinicians themselves assume (1) that they are not well prepared to do research and (2) that research does not necessarily help them or their colleagues. Both of these assumptions may have some empirical validity. It is possible that many speech–language pathologists have not had sufficient academic and practical experience in research methods. In order to do research, one should also be up to date in the slowly but surely changing field of knowledge in the discipline. The pressures of day-to-day professional practice may not be conducive to spending a considerable amount of time and energy on reading the literature. Though significant advances in communicative disorders have been few and far between, the "information explosion" has been tremendous in recent years. It does take much time just to keep up with published research. Therefore, many clinicians may think that they lack the technical knowledge of scientific procedures and current information needed to do research.

The second assumption that research is not necessarily of practical help may also be based on experience. There is some question regarding the extent to which research affects day-to-day clinical practice (Barlow, Hayes, & Nelson, 1984). In treating clients, most clinicians probably depend upon their past training and clinical experience. Experimentally evaluated new techniques advocated by research clinicians are not automatically applied in a wide variety of professional settings. Often, popular but unsupported theories have a greater influence on clinical practice than technical research reports.

As in clinical psychology (Cohen, 1979), speech–language pathologists may also be influenced to a great extent by workshops, presentations, discussions with colleagues, and lectures on the "latest" techniques. However, those who have given frequent workshops may think that clinicians rarely apply exactly what they learn in workshops and seminars. Some individuals who attend workshops frequently tend to agree equally well with totally contradictory approaches. Most clinicians assimilate what they hear (or read) in terms of their past experience and apply new techniques in modified ways. Such modifications are not necessarily undesirable. The only problem is that it is difficult to identify successful techniques because of unspecified and varied modifications of published techniques. In any case, the disturbing possibility remains that controlled and technical research does not affect clinical practice to the extent it should.

A more serious and valid reason for the belief that research does not necessarily help clinical practice is that there is a significant body of research that does *not* help clinical practice. I am not referring to basic research, which is not expected to give immediate solutions to practical problems. I am referring to the kinds of research that *are* expected to solve clinical problems. Purported clinical research may also frustrate clinicians. Clinicians who read and evaluate such research to sharpen their clinical skills may be disillusioned about the usefulness of all kinds of clinical research. In other words, certain research practices may generate a justifiable skepticism regarding the relevance of research to clinical practice.

PROBLEMS ASSOCIATED WITH CERTAIN RESEARCH PRACTICES

There are multiple modes of clinical research, and not all of them are equally helpful to the clinician in solving *current* practical problems. In Chapter 4, I shall describe different types of research in some detail. Here it may be noted that experimental–clinical research is likely to produce results that help solve immediate practical problems of clinicians. Many other types of research may lead to solutions to practical problems, but only in the future.

At the very outset, it must be clear that clinical usefulness is not the only criterion by which the value of research is determined. Basic research often does not have immediate practical significance. However, it is valuable because it might help explain a phenomenon, put unrelated observations in a single perspective, suggest new lines of experimental analysis, or produce a discovery with profound clinical impact. Thus, in the long run, basic research may produce data that can help solve the practical problems. Every discipline needs basic research, and if there is a problem in communicative disorders in this regard, it is that we do not have enough basic research.

The main problem with current research practice is that much of the research is neither basic nor experimentally clinical. Basic research can help secure the future of a discipline, while experimental–clinical research can help solve the current practical problems. Basic research creates a strong scientific base for a profession and experimental–clinical research focuses on disorders and variables that can change them. However, when not enough time and energies are devoted to these two kinds of research, we can neither solve current clinical problems nor be confident that the problems will be solved in the future. In such a situation, skepticism regarding research is inevitable.

It should also be recognized, however, that the clinical irrelevancy of "clinical research" is not the only reason why some clinicians may have a negative approach to research in general. Other factors may also contribute to clinicians' negative evaluation of research. First, if clinicians do not appreciate basic research, then their inadequate education and training in the philosophy and methodology of science may be blamed. This situation does exist to a certain extent. Second, if clinicians do not appreciate experimental–clinical research that shows better methods of treating disorders of communication, their education must be blamed somewhat. Probably this situation also exists to some degree. A majority of clinicians are slow in using techniques that have been evaluated experimentally. Instead, they may continue to use techniques that have an inherent appeal to them. Third, if clinicians do not find a significant body of clinical research that can be applied in clinical work, then the research practices within the field must take the blame.

Education and training programs must be concerned with the first two reasons, and research scientists and clinicians must be concerned with the third reason. To assess this problem, we must consider the type and quality of clinical research and the education and training of clinicians.

Possibly, clinicians who can evaluate current clinical research find very little that is applicable. This is because much research in the field is not directed toward developing new treatment procedures and evaluating the effects of existing techniques. Even journals such as *Language, Speech, and Hearing Services in Schools* (LSHSS), which one would expect to publish treatment research, may disappoint clinicians. A majority of papers published in many issues of LSHSS relate to description and assessment, not treatment (Kent and Fair, 1985). To some degree, this is true of the *Journal of Speech and Hearing Research* and the *Journal of Speech and Hearing Disorders*. Under the editorship of Perkins and Costello, there has been an increase in the publication of treatment-related research in the *Journal of Speech and Hearing Disorders*, but still not to the extent needed, simply because not many studies of this kind are submitted. On the other hand, there is plenty of speculatively theoretical writing in the discipline, and much of the research is concerned with finding differences between "normal" and "disordered" groups of subjects. Many studies attempt to establish norms of various communicative behaviors. In addition, classifying speech and language behaviors with no regard to their causal variables (structural analysis of language and speech) is very popular. This kind of research is typically justified because of the "clinical implications," but the research does not necessarily provide for more effective treatment procedures. Some clinicians who begin to read research reports of this kind may eventually stop reading them. Clinicians decide to wait until the promise of the "implications" is fulfilled in newly developed and experimentally evaluated treatment or assessment procedures.

An unfortunate research trend in communicative disorders is that those who suggest clinical implications of their nonclinical research do not take time to test those implications using clients seeking professional services as subjects. There seems to be an implicit assumption on the part of many research specialists in communicative disorders that to hypothesize is their job, but that to verify is someone else's. Many researchers betray a striking lack of curiosity about the clinical validity of their own hypotheses. Consequently, they have created a new division of labor: some researchers generate hypotheses and other researchers verify them. Unfortunately, this division of labor has not worked well because many researchers are more interested in generating their own hypotheses than in verifying their own or anybody else's.

It is possible that if studies of a different kind were to be frequently published in journals, the clinicians' evaluation of research would be more favorable. This kind of research is experimental *and* clinical. It addresses issues of immediate practical significance. This strategy involves current clinical action, not a promise of some future clinical possibility. For example, research may be concerned with different target behaviors and their clinical relevance, different treatment variables and their experimental effects, different tactics of response maintenance after treatment, issues in the measurement or assessment of disorders and behaviors, and independent variables that may be responsible for normal as well as disordered speech and language behaviors, just to sample a few. Not only are research studies like these of immediate clinical significance, but in many cases they are identical with clinical services. Clinicians who are trained to understand and appreciate this kind of research are likely to keep in touch with clinically relevant research.

Of the kinds of research that are of immediate clinical value, one kind must be singled out because it provides the most vivid example of an integrated research and service model. This is the type of research in which (1) the relevance of alternate behaviors to be treated and (2) the techniques by which behaviors can be treated are evaluated under controlled conditions. Research concerning the relevance of behaviors to be targeted for clinical intervention has barely begun in our field. This is the question of dependent variables; it is often thought that the only significant question is that of the independent variable. In other words, we may think that we know what the targets are, but we do not know how to train them. Both are important questions, however. For example, in the area of language disorders, what are the clinical targets: Communicative competence? Knowledge of the universal transformational grammar? Grammatical features? Grammatical rules? Semantic notions? Semantic rules? Pragmatic notions? Pragmatic rules? Empirical response classes? Similarly, what is (are) the dependent variable(s) in the treatment of stuttering? Self-confidence? Self-image? Approach–avoidance conflict? Anxiety reduction? Correction of feedback problems? Appropriate airflow? Correct phonatory behaviors? Reduction in speech rate? Reduction in the dysfluency rates? It is clear that there are no generally accepted answers to these questions, which means that there is no agreement on the discipline's dependent variables.

Specification of a valid dependent variable is crucial to the development of a science. If biologists were as confused about their dependent variables as we are about ours, biology's progress to date would be unthinkable. Because we are a clinical science, we need dependent variables that can be changed by the manipulation of their independent variables. Therefore, research on the valid dependent variables that can be successfully taught to the communicatively handicapped would be useful. Besides, in the course of this kind of research, the clinician would simultaneously provide clinical services.

Another area of investigation that is synchronous with clinical service concerns the effects of various treatment strategies. The value of treatment research in communicative disorders is obvious but is often taken for granted. When a clinical researcher designs a study in which a given treatment is applied and evaluated with adequate controls, the clients who serve as subjects are exposed to one possible treatment. If the treatment effects were not significant, the same clients may be experimentally treated with another technique that may prove to be more successful. In more advanced stages of research, the relative and interactive effects of more than one treatment technique or components may be evaluated. Here, too, the subjects are the clients who receive treatment during the course of research.

A paucity of treatment-related research in communicative disorders often supports the notion that research and clinical services are unrelated, and that training in research methodology and philosophy of science is a waste of time. Contrary to this notion, research and clinical activities are more similar than different. As pointed out by Perkins (1985), "Each clinical encounter epitomizes the essence of experimental research" (p. 14). Basically, treatments are a manipulation of cause–effect relations. A treatment is expected to produce changes in a client's communicative behaviors. To be accountable, the changes must be causally related. In other words, some other variable or someone else's treatment must not be responsible for the client's improved communicative behaviors. Such demonstrations are the essence of experimentation.

What is suggested here is that treatment-related research makes research *immediately* attractive to the practitioners, and therefore, they may be more likely to read and evaluate research. It is *not* suggested that basic research unrelated to immediate clinical concerns is less valuable or that there is no reason for clinicians to study basic research reports. Possibly, clinicians who do not understand or appreciate treatment research are less likely to understand or appreciate basic laboratory research. Therefore, one way of attracting clinicians to research of all kinds is to offer them initially treatment-related research that can make a difference in their day-to-day professional activities. Skills necessary to understand and evaluate treatment-related research, once mastered by clinicians, can help them understand basic research as well. In any case, the task of attracting clinicians to research is that of the clinical researcher, not that of the basic researcher.

PROBLEMS ASSOCIATED WITH
THE EDUCATION AND TRAINING MODELS

As noted before, if at least a certain number of clinicians are involved in research, the amount of in-house knowledge can be increased tremendously and in a fairly short time. However, assuming that other conditions are equal and favorable, clinicians can do research only if they are properly trained in the kind of research that is synchronous with clinical services. It would be impractical to expect a majority of clinicians to do basic research. It would be equally impractical for them to engage in clinical research that does not involve direct assessment, treatment, or maintenance strategies. Even the clinical research of "implications" cannot fulfill the service requirements. Clinicians will have to investigate questions that can be answered while providing services to their clients. In other words, communicative disorders must adopt an integrated model of education, training, and research.

If specialists in communicative disorders see their field as a clinical profession based on scientific knowledge and research, a number of much-debated pseudo-issues (such as "do we need to know scientific methods?" or "do we need to engage in research?") are dissipated. The education of clinicians must include an understanding of existing knowledge and technology, methods of producing new knowledge and technology, and methods of evaluating all knowledge and technology. Producing as well as evaluating knowledge and technology is a matter of education and training (Costello, 1979; Kent, 1983; Minifie, 1983; Moll, 1983). It is thus evident that training in research and science can be relatively unimportant only when the goal of professional education is simply to impart existing knowledge and provide training in extant technology. No one, of courses, believes that such a training model gives us scientific or professional strength.

It is often thought that education in the philosophy and methods of science takes time away from clinical training. Some may argue that since we practice a clinical profession, we should spend all the time necessary to educate ourselves in clinical methods and service delivery models. In recent years, it has even been suggested that we should develop a new *professional* doctorate with a greater emphasis on advanced clinical training than on science and research (Feldman, 1981, 1984). The issue has been debated extensively in clinical psychology and now in speech–language pathology. (For a collection of arguments on this issue, see the November 1984 issue of *Asha*, which contains two leading articles by Feldman and Ringel and comments by Goldstein, Hochberg, Koenigsknecht, and Loavenbruck.) Those who support a professional doctorate believe that the traditional PhD programs do not adequately address the clinical issues. Those who do not see a need for the new degree think that the traditional PhD programs are both strong and flexible enough to serve the needs of the profession.

The assertion that students in clinical programs should receive the best possible training in clinical methods is noncontroversial. At the same time, during their education and training, future clinicians should certainly not spend time on science and research if that is not expected to be useful. However, time spent on science and research in the training of practitioners can be a waste only when clinical service and scientific work are conceptually and methodologically divorced. The argument is not relevant when it is thought that communicative disorders is a scientific discipline and a clinical profession that adopts an integrated model of research and clinical service.

Unless clinicians are educated within an integrated model of research and clinical service, time spent on training clinicians in research will not be productive. But what is not so frequently recognized is that under the same circumstance, even researchers—with or without doctorates—are not likely to make a significant impact on the clinical issues of the profession. The existing models of research in our profession need to be revised. If the same model is used to give more information on research at the master's level or at the doctoral level, then we do not have much reason to expect that in-house clinical treatment-related knowledge will be increased by research. Creating a professional doctorate with the same clinical and research philosophy will also be of questionable value. What is needed is an emphasis on, and training in, the concepts and methods of science. The clinician must have a thorough understanding of the experimental methodology used to develop and evaluate treatment techniques as well as scientific theories.

It can be argued that historically we have not tried to develop a *clinical science*. We seem to have had the dual objectives of producing researchers and therapists. Neither objective seems to have been achieved to a satisfactory degree because of a misunderstanding of the roles of clinicians as well as of researchers. As warned by Minifie (1983), "our future role in professional service will only be as strong as the quality of our science" and we need both "clinical scientists" and "scientific clinicians" (p. 32). Kent (1983) has also stated that "we need basic scientists who study the work of applied scientists, we need scientists who do both basic and applied research, and we need collaborative research by basic and applied scientists" (p. 77).

A productive interaction between clinicians, clinical researchers, and basic researchers is possible when the education and training model combines the logic and methods of science with the concerns of clinical treatment evaluation. Such an education and training model will more successfully produce a clinical science (Perkins, 1985).

Such a training model needs to be implemented from the very beginning. At different levels of complexity, students should learn various aspects of this model at appropriate levels of their education. Within this viewpoint, the need for a new model of training is evident in the training of clinicians as well as researchers. The model must be used in training undergraduates as well as graduate students at both the master's and the doctoral levels.

It can be argued that what little training most graduates receive in science and research may not be consistent with clinical work, and therefore, that clinicians are not prepared to do research. Often, courses on research methods offer nothing but statistics (Kent, 1983). Science and its concepts and designs of research may be presented only inadequately, or not at all. Information presented on research designs may be restricted to the traditional group designs. Clinicians quickly find out that in order to do any kind of clinical research, they should be thorough in statistics, have access to a large population of clients who are willing to participate in a study, select a sample large enough to be justified statistically, select it randomly, assign subjects to treatment groups randomly, and deny treatment to a control group even if only temporarily.

Each step in this research process seems formidable, unacceptable, or both to clinicians whose immediate concern is professional service. First, most clinicians find that forgetting the basic statistics that they learned with great difficulty is surprisingly easy. Even if they remember most of it, their sophistication in statistics is rarely adequate to design statistically based research studies. Second, in their everyday work, clinicians typically deal with a small number of clients. As a result, they cannot find a population (a large group of persons with defined characteristics) of language-disordered or stuttering clients all of whom are accessible and willing to participate in a study. Therefore, they cannot draw random samples as the theory says they should. Third, even if the clinicians did draw random samples, they find it ethically unattractive to have a control group to which treatment must be denied or postponed. In essence, what clinicians learn about research in most graduate schools is not easily applied in most professional settings, where the immediate concerns are assessment, treatment, maintenance, parent counseling, case conference, and other such clinical activities.

The popularity of traditional research philosophy and methodology based on statistics and probability theory is at least partly responsible for the paucity of treatment-related research, whether by practitioners or by those who consider themselves clinical researchers. If the graduates in our discipline are exposed to different traditions of research, they may be able to select strategies to suit the kind of problems they wish to investigate. Clinicians who know of a strategy that is useful in dealing with individual clients or clients in small groups and in conducting treatment-related research may be more likely to gather experimental evidence in their day-to-day work. Such a strategy, known as the single-subject strategy, is available, and it is eminently suitable for developing a clinical science (Bauer, 1985; Connell & Thompson, 1986; Costello, 1979; Hegde, 1985; Kearns, 1986; Kent, 1983, 1985; McReynolds & Kearns, 1983; McReynolds & Thompson, 1986; Perkins, 1985; Vetter, 1985). Unfortunately, this strategy is not well represented in the education of speech–language pathologists. An encouraging sign, however, is that the single-subject strategy, described in Chapter 8, is receiving increasingly greater attention from educators, clinicians, and researchers. Clinicians who are capable of using this approach will be able to investigate questions while providing clinical services. This will also increase the amount of in-house knowledge, which may have the utmost clinical relevance.

EVALUATION OF RESEARCH

Evaluation of old as well as new knowledge is about as important as the creation of new in-house knowledge. Professionals who cannot evaluate research data and theories are not able to make effective use of appropriate information. Critical evaluation of research is a part of the clinician's repertoire. However, critical evaluation of research data requires the same knowledge needed to do meaningful research.

The process of evaluating research data follows the same logical steps as the process of designing experiments. Therefore, evaluation of research is possible only when clinicians understand how research is done. Clinicians who are not knowledgeable in science and their field of study are likely to have difficulty in judging the meaningfulness of questions researched by their colleagues, the validity and reliability of observations, the relation between results and conclusions, the transition from evidence to theory, and the distinction between theory and speculation.

Furthermore, clinicians who are not sophisticated in the philosophy of science may not see logical and empirical mistakes in designs. When they are also naive in the methods of research, they cannot critically examine the reliability, validity, and generality of results of research studies. In such cases, clinicians who read research have no choice but to uncritically accept the author's interpretations. Unfortunately, bad interpretations are about as prevalent as bad experimental designs, and clinicians who cannot detect inconsistent relations between interpretations and results are unable to separate data from conclusions. Data that are based on sound methodology are always more valuable and durable than the author's interpretations imposed on them.

Even with the most ideal condition, in which a considerable number of practitioners are involved in treatment-related research, a majority of clinicians will be concerned with research to the extent that it can help them improve their practice. The popular phrase "clinicians are consumers of research" has a ring of validity in that most clinicians will be users, not producers, of research. It is well known that naive consumers are victims of bad products. What is not equally well known is that clinicians who are naive in the methods and philosophy of science are likely victims of bad research. Unfortunately, in this process, the clients also become victims.

It is thus clear that clinicians who do not do research still need to understand science and research methods. Even if there is much research that cannot be applied, clinicians will have to keep reading and evaluating research because that is the only way they can find out what is useful and what is not. Those who avoid reading the research literature because it may be irrelevant to clinical practice are sure to miss what is relevant to them. Meanwhile, when research practices improve and clinically relevant studies are published, clinicians not only will be unaware of them but also will be unprepared for them. ■

S T U D Y G U I D E

1   What were some of the early concerns of the discipline of communicative disorders? Did those concerns include experimental evaluation of treatment procedures?

2   What legal and social considerations are prompting the profession to be more scientific in its orientation and activities?

3   What are some of the reasons to develop a scientifically sound clinical practice?

4   How can a profession draw attention to itself?

5   What kinds of professions generally have better reputation and higher social visibility?

6   What are some of the problems of wholesale borrowing of knowledge and methods from other subject matters?

7   What is meant by custom-produced information from outside a profession?

8   Why should specialists in communicative disorders produce their own data base?

9   What are some of the reasons why many clinicians do not do research?

10   What are the two possible assumptions made by some clinicians regarding research?

11   What are some of the popular sources of influence on clinical practice?

12   What is the main problem with current research practice?

13   How is basic research distinguished from experimental–clinical research?

14   What are some of the reasons why some clinicians have a negative view of research?

15   What are the strengths of the experimental–clinical research strategy?

16   What are some the problems associated with the education and training of clinicians?

17   Why were the questions such as "do clinicians need to know research methods?" or "why should clinicians do research?" described as pseudo-issues?

18 Summarize the arguments for and against the professional doctorate.

19 What is an integrated model of research and professional service?

20 From a clinician's standpoint, what are the problems of not being able to evaluate research?

■ C H A P T E R   **2**

An Introduction to Research: The Formal and Formative Approaches

■ What is research?, 22

■ Why do scientists do research?, 23

■ How is research done?, 31

■ Serendipity in research, 37

■ Concluding remarks, 40

■ Study guide, 41

The terms *science* and *research* have an air of extreme formality. Many students and professionals alike think that research is formidable, mechanistic, difficult, and somewhat boring. In addition, some practitioners may think that research is an esoteric activity, irrelevant to clinical service. Graduate students who are not involved in research may look upon those who are doing theses or dissertations with admiration totally devoid of envy. Undergraduate students may consider research as a mysterious activity, which they will understand better in graduate school. In time, the mysterious activity may reveal itself to be both arduous and uninteresting.

To a certain extent, most of these stereotypic reactions to science and research are understandable. Textbooks on research methods are written in a formal, precise, and somewhat dull style. The books are often full of statistics in which many students and clinicians do not find much joy. Statistics are only one of several and by no means inevitable methods of analyzing data, but many textbooks give an impression that statistics *is* research. Typical textbooks also describe research as a highly organized, thoroughly planned, and mechanistically efficient activity that most clinicians think they are not capable of. Clinicians and students may have heard or known of graduate students who have worked so hard on their theses or dissertations that those budding researchers "stopped living" until their project was complete. They may have seen professors and scientists who also seemed to have no fun doing research but went on with the drudgery for apparently no good reason. Finally, there is the reality of science and research itself: science is restrictive and research can be hard work. There are formal aspects to science, and there is no way of getting around them.

Nevertheless, it must be emphasized that science can be provocative, even refreshing. The logic and the framework of science constitute one of the most elegant of the abstract structures human beings have ever built. Once that logic and abstract structure are understood, organizing one's own activity within the scope of science is not very difficult. It can even be enjoyable. The logic of science can prompt the most stimulating intellectual pursuits. Much of scientific creativity, though difficult, can be highly reinforcing. A scientist's immense reward comes when his or her work throws new light on a perplexing problem that suddenly becomes a little bit more understandable.

In our effort to gain a more favorable view of research, we can find encouragement in Bachrach's (1969) comment that "people don't usually do research the way people who write books about research say that people do research" (Preface, p. x). Though research can be hard work, it need not be a drudgery because doing research can be fun. There are rewards even when it is not much fun. As we shall see later, research is at least not as formal an activity as most textbooks make it appear to be. Research scientists are people, too, and they make mistakes like anyone else. Certainly, there are people who do research not necessarily because they are especially good at it, but because they are required to. However, there are also people who may or may not be required to do research, but love to do it any way. They may not be good researchers in the beginning, but soon they learn from their mistakes and improve the quality of their work. In this process, they will have had their frustrations and pleasures.

What is needed is a more balanced view of research and science that puts both the pleasures and the frustrations of research activity in a proper perspective. When the research process is described the way it is normally implemented, one gains a more realistic picture. In a later section, we shall examine two ways of describing research activity in some detail.

WHAT IS RESEARCH?

Sometimes the terms *science* and *research* are used synonymously. Though the two terms have overlapping meanings, they do have different connotations. Science is inclusive of research, but the term *research* may not capture all the nuances of science. In the next chapter, we shall consider in detail the different meanings of science. In its broadest sense, science is a certain philosophy, a viewpoint concerning what the natural phenomena are and how they are interrelated. Science can also be viewed as a set of methods designed to investigate research questions and thereby produce reliable and valid knowledge. Finally, science refers to the actions and behaviors of scientists.

Research, on the other hand, refers to what scientists do in order to put science into practice. While science is a description of certain philosophies, viewpoints, and activities, research is mostly a description of the steps taken by scientists in their quest for order and uniformities in nature. Research is the *process* of investigating scientific questions. Research is science in action.

It is only in the sense that science includes certain methods of investigations and actions of scientists that it is synonymous with research. As such, research refers to those activities by which science achieves its goals. Even as a set of methods, science is conceptual, whereas research is mostly action. Science is the unifying theme and philosophy of research. It permeates all empirical research. Science gives the scientist both the conceptual and methodological means of doing research, but research refers to the behaviors of scientists in action.

It is probably not very useful to expand upon the various definitions of research. Within the realm of science, different strategies of research have been devised. The full range of meaning of the term *research* can be appreciated only when different types, strategies, and designs of research are understood along with the major reasons for doing research. In this sense, this entire book is about research. Therefore, we shall now turn to a discussion of some of the major reasons why research is done.

WHY DO SCIENTISTS DO RESEARCH?

Research is done for a variety of reasons. In considering this issue, we shall ignore bureaucratic reasons for doing research, although they are real. Bureaucratic reasons are those that require research on the part of scientists as a matter of employment policy. For example, research is required of faculty members in many universities. Their tenure and promotion may depend upon the amount and quality of research they publish. Scientists my be paid to do research in several organizations, in which case doing research becomes their duty. These are intermediate reasons for doing research, however. Even when a research scientist has to do research for bureaucratic reasons, he or she will have to consider the more basic and universal reasons why research is considered necessary.

Curiosity About Natural Phenomena

Philosophers of science have long recognized that one of the classical reasons for doing research is people's curiosity about natural phenomena. The scientist is prone to be curious, and once questions arise, he or she tends to do something that has a chance of satisfying that curiosity. In fact, Sidman (1960) has defined a scientist as a "person whose indulgence of his curiosity is also the means by which he earns his living" (p. 7).

People are curious about things they do not understand, causes that are hidden, and effects that are unknown. Of course, curiosity is not an exclusive characteristic of scientists. Most people are curious about various natural and social phenomena. Often, everyday curiosity is satisfied when things are explained to them, which means they now understand why someone behaved in a certain way or why a certain event happened. Scientific curiosity, on the other hand, is not satisfied by such answers. It is satisfied only by certain kinds of answers produced by certain methods. Therefore, it takes a relatively long time to satisfy scientific curiosity, which seeks special answers to complex questions.

While everyday curiosity may be concerned with private events, scientific curiosity is almost always concerned with objective events. Even when subjective experiences such as feelings or emotions become the object of curiosity, scientific curiosity treats them as objective and natural events. Answers produced by scientific curiosity are subject to public verifications, whereas those produced by private or personal curiosity are not.

Private curiosity tends to produce answers with private implications, but scientific curiosity compels answers with public implications. Everyday curiosity may not necessarily lead to answers that have great social impact, whereas the answers scientific curiosity seek have significant social consequences. In this sense, the scope of scientific curiosity is larger than that of private curiosity. In addition, scientific curiosity is always concerned with explaining natural phenomena, whereas private curiosity may be concerned with phenomena that cannot be investigated by scientific methods at all. For example, curiosity about why people have speech disorders can lead to empirical investigations using acceptable methods of science, whereas curiosity about supernatural phenomena may not lead to such investigations. However, interest in supernatural phenomena can itself be an object of scientific curiosity. A behavioral scientist may wonder why so many people exhibit certain kinds of behaviors toward supernatural phenomena and then proceed to find out by scientific investigations.

In many respects, scientific curiosity is insatiable. An answer to one question may contain the seeds of several more questions that need to be investigated. A curious scientist can go on from one research activity to another, since every piece of work satisfies some curiosity while arousing some other curiosity. In fact, good research typically raises important questions for further empirical investigations. Some investigations may not produce any answers at all. Instead, they may raise important questions for research. Such investigations keep the proverbially curious scientist busy for a long time. It is this type of insatiable curiosity that sustains a chain of investigations and a lifetime of scientific research.

Research driven by curiosity is often not designed to test formal scientific hypothesis (Sidman, 1960). When a scientist wonders what causes an event, he or she may begin to arrange conditions under which that event can be systematically observed. A hypothesis is a tentative answer to a research question, but one may not have a tentative answer, only a desire to find out. After some observations, the scientist may manipulate some aspect of the situation under which the phenomenon occurs reliably. This is the stage of experimentation, which can also be devoid of formal hypotheses. The history of both natural and behavioral sciences is full of examples of research that was done to see what happens when some specific variable is introduced, increased, decreased, or withdrawn.

The contrasting features of everyday and scientific curiosity should not suggest that the two are unrelated. Possibly, everyday curiosity is cultivated and modified into scientific curiosity. That science is a human activity is illustrated by all research, but it is best illustrated by research done to satisfy one's own curiosity.

Explain Events

A well-recognized reason for doing research is to explain events and effects. Scientists wish to offer explanations as to why certain events take place and why certain effects seem to be produced by variables not yet identified. In fact, it is often said that one of the goals of science is to explain natural phenomena. Therefore, a need to explain events is a significant reason for doing scientific research.

An event is explained when its cause is experimentally isolated. When it is demonstrated that a certain treatment procedure can produce language in a client with no language, we understand how language behaviors can be modified. Similarly, when animal experiments successfully produce a certain disease condition by introducing a chemical into the animal's body, that disease is explained at some level of generality and confidence. Procedurally, experiments arrange certain conditions to see if a variable produces a measurable effect. If certain steps are taken, the influence of other potential variables is ruled out or controlled. In this manner, a cause–effect relation between two events is established.

Research aimed at explaining events can follow one of two approaches. One of the approaches is to first offer a comprehensive deductive theory of an event and then test various deductions of that theory in a series of experiments. In other words, first the event is explained and then the attempts to verify that explanation are begun. This explain-first-and-verify-later approach is known as the deductive method. In the second approach, the investigator refrains from offering a theoretical explanation of an event until he or she has had a chance to conduct a series of experiments that can support a theory. This experiment-first-and-explain-later approach is known as the inductive method. Each of these two approaches has its advantages and disadvantages, and they are discussed in Chapter 3.

In science, a valid explanation of an event is worthwhile in and of itself. However, in many branches of science, a well-supported explanation suggests other possibilities. In most empirical sciences, the course of the event successfully explained can be altered. This means that scientists can gain some control over the events they explain. Typically, events not yet explained are difficult if not impossible to control or alter. An access to causes of events will make it possible to change the event by manipulating those causes. The applied implications of a valid explanation, then, are self-evident. Valid explanations make it possible to control diseases, disorders, and undesirable social and personal conditions.

Research done to explain events poses several risks to scientists, however. Within the inductive framework, scientists must constantly control their tendency to offer an explanation too soon. Whether sufficient evidence has been gathered so that a reasonably valid explanation can be offered must be judged by the scientist. Within the deductive framework, the scientist must make sure that after a theoretical explanation has been offered, the research program to verify it is promptly initiated. Furthermore, the scientist must make sure that the initial explanation is suitably modified in light of the data that are produced by systematic experimentation.

It is worthwhile to remember that the validity of scientific explanations is a matter of degree and that no explanation is 100 percent valid. This is because no group of scientists can claim that all possible observations of a phenomenon have been made. There is always a possibility that some new observations will produce new data that may question the old explanation. Therefore, science treats all explanations as more or less tentative. Explanations with adequate support are sustained only until data indicate otherwise.

Solve Practical Problems

Another reason to do research is to solve practical problems. There are many varieties of practical problems that scientists try to solve, but they can be grouped into two broad kinds for the sake of discussion. One kind of problem is found in the physical, chemical, social, and behavioral realm of the scientists' milieu. These are the problems that people, including scientists, face in their day-to-day living. Much of applied research is designed to solve practical problems of this kind. For example, research on better ways of constructing houses; developing more effective fertilizers to improve crops; new methods of reducing energy consumption; reducing highway accidents; and treating cancer, stuttering, or language disorders falls into this category of research. Obviously, this kind of research has the most immediate and highly visible social impact, and therefore, it is the better known of the two kinds of research designed to solve practical problems.

Research done to solve practical problems is crucial for clinical sciences because research done to evaluate treatment procedures falls into this category. Systematic experimental evaluation and modification of existing treatment procedures, and development of new and more effective procedures, are important for any clinical profession. One would think that a significant part of research in communicative disorders is of this kind. Unfortunately, this is not the case. Other kinds of research dominate the field. There are many reasons why this kind of research is not done to the extent it is desirable, and most of these reasons were discussed in Chapter 1.

When research done to solve practical problems is successful, it gives rise to *technology*. Technology is the application of the results of certain kinds of scientific research in further solving problems, improving living and working conditions, saving natural resources, enhancing the behavioral potential of people, treating various disorders and diseases, and so on.

The second kind of practical problem that scientists address can be described as in-house problems. Scientists face many practical problems that impede or even prevent a scientific analysis of a problem under investigation. Most scientists are handicapped if effective methods of observation and measurement are not available. Before conducting a conditioning experiment involving rats, for example, early experimental psychologists had to build the needed experimental chambers themselves. When available methods of measurement are found to be inadequate for certain scientific purposes, new methods of measuring the phenomenon of interest must be developed. When the phenomenon of interest cannot be directly observed, one has to solve this practical problem of not having a means of observation before further research can be initiated. The invention of a microscope, a telescope, a physiograph, an audiometer, or a flexible fiberscope illustrates the need to solve the practical problems of observation. Such instruments extend the range, the power, or the precision of scientists' observations. New devices make it possible to observe events that were never directly observed before. For example, the laryngeal behaviors during stuttering were a matter of speculation for a long time, but the behaviors themselves were not directly observed until such techniques as fiberscope and cineradiography were used.

In addition to new instruments, scientists also develop new methods of controlling their phenomena. New experimental designs are often tried to see if they afford better control over the variables under study. When existing methods of arranging experimental conditions prove inefficient or in some ways unsatisfactory, new arrangements may be tested to find out if they help overcome the problems with the existing arrangements. Behavioral research contains many examples of new experimental arrangements that were developed to overcome some of the problems of the statistical approach to research. Skinner (1953), for example, found that the traditional method of studying a large number of subjects, each somewhat superficially, was not suitable for an experimental analysis of behavior. He therefore devised the method of intensive study of individual subjects. When methods of averaging group performance to see a fake order in diverse behavior patterns were given up in favor of controlling conditions under which an individual organism could be studied, a true order and patterning of behaviors emerged. In essence, Skinner was able to gain a better control over the behavior because he could then alter patterns of behavior by changing the conditions under which the organisms behaved. As a result, Skinner's experimental analysis of behavior was able to offer a new view of behavior simultaneously with new techniques of controlling behavioral phenomena.

The emergence of new experimental designs illustrates how scientists solve their methodological problems. In recent years, applied behavioral research has witnessed the development of many new experimental designs. For example, when it became evident that the single-subject ABA design (see Chapter 8) was undesirable for clinical research, the multiple-baseline design was developed as an alternative (Baer, Wolf, & Risley, 1968). In the ABA design, first a behavior is baserated, then a variable that will change that behavior is introduced, and finally that variable is withdrawn. With these operations, the investigator hopes to show that the behavior changed from the baseline when the variable was introduced and that the change was nullified when the variable was withdrawn. However, the design that served well in laboratory experiments proved undesirable in treatment evaluation because the experiment would end with no treatment and the clients would be where they were before the treatment was started.

The multiple baseline, which was designed to overcome the problems of the ABA design, afforded an opportunity to demonstrate the effect of treatment without neutralizing it. In this design, several behaviors of a client are baserated and the behaviors are treated in sequence. Every time a behavior is treated, the remaining untreated behaviors are baserated to make sure that only the treated behaviors changed while the untreated behaviors did not. This strategy has been used extensively in clinical treatment research.

An experimentally active discipline is constantly seeking new ways of observing, measuring, and controlling the phenomena of interest. Efforts to extend the control techniques to new range of phenomena are also made continuously. In fact, the amount of successful research done to solve practical problems and bring new range of phenomena under experimental control is often an indication of the degree of scientific progress made by a discipline.

Demonstrate Certain Effects

Finally, research may be done to demonstrate the effects of newly discovered variables. Research of this kind often results in the observation of new phenomena. Generally speaking, science starts with a certain effect and then proceeds to find out what caused it. The experimental search of the cause of an event involves the active manipulation of selected variables. If the event changed, then the manipulated variable may be the cause; if it did not, then some other factor may be the cause. In this manner, and with appropriate control procedures, the scientist determines what caused an event. It must be noted that in all such cases, the scientist has a clear idea of the effect but is not sure of the cause.

The research study designed to demonstrate the effects of a certain variable, on the other hand, starts with a causal variable. What is not clear in this case is the effect of that variable. This kind of research situation arises frequently, although it takes a keen observer to notice new variables whose effects are yet undetermined.

A new variable that may produce new effects is often discovered accidentally. In the field of stuttering, for example, Lee (1950, 1951) accidentally found that a speaker's speech becomes disturbed when a delay is introduced in the auditory feedback of one's own speech. Lee, an engineer, was working on some audiotaping systems that accidentally introduced a delay in feedback, and he found himself "stuttering" under this condition. He and other researchers then began to investigate the effects of delayed auditory feedback more thoroughly in order to determine the full range of its effects on speech. It must be noted that in the beginning, Lee was not at all studying the effects of delayed auditory feedback on speech. The variable emerged accidentally, and its effects were then evaluated.

The literature on behavioral research contains many examples of accidental discovery of certain variables whose effects were later investigated in several experiments. Skinner (1956) has documented several of these examples in his own research. The now well-documented effects of intermittent reinforcement on behavior was discovered entirely accidentally (Skinner, 1956). At a time when Skinner was reinforcing rats with custom-made food pellets, he had to manufacture his own supply of pellets with a hand-operated machine that he himself had constructed. He was also reinforcing every lever press response (continuous reinforcement). As Skinner tells the story:

> One pleasant Saturday afternoon I surveyed my supply of dry pellets and [found] that unless I spent the rest of the afternoon and evening at the pill machine, the supply would be exhausted by ten-thirty Monday morning . . . [This] led me to . . . ask myself why every press of the lever had to be reinforced. . . . I decided to reinforce a response once every minute and allow all other responses to go unreinforced. There were two results: (a) my supply of pellets lasted almost indefinitely; and (b) each rat stabilized at a fairly constant rate of responding. (p. 111)

The above story points out several interesting aspects of the research process. Skinner did not *hypothesize* that intermittent reinforcement causes a more constant response rate than continuous reinforcement. At least initially, he did not *design* a study to evaluate the effects of not reinforcing every response. Of course, he knew well what he had done that Saturday afternoon: he had changed the way the rats were reinforced. But he had no clear idea of what it would do to the response rate. He probably did not think that it would make a big difference in response rates. But the data he saw on Monday morning were different. This led him to start a series of studies on the many different ways in which a response could be reinforced. These studies by Skinner and others (Ferster & Skinner, 1957) have shown that different reinforcement schedules have characteristic effects on response rates and patterns. This area of research contains one of the most well-controlled and replicated evidence in behavioral research. More importantly, it shows how a variable discovered accidentally suggests a new line of investigation to assess its effects more fully.

Physical and biological sciences are also full of examples of accidental discoveries of certain variables whose effects were studied subsequently. It is well known that penicillin was discovered accidentally (Batten, 1968; Wilson, 1976). It was in the process of culturing certain bacteria for some other research purposes that Sir Alexander Fleming repeatedly found that a certain green mold that developed in the dish routinely killed his colony of bacteria. Some other scientist probably would have ignored the green mold, considered the death of the bacteria an accident, and perhaps proceeded to develop a fresh colony of bacteria. Although Fleming did this to a certain extent, the repeated deaths of bacteria forced him to take a closer look at the effects of the green mold. Eventually, the presence of the unexpected green mold led to the discovery of penicillin, whose effects were studied extensively in later experiments.

When the effects of a newly discovered variable are experimentally analyzed, the existence of new phenomena are simultaneously documented. When Lee analyzed the effects of delayed auditory feedback on speech, several interrelated phenomena concerning speech production and its continuous monitoring through auditory mechanism were documented. Skinner's discovery of the effects of reinforcement schedules led to demonstrations of new phenomena of response patterns under different arrangements of consequences. Fleming's discovery of penicillin led to the documentation of a host of biological phenomena relative to the treatment of various disease conditions.

The four kinds of reasons for doing research described here are not exhaustive, but they include the major factors that typically lead scientists to research and experimentation. Also, the four reasons are by no means mutually exclusive; they are in fact interrelated. Research done to satisfy one's curiosity may explain an event. Often, curiosity compels one to ask why a certain event is happening, and an answer to that question may also isolate the cause of the event. Curiosity can initially draw a scientist to a field of investigation. But soon, the scientist may be doing research to explain events (develop theories), solve practical problems, or demonstrate certain effects. It should also be clear that research done for any other reason will also satisfy the scientist's curiosity.

Research done to explain events can serve as a basis for additional research done to solve practical problems. For example, an experimentally based explanation of language disorders should also suggest ways of controlling or eliminating them. Because an explanation always points to at least one cause of an event, one can then assume that additional research on the methods of manipulating that cause should provide a means of controlling that effect. Such controlling techniques are the same as treatment procedures.

In a similar manner, research done to solve practical problems can eventually lead to an explanation of certain phenomena. For example, successful treatment of language disorders through certain environmental manipulations may suggest that certain variables may be necessary for normal language acquisition. The absence of those variables may be responsible for an absence of normal language. Unfortunately, a widely held assumption is that applied research cannot explain phenomena but can only manipulate them with the knowledge derived from basic research. However, well-controlled experimental treatment research can offer excellent suggestions on the controlling variables of phenomena treated successfully. This is because in solving practical problems, one often has to isolate the independent variables of the phenomenon of interest. The same variables can be used to explain the phenomenon.

HOW IS RESEARCH DONE?

In this section, I shall not address the actual mechanics of doing research, for that is the running theme of this book. Besides, the final part of the book contains more specific suggestions on how to do research. In this section, I shall present two approaches to *describing* research activity. Different ways of conceptualizing and describing research activity may impede or retard a favorable understanding of it.

It was noted earlier that the traditional viewpoint of research is that it is an extremely well-organized, formal activity and that this viewpoint may be largely mistaken. A different viewpoint of research is that it is always a formative, not formalized, activity. We shall take a closer look at the research process and contrast these viewpoints in order to appreciate the fact that research is what some *people* do.

The Formal Viewpoint

It is *not* proposed here that there are two ways of doing research, one more formal and organized than the other. What is proposed is that research is *described* in two ways, and that *all* research is less formal and organized than what is indicated by the end product, published articles, or descriptions of research as found in most textbooks. The popular view that research involves an invariable, systematic, and step-by-step progression from the literature review to the problem, methods, results, and conclusions is simply due to the *format of published research.* Those who write textbooks on research support that view by omitting the process of research while describing the *mechanics of organizing research already done*, regardless of how it was done.

When a student of research methods reads an article published in one of the journals to understand the *process* of research, he or she may gain the impression that the researcher knew everything from the beginning and that all that needed to be done was to simply take the predetermined and incredibly clear steps of conducting the research. The student is apt to think that the experimenter had read everything about the past research well before he or she ever thought of the problem. Existing research being clear, the brilliant researcher suddenly and inevitably generated the question that needed to be researched. The question as originally conceived must have been clear cut and well formulated, for there is no indication in the article that the question was modified, was rewritten, or was not at all the original question considered for investigation. There is certainly no hint that the question investigated was one of several similar ones considered, or that it was initially quite fuzzy.

The student might then think that as soon as the problem was posed, the researcher knew what kind of results would be obtained, so a hypothesis was formulated. However, in order not to give the impression that the investigator had a personal stake in supporting his or her guesses, a null hypothesis, which is essentially a prediction that nothing significant will come out of the research, was proposed (see Chapter 3). The investigator then knew what exactly to do in order to test the hypothesis. It might appear to the student that there was no question as to what kind of design to use in the study. The design used must have been the only one available. If alternatives were available, the choice must have been easy and clear. The procedure of subject selection must also have been clear from the very beginning, since there is no indication of troubled decisions on this matter. All subjects must have been readily available, and all the experimenter had to do was ask them to participate in the study. Furthermore, it may appear that the investigator was sure of the best method of measuring and manipulating the variables. In this manner, the student is likely to imagine that the scientist simply moved through a series of well-defined steps, which resulted in the conclusion of the study.

Once the study was completed, the predetermined method of analysis was simply applied to the results. Apparently, the meaning of the results was also unambiguously clear to the scientist, since the article talked about a definite number of implications that seem to have emerged full-blown in the order in which they were presented. Apparently, it was with great ease that the scientist was able to relate the findings of the study to those of other investigations.

In essence, a typical journal article gives the student the impression that research is possible only when everything is brilliantly clear to the scientist. Since the student has not heretofore seen anything so complex and yet so clearly and beautifully organized, research seems to be both an entirely unique and personally formidable task.

The fact that a student gains such an impression of the research process is not a fault either of the student who reads research reports or of the scientist who writes them, because doing research and organizing it for publication are two separate activities. When the concern is to communicate what the research question was, how it was investigated, what results were obtained, and what the author thinks are the implications of those results, it is best to omit the details of the research process. The process of doing research is full of various personal, practical, ideational, emotional, and organizational details that may not be entirely relevant to an understanding of what was done and what results were obtained. These factors, if chronicled in an article, may confuse readers. Besides, no journal will have the needed additional space to print the story of research in addition to research, no matter how interesting the story might be. Therefore, the preceding characterization of the research process that can be gleaned from journal articles is not meant to suggest that the reporting itself should reflect the actual process of doing research.

One would expect, however, that when research scientists talk about how they did their research or when authors write books on how to do research, the actual process would be reflected. Unfortunately, many authors who talk or write about research paint an unreal picture of the research process. The textbooks on research procedures, especially those based on statistics, are particularly vulnerable to this criticism. Textbooks typically reinforce the questionable notion of the research process that the students gain from reading journal articles.

The Formative Viewpoint

A research report documents (1) several decisions made by the investigator, (2) how those decisions were implemented, (3) what results followed that implementation, and (4) what the author thinks of those results. Decisions are made concerning the problem of investigation, what the previous research suggests, how the problem will be investigated, and how the results will be interpreted. However, these decisions should not be confused with the actual process of arriving at those decisions. Students who wish to know how to do research should gain an understanding of how such decisions are made.

It is possible that scientists who describe the process by which they made their own discoveries tend to give the process an unnecessary air of formality, clarity, logical precision, and inevitable movement through specific steps. In an article entitled "A plea for freeing the history of scientific discoveries from myth," Grmek (1981) has expressed skepticism about the validity of many famous scientists' autobiographical accounts of the *process* of scientific discovery. Grmek believes that in describing their own past discoveries, many scientists resort to "rationalizing readjustment, whereby the actual sequence of events is transmuted in favor of logical rigor and coherence" (1981, p. 15).

Many authors who consider themselves competent researchers may be somewhat reluctant to talk about the typically uncertain, sometimes confusing, and generally groping nature of doing research. There may be an implicit assumption that *science* cannot be anything but utter clarity, beautiful organization, and superb efficiency. Scientific research may be thought of as entirely official, proper, prim, and uncompromising. However, when science is viewed as something people do, the emerging picture of the research process may be less magnificent, but it will be more real.

Research is more formative than formal. It is a process in which concepts, ideas, procedures, and skills are formed slowly. The movement from *problem* to *discussion* is not as certain, neat, and linear as a published article might imply. We think that there is a beginning and an end to a particular study, but the boundaries are not always clear. More importantly, everything in between may involve many back-and-forth movements. Grmek (1981) states that the typical textbook depiction of the linear ascent towards truth is a myth. In addition, he stated that 'neither the meanderings of individual thought, nor the advances of scientific knowledge within a community, proceed by successive approximations, always in the right direction, towards truth. The path to discovery is a winding one" (p. 20).

Patterns that can be found in research activity are broad and flexible. There are broad conceptual and methodological patterns. There are patterns pertaining to theory and practice. Unfortunately, the textbooks turn those broad and flexible patterns into specific and rigid steps of doing research. Research is a continually evolving process, which stays sensitive to changing conceptual, methodological, practical, and evidential bases. The formal and clearly stated research question as it finally appears in a published article may barely resemble the early troubling but uncertain, vague yet haunting sensations that are often a coalescence of thoughts, images, and feelings about the phenomenon of interest. If one were to question the scientist at this stage as to what he or she is doing, the answer might be more confusing than illuminating. The scientist's thoughts may appear not well organized at all. In all likelihood, the problem at this stage is that some phenomenon is bothering the scientist but there is no clear *research* problem that can be investigated. At such a time, the scientist's speech, if he or she at all is willing to talk about the problem, will certainly not resemble the convention lecture given on the completed research a year later.

There may be a few exceptional scientists who, without much effort and time, can formulate significant research questions that, when investigated, yield meaningful data. In most cases, however, the emergence of research questions is a slow and formative process. Generally speaking, the beginnings of a research question may be felt after a lot of reading on the issue, or on rare occasions without much reading. Some researchers may think of questions while talking about an issue or a topic. Others may sense potential questions while engaged in some practical work, such as working with a client.

Research itself is probably the most productive locus of additional research questions. Tentative research questions may emerge during observation of a phenomenon or during the course of some empirical research. The results of an experiment might suggest additional questions for future investigation. The researcher may have found out that the method selected was not effective and that a different tactic might prove more useful. Thus, both effective and ineffective research can suggest valid questions to be investigated. Descriptive research might suggest questions for experimental research. A basic analysis of a phenomenon might suggest applied research questions.

A clinician who is a keen observer may think of many questions during treatment sessions or simply while watching client behaviors. An inefficient treatment should be an excellent source for treatment-related research questions. The clinician who has carefully broken down the treatment into separately manipulated components may be able to observe differential effects of certain components. This might be something that the clinician can pursue in a research study.

In most cases, a lot of reading, keen observation, critical analysis of existing research literature, some experience in research, an understanding of logic and the philosophy of science, and critical thinking are all necessary to formulate significant research questions.

As noted before, most research questions are not very clear in the early stages. Furthermore, upon further thinking and reading, those that were clear to begin with may be judged the wrong kind of questions. The refinement of the question takes a considerable amount of thinking, and most questions undergo several revisions before they are ready for investigation. The relative emphasis on the variables within a question may be changed when the investigator begins to think of a strategy to implement the experiment.

Once the question becomes reasonably clear, the scientist begins to think about the ways of answering it. At least theoretically, different methods can be used to answer the same research question. For example, the effects of a new stuttering treatment program can be tested within a single-subject design or a group design. In the former, all subjects experience all conditions of the experiment. In the latter strategy, subjects in one group receive treatment and the members of the other group do not, thereby serving as a control group. Of course, the investigator selects what he or she considers the best strategy to answer the particular research question. But the scientist's own investigative history probably plays a key role in that selection. Here too, and in all probability, the investigator goes through a period of vacillation. Finally, a design may be selected for certain practical reasons. A group design, for example, may be selected simply because a certain number of subjects happen to be available.

Various other aspects of the procedures of a study are decided one way or the other, often without any clear-cut guidelines or requirements. When there are no stringent guidelines, the investigator judges whether the selected procedure can be justified on some grounds. Also, a given course of action may be taken because no other option is available. For example, how many subjects should be selected for the study? A group design would require more subjects than a single-subject design, but in many cases, the answer depends simply on the availability of subjects, especially in clinical fields. If ten stutterers are available for a study, the investigator decides to go with that number. It may happen that only six stutterers were willing to participate and the study had to be completed with them. When the report is written, however, it may indicate that the planned and well-considered number of subjects was six. As such, planning may have had nothing to do with the number of subjects used in a particular study.

Answers to many other questions may be similarly determined. What kinds of equipment will be used? In what physical facility will the experiment be conducted? Investigators construct new mechanical devices and buy new instruments when funds are available. Ideally, the best available instrumentation must be used for the study. But in practice, most investigators use what is available. Sometimes, a problem already defined may have to be redefined or modified to accommodate the only available instrument. For example, an investigator who wanted to monitor different physiologic variables such as heart rate, muscle potential, cortical electrical potential, blood volume, and breathing patterns in stutterers during treatment sessions might drop one or more of those variables simply because a multichannel polygraph that measured all of them was not available. Once again, practical exigencies, not planning, would have determined the variables selected for the study.

Many times, research problems literally sit on the shelves collecting dust because the investigator did not have the necessary time, subjects, or money. Other problems may not be investigated because of methodological difficulties. However, a problem that has been forgotten or neglected may suddenly be revived because a certain number or type of clients become available. The investigator will somehow make time and convince himself or herself that the existing equipment, though not ideal, will do. During an incidental and entirely informal conversation with a colleague, a way to study one of the methodologically difficult problems may emerge. Or, a recently published article containing some methodological innovations may suggest a procedure. Not infrequently, the investigator may think of a procedure while taking a walk or while just sitting and thinking about the problem. Suddenly, the problem lying on the shelf is picked up and dusted off, and the investigator drops everything else and becomes immersed in the new study. Meanwhile, other research ideas maybe neglected.

In any discipline, there is probably no objective count of studies that are half-finished or abandoned soon after they were begun. But the number cannot be too small. Many investigators are likely to have a few studies that were implemented to varying degrees and discontinued for a number of reasons. Maybe the investigator found out that after all, it was not a great study (meaning it was bad). Maybe the researcher came across a more interesting study, or obtained some grant monies that forced the attention into some other area of investigation. Perhaps the investigator got sick during the course of the study and never again had time to finish it. Furthermore, subjects may drop out, equipment may break down, and the investigator may move to another position. All of these not-so-formal reasons for discontinuing research are real and more common than the books on research methods lead us to believe.

A certain number of research studies that are completed may never be published. Again, objective data are lacking, but editors of journals can testify to the number of rejected articles. An article rejected by one journal may be published in another journal; but still, a considerable number of articles prepared for publication may never be published. Besides, a completed research study may never be written up for publication. A study may have been completed without its flaws having been realized, but one look at the data may convince the investigator that the study is not worth publishing.

The sequence of research found in published articles gives an impression of an orderly progression through an invariable sequence. Most empirical research articles have a rigid sequence because scientific journals require it. An article starts with the *Introduction* or the *Review of Literature*, proceeds to the *Method* and then the *Results*, and finally to the *Discussion* or

Conclusion. The article is ended with *References*, *Appendixes*, or both. But this rigid sequence is rarely a reflection of how the research itself was conducted. In some cases, investigators have sufficient reason to do a study with only a minimal survey of literature. This is especially true when an investigator knows that no study of the kind being considered has been made. After the study has been made, a more thorough search of the literature may be conducted to determine if the new findings can be related to any of the old findings. Often, methodological considerations precede a more thorough analysis of the research problem itself. One may have a general idea of the research problem, such as an evaluation of two language treatment programs, but the more critical factor to be assessed at the very beginning may be the number of subjects that are available for the study. This may then determine the particular design strategies. An author may not wish to use statistical methods of analysis, in which case considerations of data analysis may determine the design to be used. In this manner, the investigator considers factors sometimes in the sequence in which the paper is written but many times in a sequence dictated by the practical contingencies that affect the researcher as a person.

It must be recognized, though, that some research practices are more rigid than others. The statistically based group research designs are relatively more rigid in their strategies than are the single-subject designs. Typically, within the group research designs, the study is completed the way it was planned even if it becomes evident that something is wrong with the study. The design itself is rarely, if ever, modified in the middle of an investigation. Within the single-subject approach, on the other hand, a design can be modified when the data warrant a change. For example, if found ineffective, a treatment procedure in clinical research may be changed within a single-subject strategy, but usually not within the group strategy. The number of days for which the experimental manipulations are done may also be predetermined in the group approach but not within the single-subject approach. For instance, stutterers may be treated for a fixed duration in a group design study. On the other hand, in a single-subject study, the same treatment may be continued until stuttering is reduced markedly or until it becomes evident to the researcher that it is no use to continue the experimental treatment. Such judgments, made *during* the course of the study, are considered undesirable in the group research strategy. However, the same judgment or similar judgments made *prior* to the implementation of the study are considered a part of good planning.

SERENDIPITY IN RESEARCH

We noted earlier that accidental events have often helped scientists discover new phenomena. The very fact that "accidents" lead to significant scientific findings makes one wonder about the validity of the typical assertion that all research must be totally planned. By definition, accidental discoveries are unplanned, but they are scientific discoveries nonetheless. Some accidental discoveries have proved more valuable than the planned research during which such accidents happened.

Walpole's story *The Three Princes of Serendip* has given rise to the term "serendipity" in research (Cannon, 1945). The story goes that three princes, while looking for something that they never found, nevertheless found many interesting things that they had not thought of finding. Often, when looking for something, scientists may find something else. Such accidental discoveries may help scientists initiate an entirely new line of highly productive investigations. We noted earlier that Fleming's discovery of penicillin was accidental, as was Skinner's discovery of the effects of intermittent reinforcement on response patterns.

A particularly fascinating story of accidental discovery in medical sciences is that of Ignaz Semmelweis, a Hungarian physician who worked in a maternity ward of the Vienna General Hospital from 1844 to 1848 (Sinclair, 1901). The hospital had two maternity wards, and Semmelweis worked in the first ward. An anguishing puzzle he faced was that in his ward, the death rate due to childbed (puerperal) fever among women after delivery was as high as 11 percent; but in the other, identical ward, the death rate was around only 2 percent.

Like most investigators, Semmelweis began to test various logical possibilities and opinions about the causation of the unusually high mortality rate. Unfortunately, none of the logical possibilities proved to be the cause of the death rate. He found that such variables as overcrowding, unexplained "epidemic influences," rough examination by medical students, the posture women assumed during delivery, and a variety of psychological factors all proved to be inconsistent with facts or specific manipulations. For instance, overcrowding was common to both the wards and hence could not explain a differential death rate. Reducing the number of examinations by medical students did not reduce the death rate. Semmelweis reasoned that unexplained epidemic factors must be common to both the wards.

The puzzle was eventually solved in 1847, but the solution did not come from any of Semmelweis's rigorous hypothesis testing. It came from an unfortunate accident. While performing an autopsy, a student's scalpel punctured a wound in the finger of his instructor, Kolletschka. Soon Kolletschka became violently ill with the same symptoms of childbed fever. He died, just like many women with childbed fever. This led Semmelweis to think that perhaps the "cadaveric matter" the student's scalpel had introduced into Kolletschka's bloodstream must be the cause of the disease. The medical students were not trained in the other ward that had the low death rate. In that ward, midwives who did not dissect cadavers delivered babies. It then dawned on Semmelweis that he, his colleagues, and the medical students regularly came to examine the women in labor soon after completing dissections. Possibly because they did not wash their hands thoroughly, the physicians and medical students themselves were the carriers of the deadly microorganisms that were introduced into the bloodstream of women in labor.

Semmelweis solved the problem when he ordered that before examining the women in the ward, all physicians and medical students wash their hands thoroughly with a solution of chlorinated lime. As a result, the death rate in Semmelweis's ward declined to the level found in the other ward.

The Semmelweis story suggests that a problem is not always solved by a planned test of a formal hypothesis. An accident that reveals an unsuspected relation between events can solve a problem that had proved frustrating.

A not well recognized source of accidental discovery is the apparatus failure. All scientists know that instruments do break down and that in most cases they create problems for the scientist. Most scientists dread apparatus failure in the course of an experiment. Nevertheless, important discoveries have been made when apparatuses broke down in the middle of experiments. Two examples from behavioral research illustrate this. First, the discovery of operant extinction was aided immensely by a breakdown in the equipment Skinner was using to reinforce responses. In fact, one of Skinner's (1956) unformalized principles of scientific practice is that "apparatuses sometimes break down" (p. 109). As it happened, one day the food magazine, which was a part of the mechanical device used to automatically reinforce the bar press responses in rats became jammed. As a result, the rat's responses went unreinforced against the plan of the experiment in progress. The result was an extinction curve, which led to a series of experiments on the properties of extinction and on the functional relations between the prior reinforcement contingencies and later patterns of extinction.

The second example also comes from the experimental research on conditioning and is provided by Sidman (1960):

> An experiment on avoidance behavior was in progress in which an animal was scheduled to receive only 20 per cent of all the shocks that became due when it failed to make the avoidance response in time. A relay failure in the automatic programming circuit altered the procedure one day in such a way that every fifth shock was delivered *regardless* of whether or not the animal had made an avoidance response. The apparatus failure was discovered when the animal's usually stable rate of lever pressing began to accelerate, and continued to increase throughout the experimental period. The increased rate of avoidance responding in the face of unavoidable shock was so unexpected that a new research program was immediately launched, a program which has been productive for three years and is still continuing. (p. 9)

The phenomenon Sidman discovered because of an accidental failure of apparatus has come to be known as the Sidman avoidance, in which an organism has no prior signal of an impending aversive stimulus, and there is no escape, but each response postpones the aversive stimulus for a fixed period of time. It is known that the Sidman procedure produces a high and consistent rate of response, which is unusually resistant to extinction. Sidman's original finding has been replicated widely, and its human behavioral and clinical implications are extensive. But, the point to be made here is that the discovery of this important phenomenon of aversive conditioning was entirely due to a break down in instrumentation.

When experimental apparatuses break down, many scientists may be tempted to discard the data collected up to that point because of the "contamination caused by equipment failure." After having cried on the shoulders of a friendly colleague for a brief period of time, the scientist will rebuild the apparatus and start all over again. In many cases, equipment failure can be a cause of worry, especially when all the data are lost and there is nothing to discover. However, the results produced by failures are always worth a serious examination. The investigator may find new problems for exciting research in those unexpected results.

Serendipity in research also casts doubt on the validity of the common assertion that all meaningful research should involve hypothesis testing. If this is true, the chances for accidental discoveries are virtually eliminated. In hypothesis testing, the scientist asks a question and then formulates a tentative answer, which is then put to experimental test. The results of such research studies are always evaluated in terms of their relation to the hypothesis. Anything not relevant to the hypothesis is not of interest. Because "accidental confirmation of a hypothesis" is a contradiction of terms, accidental discoveries must be necessarily useless.

CONCLUDING REMARKS

The viewpoint that research is more formative than formal does not imply that research is casual and there is no need for planning or preparation. It must be noted that even accidental discoveries happen in the process of investigation, many of them well planned. The scientist needs to be an intellectually prepared person. A thorough knowledge of existing research is usually necessary, if only to avoid the same conceptual or methodologic mistakes committed by other scientists. Research is a process in which evidence accumulates slowly and as a result of the collective efforts of all scientists involved. The building blocks of scientific knowledge are the little pieces of research done by a variety of researchers past and present. As such, any researcher must be able to see interrelations between research findings, and this takes painstakingly achieved scholarship.

Good research also requires a working knowledge of the methods of manipulating and measuring variables. Good research also requires some skill and experience in looking at data and thinking about their importance.

Undoubtedly, many questionable investigations are due to poor scholarship, inadequate technical skills, and lack of sufficient planning on the part of researchers.

The formative viewpoint does suggest, however, that research is a more flexible, open, human, sensitive, and practical activity than it is often depicted to be. At both the conceptual and methodological levels, research is formative in the sense that different contingencies continuously affect the process. A good research scientist is always willing to go back and forth, and to change ideas or plans of experiment. A scientist is not necessarily bound by rigid sequences that may not promote creativity. Such a scientist is sensitive to unplanned events that happen during the course of research and does not have the great investment in his or her own guesses (hypotheses) that seems to create a scientist's affliction called "hypothesis myopia" (Bachrach, 1969). Though he or she is knowledgeable regarding previous research findings, the scientist's thinking is not limited by those findings. The scientist knows that nature is likely to display events not suggested by previous research or predicted by hypotheses and theories. As a result, such a scientist is fully prepared to seize an unplanned and unexpected moment of creativity. ■

S T U D Y   **G U I D E**

1   Distinguish between research and science.

2   Define research.

3   What are the "bureaucratic" reasons for doing research?

4   Describe the various reasons for doing research.

5   Explain why research done to satisfy one's own curiosity may not involve hypothesis testing.

6   What is the difference between private curiosity and scientific curiosity?

7   What is a scientific explanation?

8   Write a (hypothetical) statement of explanation of a selected disorder of communication.

9   What are the two kinds of practical problems scientists try to solve?

10 What is the name of the by-product of research that is successful in solving some practical problems?

(continued next page)

Study Guide *(continued)*

11   Give two examples of scientists' in-house problems.

12   What kind of research results in the observation of new phenomena?

13   What are the two approaches to describing research activity? Compare and contrast the two approaches.

14   Why do students tend to have a formal view of research?

15   What is meant by the statement that "research is more formative than formal"?

16   Give an example of accidental discovery in scientific research. Find an example not given in this text.

■ CHAPTER   **3**

Science and Its Basic Concepts

■ Popular misconceptions about science, 44

■ What is science?, 45

■ Outcome of scientific activity, 50

■ Variables and their types, 52

■ Causality and functional analysis, 56

■ Experiment and experimental control, 60

■ Hypotheses in scientific research, 61

■ Theories and scientific reasoning, 65

■ Theories and scientific laws, 69

■ Data and evidence, 70

■ Study guide, 72

W e all seem to know what science is, but a formal question "what is science?" is not always easy to answer. Experts have approached the question from different viewpoints, and therefore, there are many different answers, each of them accurate within its own frame of reference. However, there are many popular misconceptions about science, and it is instructive to know what science is not. Some of these misconceptions may be entertained by persons who are otherwise educated but have not formally studied the philosophy and methods of science.

POPULAR MISCONCEPTIONS ABOUT SCIENCE

Probably the most common misconception about science is that it is certain subject matters. Many people think that science is physics, chemistry, or biology. Traditionally, certain subject matters have come to be regarded as sciences. Therefore, the popular opinion has equated science with those subject matters. Certain other subject matters, such as sociology or speech–language pathology, may not be regarded as sciences.

The misconception is understandable because scientists themselves have often defined science in terms of a "body of knowledge" that is systematic and verified. Some disciplines have more of a systematic and verified body of knowledge and therefore are more likely to be equated with science. Other bodies of knowledge may not be as systematic, or may still be under verification, and therefore may not qualify for the title science. The metaphoric notion of the "body of knowledge" is misleading if it is equated with science but appropriate if it is thought of as a product of science. Years of scientific activity on the part of a group of people investigating certain phenomena may result in knowledge that is consistent with the philosophy and methods of science.

Science is not the same as particular subject matters such as physics or biology, though it may be appropriate to say that some subject matters are more scientifically oriented than others. A subject matter is more or less scientific depending upon the extent to which it applies the methods of science in investigating its phenomena.

A second misconception equates science with activities carried on in certain physical settings such as laboratories involving complex instruments. While several scientific disciplines do make use of laboratories and instruments, such facilities are not always necessary or sufficient to make a piece of investigation scientific. Scientific experiments can be conducted in many nonlaboratory situations. They can be conducted in playgrounds, shopping centers, or living rooms. Experiments can be done in classrooms, in industrial assembly lines, in outer space, or under water. Many experiments can be conducted with no complicated instruments.

A third misconception about science is evident in a confusion between science and technology. Designing and building machines such as computers or spacecrafts, and constructing bridges or buildings, are technological in nature. Technology is often the application of science in solving problems, but it is not necessarily the science itself. The confusion is understandable because technology provides highly visible examples of the application of science.

WHAT IS SCIENCE?

As suggested earlier, science can be defined from different but relatively valid viewpoints. There are three basic viewpoints that stress different aspects of science. Thus, science can be defined in terms of (1) a philosophy, (2) a certain kind of behavior, and (3) a set of methods. I shall briefly describe each of these viewpoints. All three of them are necessary to obtain a comprehensive view of science.

Science as a Philosophy

Science is a certain philosophical position regarding nature and the nature of events. The philosophic foundations of science include *determinism* and *empiricism*. Determinism means that events are determined by other events. Events do not happen haphazardly; they are caused by other events. Without this basic philosophy, scientific activity would not be meaningful, for as we shall see shortly, that activity is essentially a search for the causes of events.

The early history of science shows that the laity as well as learned people had difficulty accepting the philosophy of determinism. People in most societies believed that events happen because of a divine design that is beyond the scope of human observation and investigation. Science, on the other hand, insisted that causes of events are other events and that the causes can be observed, studied, and in many cases controlled. Before the advent of science, scholasticism and religion ruled the world of knowledge, understanding, and explanation. Both scholasticism and religion had their explanations of the physical, chemical, biological, and human world. Often, science found itself in conflict with this traditional wisdom. Both science and scientists have suffered because of this.

It is well known that the physical, chemical, and biological phenomena were among the very first to come under the scope of the philosophy and methods of science. Science replaced the notion that the earth is flat and that it is the center of universe. It challenged the notion that human beings suddenly emerged because of divine creation. It showed that the behaviors of physical, chemical, and biological phenomena are lawful and that those laws can be discovered. The progress in such basic scientific analyses eventually led to technology, which helped solve many problems of living. Technology began to make life a little easier and thus reduced some of the resistance to science. Nevertheless, every new invention or discovery has also provoked social resistance (Johnston & Pennypacker, 1980).

Generally speaking, resistance to the philosophy of science is less marked when it comes to physical and chemical phenomena. As applied to biological phenomena, scientific philosophy still provokes considerable resistance. The recent and continuous controversies over science and creationism in American public schools testify to this persistent resistance to the philosophy of science.

The resistance to determinism is even more vocal with regard to the study and explanation of human behavior. Human behavior has been the last stronghold of antiscientific philosophy. Traditional philosophies that assert that human beings are created also tend to discredit the possibility that human behavior is determined. Human actions are supposed to be due to inner forces such as free will. Many people who readily accept the philosophy that natural events are caused by other events may vehemently oppose the notion that human behavior has its causes that can be studied and controlled by the methods of science. In recent years, the science of human behavior has been one of the most attacked of sciences.

Within the domain of human behavior, language, thinking, and "higher mental functions" have been a particularly strong sanctuary for the traditional, nonscientific philosophies of rationalism, mentalism, and scholasticism. When the evidence that most forms of human behaviors can be analyzed by the methods of science became overwhelming, language and creativity seemed like an urgently needed exception to maintain the traditional concepts of human behaviors. The nativists' strong rejection of the behavioral analysis of language in the late 1950s and 1960s was but one indication of this tendency.

The history of science makes it clear that it has been relatively easy to look at physical and chemical phenomena and analyze them objectively. Because scientists are also behaving organisms, a science of behavior requires that we analyze our own behaviors objectively. Unfortunately, looking at ourselves and analyzing our own actions has been one of the most difficult of the scientific activities. The historical resistance to the concept of determinism as applied to human behavior may just be a part of this difficulty.

Another philosophical cornerstone of science is empiricism. Empiricism is a philosophical position that sensory experience is the basis of knowledge. Traditional (nonscientific) thinking would suggest that knowledge may be derived from rational thinking and intuition, or by mystical, religious, and divine revelations. Science, on the other hand, insists that valid knowledge is based on sensory experience. This experience must be socially and objectively verifiable, for after all, even divine revelation can be an "experience." The process involved in making experience acceptable to science is what is known as scientific methods.

It is the philosophy of empiricism that requires observation and measurement of what is being studied. For the most part, observation is a sensory process. Observation requires that we come into sensory contact with the phenomenon under study. If different scientists establish contacts with the phenomenon and arrive at the same or similar values of measurement, then the probability is high that the phenomenon exists and does so in the manner measured. Once the existence of a phenomenon is confirmed through observation and measurement, the scientist is ready for the next step in which the phenomenon is manipulated. Such manipulations are called scientific experiments. In later chapters, we shall take a closer look at both observation and experimentation.

Science as Behavior

The term *science* also includes the actions and behaviors of scientists. Obviously, science is the result of what people called scientists do. The viewpoint that science is a certain kind of behavior is not well known because of the emphasis on objective methods, procedures, and philosophies in describing science. While such an emphasis is entirely valid, the need to understand the behavior of scientists in order to appreciate the full meaning of science should not be ignored. Approaching science from the standpoint of scientists' behaviors may have the best pedagogical value. Young people may understand science better when told how accomplished scientists tend to behave.

The viewpoint that science is a certain kind of behavior is relatively new. Behavioral scientists such as Skinner (1953, 1974) have insisted that the behavior of scientists is also a subject matter of the science of behavior. Systematic analysis of the behavior of scientists has barely begun, partly because of the traditional notion that both scientific and literary creativity are mysterious and unique, and thus beyond the scope of scientific analysis. There is some fear that an objective analysis of the process of writing a poem, painting a picture, or discovering some lawful relations in nature will adversely affect such valuable (but poorly understood) activities. Possibly, the resistance to a scientific analysis of the behavior of scientists and artists may simply be a part of the historical skepticism regarding determinism of human behavior.

Consistent with some of the misconceptions of science, there are also several misconceptions about scientists as persons. Scientists are popularly depicted as impractical, fanciful, and unsociable. They may be considered maniacs who wish to control the world and all humanity. Scientists are thought to be absentminded and slovenly. They may be considered cold, mechanical, and lacking in feelings and warmth.

As Bachrach (1969) put it, such a stereotypical notion of scientists is "arrant nonsense" (p. 111). More sensibly, scientists are described as curious people who are often dissatisfied with existing "explanations" of events they wish to study. Skinner (1953) has stated that scientists are disposed to "deal with facts rather than what someone has said about them" (p. 12). Curiosity, dissatisfaction with existing "explanations," and a tendency to deal with facts, all lead to a disposition to reject authority. The history of science shows that science "rejects its own authorities when they interfere with the observation of nature" (Skinner, 1953, p. 12).

A scientist is more willing than other people to set aside his or her wishes and expectations and let the facts and results of experiments speak for themselves. The scientist is interested in having objectively demonstrated relations replace subjectively held opinions and convictions. As pointed out by Skinner (1953), intellectual honesty—which is the opposite of wishful thinking—is an important characteristic of scientists. A scientist may find out that the results of an experiment are not as expected or predicted, and may even contradict his or her own well-known theory. In such cases, an honest scientist would report the findings as they were observed, because "the facts must stand and the expectations fall. The subject matter, not the scientist, knows best" (Skinner, 1953, p. 13).

Another characteristic of scientists, according to Skinner (1953), is that they are willing to remain "without an answer until a satisfactory one can be found" (p.13). Beginning students in many fields are often surprised when told that there is no satisfactory answer to certain questions. When students are told that we do not know precisely how language is acquired or stuttering is caused, they find it hard to believe that "all those experts do not have any idea" and that the experts can live with such uncertainties. Scientists can tolerate such uncertainties because they are trained to reject premature explanations and theories. The fact that something cannot be explained at a given time is less bothersome to scientists than it is to nonscientists. Instead of accepting whatever explanations that may be available, scientists tend to investigate.

It is sometimes thought that when there is no good explanation, what is available can be, or even must be, accepted. Doing so would be dangerous, however. Unfortunately, this practice is often encouraged by investigators who, after having advanced their own explanations, challenge others to either accept those explanations or offer better ones. Good scientists do not pay much attention to such challenges. One need not propose a better explanation in order to reject a bad one. Explanations (and theories) stand on their evidence, and if there is no acceptable evidence, they just do not stand. One can examine alternative explanations and reject one in favor of the other. But one can also reject an explanation in favor of none (Hegde, 1980a).

The debate over the Chomskyan innate hypotheses in the explanation of language acquisition illustrates this issue. During the 1960s many linguists and psycholinguists who had proposed a variety of innate hypotheses to explain language acquisition had also repeatedly challenged nonnativists to either accept those hypotheses or offer better explanations. A philosopher of science who was involved in a symposium that addressed the issue of Chomsky's nativistic theory of language said that "for certain remarkable facts I have no alternative explanation. . . . That alone does not dictate acceptance of whatever theory may be offered; for the theory may be worse than none. Inability to explain a fact does not condemn me to accept an intrinsically repugnant and incomprehensible theory" (Goodman, 1967, p. 27). This again underscores the view that scientists are people who can go without an explanation.

Science as a Set of Methods

In addition to certain philosophies and behavioral dispositions, science is a set of methods. The definition of science as methods is generally better understood than either the philosophy of science or the behavioral dispositions of scientists. This is understandable because in the teaching of science and research, tangible methods receive greater attention than philosophies and dispositions.

The methods of science have many characteristics. Most of this book is devoted to elaborating them. Therefore, in this section, only a few major aspects of the definition of science as methods will be highlighted.

Science can be defined as a certain way of studying events and solving problems. Science is a set of methods designed to investigate research questions in a manner acceptable to scientists. The methods of science can also be described as rules that dictate scientists' conduct in carrying out a piece of research. Violation of these rules can produce questionable results. Therefore, scientists are trained in those methods so that they can engage in activities that produce valid knowledge.

The most important aspect of the methods of science is that they make it possible to answer research questions. The methods are a structural as well as a conceptual means of investigating research problems. The selection, formulation, and definition of research problems; selection of subjects (when appropriate); specification of variables or factors to be analyzed; the manner in which the variables are measured and manipulated; and the techniques of data analysis are all a part of the scientific method.

Probably the most basic characteristic of the methods of science is that they are *objective*. Objectivity is achieved when the methods and the results are publicly verifiable. Public verification simply means that other scientists can reproduce both the procedures and their results. Under scientific observation, similar procedures should produce similar results.

Of all the aspects of scientific methods, observation, measurement, and experimentation are the most fundamental. Observation is a basic tool necessary for all of the scientific operations. Measurement is another basic tool of science. Much of the progress that can be made in the scientific analysis of a phenomenon depends upon precise and objective measurement of that phenomenon. In Chapter 5, I shall describe observation and measurement in greater detail.

Once a phenomenon comes under systematic observation and measurement, experimentation becomes possible. It is through experimentation that scientists establish cause–effect relations between events. The concept of experiment is described later in this chapter.

To summarize, a comprehensive view of science includes the philosophical, behavioral, and methodological considerations just described. Throughout the book, I shall address these aspects of science in different practical and theoretical contexts.

OUTCOME OF SCIENTIFIC ACTIVITY

It is often said that science has certain "goals." However, when we talk about the goals of science, we are actually talking about the eventual outcome of scientific activity. The term *goal* suggests that something that might happen in the future affects scientists' behavior. Neither scientists nor others are affected by future events. The question of the "goals" of science is the question of why scientists do what they do. Scientists do what they do because of their past and the present contingencies, not because of some future events called "goals." Why scientists do research cannot be answered by listing the "goals" of science. Therefore, it is more meaningful to consider the typical outcome of scientific activity. It is only in a nontechnical sense that scientists are "after such outcomes."

A basic outcome of scientific activity is *description* of natural phenomena. After having observed a phenomenon, scientists describe its characteristics. Therefore, describing a phenomenon is usually the first step in scientific analysis. An adequate description of the characteristics of an event is often useful in taking additional steps such as experimentation and prediction. At this stage, mostly the observable properties of the event under study are described. A researcher observing the language behaviors of a 2-year-old child may note the conditions under which specified language behaviors are produced. The observation might answer questions about the amount and types of language behaviors a 2-year-old child is able to produce under specified conditions of stimulation.

Some disciplines rely heavily on naturalistic observations. Ethology, for example, is a study of the behavior of animals in their natural habitat. Ethologists typically do not manipulate the animal's natural environment to see what effects follow. The goal is to understand the relation between animal behavior and its habitat, including the animal's social milieu. Similarly, astronomy is mostly observational, not necessarily because of choice but because of necessity. Nonexperimental, observational sciences do not seek to effect changes in the phenomena they study. However, in many branches of science, mere description of a phenomenon is not sufficient for a complete scientific analysis. This is because in the case of many complex events, descriptions tell us what is happening, but not necessarily why. Therefore, a description often leads to experimentation designed to find out why the event is taking place.

In communicative disorders, there is a considerable emphasis on descriptive studies and models. This is partly understandable because other kinds of studies, especially those designed to develop theories or find the instigating causes of speech–language disorders, have been few, mostly inadequate, and therefore frustrating. This does not mean, however, that we should stop at the level of descriptive analysis. As we shall see in later chapters, experimental analysis of causal variables of speech–language behaviors is much needed. Such an analysis makes it possible to effect changes in disordered communication.

Another significant outcome of science is typically described as _understanding_ natural phenomena. We do not understand an event when we do not know what causes it. No amount of description, therefore, is sufficient to achieve an understanding of a given event. Therefore, discovery of cause–effect relations is one of the most desirable outcomes of scientific activity. Cause–effect relations are discovered through experimentation in which some presumed cause is systematically varied to see what effects are produced.

An outcome closely related to understanding an event is _explanation_. It is often said that science seeks to explain events. In a technical sense, an explanation is the specification of a cause–effect relation. Scientists explain events by pointing to their causal factors. Therefore, the two outcomes—understanding and explanation—are realized simultaneously.

A thorough understanding and a valid explanation often lead to the next outcome of scientific activity: _prediction._ In most cases, a demonstrated cause of an event will help predict the occurrence of that event. Scientific predictions are reliable to the extent the explanations are valid.

A final outcome that depends upon the other outcomes is _control_ of natural phenomena. In most sciences, scientists can control an event when they understand its cause and predict its occurrence. Events are controlled when they are changed in some manner. An extreme change is achieved when its occurrence is totally prevented. Other kinds of changes are obtained when some properties of the event are altered. The event may still take place, but at a reduced magnitude, duration, or intensity.

Control can be described as an optional outcome of science. One might understand, explain, and predict an event, but may be unwilling to change it in any way, although this is not a very likely course of a majority of sciences. To a certain extent, an option to control an event may be a matter of social policy. For example, experimental genetics might show that it is possible to create new forms of life, but the society may not wish to exert that control.

On the other hand, some sciences cannot exert significant control on most of the phenomena they study even though the scientists understand them and reliably predict their occurrence. Astronomy is a significant example. The movements of planets and resulting events such as eclipses are well understood and reliably predicted, but no control is exerted on these events.

It is clear that most of the outcomes of science depend upon one thing: the specification of cause–effect relations. From a methodological standpoint, much of the activity in matured sciences involves operations designed to isolate cause–effect relations among natural phenomena. Disciplines that do not focus upon this kind of activity usually cannot achieve such other outcomes as explanation or prediction. They are also less likely to be regarded as sciences.

VARIABLES AND THEIR TYPES

The basic method of scientific investigation is empirically analytical. That means that in many cases, the phenomenon to be studied is broken down into smaller components that can be observed more easily, measured more precisely, and manipulated more successfully. Very broadly defined phenomena are often not suitable for scientific investigation. This is especially the case during the earlier stages of investigation. In the analysis of a phenomenon, scientists first identify some specific aspect that can be defined in a narrow and precise manner. Such narrowly defined aspects (of phenomena) that can be measured and manipulated are called *variables*. In this sense, a phenomenon refers to a broad event, and variables are certain aspects of it.

It is apparent that the term *variables* refers to specific aspects of events that vary. Everything that exists varies across time and conditions. In fact, much of the methodology of science has been designed to isolate and (when appropriate) control the sources of variability in naturally occurring events. Science seeks to analyze variables. They are what the scientist observes, measures, changes, and manipulates in some way.

As phenomena, all natural events are a bundle of variables. As such, there are physical, chemical, biological, behavioral and other kinds of variables. Articulation, language, fluency, and voice are the four large classes of phenomena that communicative disorders is most concerned with. The "normal" as well as the "deviant" aspects of these phenomena create a host of specific variables that must be measured and manipulated. The phenomenon of language is a collection of such specific variables as the production of plural /s/ or two-word phrases. The phenomenon of articulation contains specific variables relating to the production of various phonemes at different levels of response topography. Similar specific variables can be identified for other aspects of communicative behaviors.

There are different types of variables, and a discussion of them can be helpful in gaining a better understanding of this important concept in scientific research and theories. The most important of the variables include the following: dependent, independent, active, assigned, and intervening.

Dependent Variables

The technical term for an effect is *dependent variable.* In many cases, scientific analyses start with some dependent variables, which are the effects of unknown causes. Confronting an effect, the scientist may try to find out its cause. In other words, the dependent variable is an event or an aspect of some event that needs to be studied and explained.

Many research questions contain at least a dependent variable. Questions such as how do children acquire language, what are the causes of aphasia or stuttering, why do some children fail to learn the correct production of speech sounds, why do deaf children fail to acquire language, what is the best way of teaching manual signs to deaf individuals, and what causes high-frequency hearing loss are some of the many questions the communicative disorders specialist typically asks and tries to answer. Thus, language, speech, fluency, voice, hearing loss, and different modes of communication are all a collection of dependent variables.

As the term suggests, the existence of dependent variables is contingent upon some other variables. Dependent variables are said to be a *function* of causal variables. It means that effects depend upon causes; therefore, no causes, no effects.

Dependent variables are typically measured and monitored by the scientist, but they are not directly manipulated. They can be manipulated only indirectly, and that only when their causes are known. Throughout a scientific study, the dependent variables are measured by the scientist to see if the effects are systematically altered when the presumed causes are manipulated.

In order to be useful in research, dependent variables must be defined in precise terms. They must be defined operationally, which means that the definition must specify how the variable will be measured. Language, for example, is too broad a dependent variable to be of use in particular research studies. Typically, some specific aspect of language, such as the production of certain morphemes, phrases, or sentences, is the defined dependent variable in research studies.

Independent Variables

These are the causes of the effects under study. Independent variables are often unknown, many times presumed, and sometimes accidentally stumbled upon. When a research question aimed at discovering a cause–effect relation is effectively answered, an independent variable will have been identified. Therefore, the specification of independent variables is crucial to any type of causal analysis. In many cases, the effect ("goal" or "objective") of successful scientific research is the description of an independent variable. Independent variables *explain* dependent variables, since an explanation of an event is nothing but a specification of its cause.

Independent variables are measured *and* directly manipulated by scientists. An independent variable is the one that when manipulated can induce systematic changes in a dependent variable. When there is no access to the independent variable of an event, the scientist cannot induce changes in that event.

There are three most important kinds of independent variables in communicative disorders. The first involves those variables that are responsible for the communicative behaviors in general. The potential causal variables of language, speech, voice, and fluency fall into this category. For example, one can ask what causes fluency or what causes language or phonological acquisition. Typically, the independent variables of this kind are concerned with the "normal" speech–language behaviors.

The second kind of independent variables is concerned with various disorders of communication. Why do children fail to acquire language, phonological responses, or fluency? The same questions can be rephrased in terms of the causes of language, articulation, or fluency disorders. Questions such as these address the causes of disorders and diseases in a clinical science. The first and second kinds of independent variables can be counterparts of each other. For example, if language acquisition is made possible by parental stimulation (whatever that means), then a disorder of language may be due to deficiencies in such stimulation.

The third kind of independent variables is the treatment techniques. Treatment variables are the causes of change in the disordered behaviors. They can help change undesirable effects (diseases or disorders). Just as a scientist cannot directly affect an event, a clinician cannot alter diseases and disorders directly. The clinician must gain access to a treatment (independent) variable to effect changes in the disorder. The treatment variable is systematically manipulated so that the effects are eliminated or modified.

Most variables can be either dependent or independent. The status a variable assumes depends upon the frame of reference of particular studies. A given variable may be independent in one study and dependent in another. For example, anxiety may be treated as an independent variable in a study designed to assess its effects on stuttering. The investigator may hope to show that systematic increases or decreases in experimentally manipulated anxiety produce corresponding changes in the amount of stuttering. In another study, the investigator might show that when stuttering frequency is experimentally manipulated, the amount of anxiety varies. In the first instance, anxiety is an independent variable and stuttering is the dependent variable. In the second instance, the position is reversed: what is analyzed is the effect of stuttering on anxiety. Similarly, hearing loss is a dependent variable when its cause is investigated, but it is an independent variable when its effect on communication or academic performance is assessed.

Active and Assigned Variables

Typically, research studies involve many variables, some of which are controlled by the researcher while others are not controlled. In experimental research, at least one independent variable is under the control of the investigator. But the investigator might suspect the existence of other potential independent variables, some of which are not manipulable. A manipulated independent variable is sometimes called an active variable.

Other suspected independent variables that may influence the dependent variable under study may be considered assigned variables. An assigned variable is typically a presumed independent variable that is not manipulated by the investigator. In fact, assigned variables are typically not manipulable. They are often inherent characteristics of subjects used in research.

In research involving biological organisms (including human subjects), assigned variables are thought to play an important role. The typical assigned variables include such factors as age, sex, intelligence, socioeconomic status, occupation, education, ethnic and cultural background, physical and mental health, "personality" characteristics, and genetic predispositions. The actual effect of an active (manipulated) independent variable may be influenced to a certain extent by one or several of these assigned variables. For example, an investigator may try to determine the effects of a parent stimulation program on the rate of normal language acquisition. In this case, the parent stimulation program is the active, manipulated, independent variable. At the same time, the rate of language acquisition may be partly determined by assigned variables such as the child's intelligence, sex, age, and undetermined genetic predispositions. Obviously, such subject characteristics are not under the control of the investigator. They are treated as assigned independent variables whose contribution is often inferred.

In experimental research, it is possible to rule out the influence of most assigned variables. For example, an investigator can show that the parent stimulation program works regardless of children's intelligence, sex, and socioeconomic status.

Assigned variables are most troublesome in nonexperimental research, in which there is no manipulation of an independent variable and none of the potential variables are controlled. In certain kinds of research, subjects are grouped on the basis of assigned variables. Subsequently, the groups may be shown to be different on some dependent variable. Then the investigator may conclude that the differences in the dependent variable are due to the difference in the assigned variables. For instance, a sample of children may be grouped according to their social class while measuring their language performance. Any difference in the performance of the groups may then be attributed to the subjects' social class. In this type of research, there is no control on potential independent variables, and therefore there is no assurance that the conclusions are valid. In Chapter 4, I shall describe and compare different types of research in greater detail.

Intervening Variables

Of all the kinds of variables researched by social, behavioral, and biological scientists, the intervening variables are the most controversial. Intervening variables refer to events or processes that are supposed to be active inside a person's body. They are informally described as "in-the-head" variables. Mind, nervous system, and cognition are among the major sources of intervening variables. These variables are thought to provide a link between observed dependent and independent variables. Such a link is considered missing when only the observed cause–effect relations are described.

The study of human behavior and particularly that of language is replete with intervening variables. The emphasis found on such presumed variables as "language processing," "linguistic competence," "internalized rules of grammar," and "knowledge of phonologic rules," in the current linguistic analyses demonstrates the use of intervening variables. The term *cognition* is an enormous collection of a variety of intervening variables. The observable, productive language behavior is thought to be impossible without cognitive "inputs" and information "processing" strategies.

The historical roots of intervening variables lie in the philosophy of mentalism. Mentalism asserts that observable behaviors are a product of internal, mental (psychological) processes that are not observable. According to mentalism, the unobservable mind is the source of observable actions. In due course, the nervous system, especially the brain, became more attractive as a source of action. Various kinds of processes are supposed to underlie observable actions. Currently, the most popular source of action in general and language in particular is cognition.

Intervening variables are attractive to theorists who believe that an explanation of observable behaviors lies in unobservable events taking place in presumed entities or processes. The main problem with intervening variables is that they are simply inferred from observable behaviors, often in the absence of any kind of experimental manipulations. The most questionable practice relative to intervening variables is that processes inferred from observable behaviors are immediately offered as explanations of those behaviors. For instance, the presence of cognitive processes is inferred from certain language behaviors; in turn, cognitive processes are offered as explanations of those language behaviors. Since they are neither directly measured, observed, or experimentally manipulated, the explanatory status of cognitive processes is highly questionable. What is inferred from an action cannot explain that action.

CAUSALITY AND FUNCTIONAL ANALYSIS

It was stated earlier that science is essentially a search for cause-effect relations in natural events. Basic and applied scientists as well as clinicians need to gain access to causes of events in order to modify, control, or eliminate them.

Diseases and disorders can be treated more effectively when their causes are known. Also, as noted before, when causes are specified, events are explained.

Multiple Causation and Levels of Causality

One of the basic assumptions of science is that events typically have multiple causes, and that an identified cause of a given event is only a reflection of the level at which the event has been analyzed. Different causes can be identified at different levels of analysis. In many cases, it is also possible to identify multiple causes at the same level of analysis. This means that causes and effects are nothing but a string of events. Depending upon the temporospatial locus of analysis, an event is a cause of the succeeding effect, which is in turn a cause of the next event in the string. At times, it may not be possible to see or analyze the entire string, since in many cases scientists may not know about all aspects of the event that constitutes the effect.

Although experimental demonstrations are rare, it is often thought that most communicative disorders are caused by a combination of genetic, neurophysiological, and environmental factors. Therefore, speech and language disorders can be analyzed at the levels of genetic, neurophysiological, and environmental events. At each of these levels, there may be multiple causes. Theoretically, there are many genetic conditions that can be causally related to a given disorder, some of which may be active simultaneously. Cleft palate, for example, can be a result of several potential genetic, teratogenic, and toxic factors. Neurophysiological variables may be genetically determined to a certain extent, but some of them may not have a clear-cut pattern of inheritance, thus making it difficult to identify potential genetic factors in given cases. Nevertheless, at the level of neurophysiological functioning, multiple factors may be involved in the causation of a given disorder. The neurophysiological mechanism may show an inherited weakness, an injury-based (environmentally induced) deficiency, or a disease-based problem. Similarly, an environmental analysis may show deficiencies in stimulation, reinforcing contingencies, or educational practices.

The nature of the cause or causes identified for a given disorder depends upon the level at which the disorder is analyzed. Different types of causes can be identified at different levels of analysis. A causal analysis may involve neurophysiological, genetic, or environmental variables. Once the independent contribution of these variables is determined, the causal analysis may be shifted to a more complex level. The investigator may now be concerned with potential interactions between different types of causes. Thus, initially, it may be found that stuttering is partly determined by a genetic predisposition. Neurophysiological research might reveal neural and muscular aberrations in stutterers. In turn, it might be shown that certain types of conditioning variables (environmental events) are also important in the etiology of stuttering. Eventually, the analysis might be concerned with how these three types of causal variables interact to produce the final effect (stuttering).

It must be understood that a tentative determination of a cause at a given level may not necessarily negate the importance of causes at other levels of analysis. For example, the strong possibility that there are some genetic factors in the etiology of stuttering does not rule out the presence of environmental factors. Similarly, experimental demonstration of environmental factors does not negate the importance of genetic influence in the etiology of stuttering. It is often believed that genetic and neurophysiological explanations of behavioral phenomena will automatically discredit explanations based upon environmental or conditioning variables. However, the philosophy of multiple causation does not support this belief. For example, the evidence that stuttering is associated with a genetic predisposition does not negate the experimentally demonstrated effects of a conditioning contingency. In the future, neurological investigations may be better able to describe what happens in the brain when someone stutters, but they would not minimize the importance of *experimentally demonstrated* effects of reinforcement or punishment contingencies. Similarly, future neurology may be better able to describe what happens in the nervous system when a child learns the alphabet or produces the very first word. Such a description, however, could not suggest that no environmental variables are involved in that learning process. The parents and teachers would still be providing certain stimulus conditions and arrange certain response consequences. In cases such as these, the only and the highly desirable outcome of more exact and sophisticated descriptions of neurological events associated with behaviors is a better and more comprehensive understanding of those behaviors at both neurological and environmental levels.

Instigating versus Maintaining Causes

Many disorders, including those of communication, may have one set of causes to begin with and an entirely different set that eventually come to control and maintain those disorders. This idea may simply be a variation of the theme of multiple causation. An event may be caused and maintained by the same multiple causes. On the other hand, an event may be caused by one set of causes but maintained by a different set of causes. Alternately, regardless of how it was started, an event may be maintained by different causes at different times.

In physical and medical sciences, the maintaining causes may not always be radically different from the original or instigating causes. Theoretically, the same infection or tumor or injury can be the original as well as the maintaining cause of a given disease. This is not to say that either the cause or the effect is static. Both are in fact dynamic, which means that they change and produce additional effects, which become new causes of new effects. Nevertheless, physical, chemical, or topographical similarities between the instigating and maintaining causes can often be identified. However, in disorders of human performance or behavior, the instigating and the maintaining causes could be entirely different.

Several hypotheses in communicative disorders could illustrate this point. For example, it may be hypothesized that parental punishment of "normal" dysfluencies causes stuttering in young children. Thus, the instigating cause of stuttering may be parental punishment. However, the very fact that stuttering might continue into adult life in the absence of parental punishment also suggests the possibility that the maintaining causes are different. One might hypothesize that the maintaining causes are negatively reinforcing events stemming from avoidance of difficult speaking situations. In this case, the maintaining causes may be diametrically opposed to the original causes (punishment versus reinforcement). To take another example, the speech and voice disorders of a child with cleft palate might persist even after an adequate surgical repair of the cleft. This persisting disorder can no longer be attributed to nonexisting cleft. A reasonable assumption in such cases is that the disorder has a different set of maintaining causes.

It is well known that searches for the causes of communicative disorders have often been frustrating. At best, such searches have led only to speculative reasoning. When parents ask such questions as "what caused my child's stuttering" or "what is the cause of my child's language delay," we often go into a discussion of possibilities and conjectures that may have some relevance only to cases at large. But such discussions are totally dissatisfying to the parents, who expect an answer relevant to their child. It is also equally well known that in the "diagnostics" of communicative disorders, clinicians do not diagnose anything, since within the medical model, diagnosis means finding a cause or causes of a given disease. Often, this failure to find causes of communicative disorders has led to a belief that clinicians should simply be "descriptive" and not worry about causes.

Description is only the beginning stage of any kind of scientific analysis. There is no substitute for a causal analysis in either a basic or an applied science. The frustrating searches in the field have been concerned mostly with original causes of communicative disorders, be they organic or environmental. Such causes of communicative disorders have been inaccessible, perhaps for several reasons. One possibility is that the original causes may not be physical or chemical conditions that are available for examination as long as the disorder persists. Another possibility is that even if physical or chemical conditions do cause communicative disorders, such conditions may not be enduring. Therefore, those conditions may not be present at the time of examination, which is typically done some time after the manifestation of the disorder. Still another possibility is that the causal physical or chemical conditions are as yet unobservable because of technical limitations. Furthermore, there may be temporary environmental causes, which are also not detected when examined later.

We know more about the maintaining, than about the instigating, causes of communicative disorders. The search for environmental maintaining causes has generally been more productive and less speculative than searches for original causes. It is known that in treating many disorders of communication, clinicians often alter possible maintaining causes and teach behaviors that are incompatible with the existing faulty behaviors. For example, when a clinician ignores misarticulations while reinforcing correct productions, he or she is trying to alter the contingencies that may have been maintaining those misarticulations. When a language clinician withholds all attention to gestures and grunts while reinforcing meaningful vocal productions, an attempt to alter the maintaining factors of inappropriate behaviors is made. Though the instigating causes of many of the communicative disorders are unknown, clinicians can still treat several disorders successfully. This suggests that clinicians generally manipulate maintaining causes of both the appropriate and the inappropriate behaviors in their clients.

It is certainly desirable to find the original causes of diseases and disorders. A knowledge of the original causes of a given disorder can be useful in preventing that disorder. In order to take the applied advantages of original causes, they must be experimentally demonstrated, not just inferred from the effects. The problem, however, is that most presumed original causes are difficult to manipulate experimentally. Johnson's hypothesis that stuttering is a result of parental negative reaction to the child's normal "nonfluency" is a case in point. For various practical and ethical reasons, negative parental reactions are not experimentally manipulable.

EXPERIMENT AND EXPERIMENTAL CONTROL

As noted earlier, establishing cause–effect relations is the key to understanding, explaining, predicting, and controlling natural phenomena. To establish cause–effect relations, scientists engage in various activities including observation, measurement, and data analysis. However, the most crucial of these activities is known as an *experiment*. Experiment is the most important of the concepts of science, and it is the most powerful of the strategies available to scientists to establish cause–effect relations.

The term *experiment* is often used loosely to indicate any type of research study. The term, however, has a technical meaning in science. Not every kind of research is an experiment. An experiment can be technically defined as the manipulation of an independent variable or variables under controlled conditions to produce systematic changes in a dependent variable or variables. There is no experiment unless the researcher has clearly identified at least one causal factor whose influence on a dependent variable is assessed while controlling for other potential causes.

Manipulation of an independent variable is the most important feature of an experiment. It means that the effects of a causal factor are studied by introducing, or in some way altering, that factor. The typical question that prompts an experiment is "what happens when I do this," and in this sense, the researcher is already clear about the potential independent variable. In clinical treatment research, an independent variable is *manipulated* whenever a treatment technique is introduced, withdrawn, reversed, or varied in some systematic manner.

A treatment is introduced when it is first applied, withdrawn when simply discontinued, reversed when it is applied to some other behavior or disorder, and varied when its frequency or intensity is altered. When the number of treatment sessions is increased or decreased, the strength of the independent variable is altered. Within given sessions, the frequency of applications of an independent variable may be changed. The frequency of reinforcer delivery, for example, can be changed within or across treatment sessions. Manipulations of an independent variable include these and other alterations introduced by the researcher.

Another important feature of an experiment is that the independent variable is manipulated under *controlled conditions*. Conditions are controlled when extraneous independent variables are systematically ruled out. In other words, when establishing a cause–effect relation, the researcher must ensure that other potential causes were also not involved in the experimental situation. When several potential causes are present, it becomes impossible to determine the cause or the causes of the effect being analyzed. Thus, the manipulation of a single independent variable under controlled conditions that results in certain changes in the dependent variable is the essence of an experiment.

In clinical research, experiments are the means by which one can demonstrate that certain treatment variables were indeed effective. Through experimental manipulations, clinicians can demonstrate that changes in disorders were brought about by particular treatment variables and that those changes were unrelated to other potential treatment variables. We shall return to this type of research in Chapter 4.

The cause–effect relation isolated by an experiment is also known as a *controlling relation*. Well-designed experiments help isolate a controlling relation between two variables: the cause controls the effects. Controlled conditions, however, should not be confused with controlling relations. The term *controlled conditions* refers to various procedures designed to rule out the potential causes other than the one the researcher is interested in. In essence, controlled conditions refer to structures of experiments, whereas controlling relations are abstract ways in which events are related to one another.

HYPOTHESES IN SCIENTIFIC RESEARCH

It is often said that scientific research starts with a hypothesis. Traditionally, research is equated with hypothesis testing. Scientists are typically supposed to formulate a hypothesis first, then design an experiment to test that hypothesis, and finally retain or reject it in light of the results yielded by the experiment. In view of the importance attached to hypothesis testing in certain philosophies of research, it is necessary to understand what they are and what role they play in scientific investigations.

Hypotheses can be defined as a priori statements about a relation between two or more variables. A good hypothesis specifies a dependent variable and at least one independent variable. Therefore, all hypotheses are statements of cause–effect relations between specified phenomena. Because hypotheses are typically formulated prior to the actual experimentation, they are in fact predictive statements. A hypothesis predicts that when a certain event is present, a certain other event will follow as a consequence.

Scientific hypotheses contrast with everyday guesses, predictions, and assumptions about cause–effect relations. For the most part, hypotheses of everyday life are informal, sometimes vague, and rarely expressed in measurable terms. As a result, popular hypotheses are difficult to verify. Scientific hypotheses, on the other hand, are more formal, specific, and expressed in operational (measurable) terms. Since they are stated in measurable terms, scientific hypotheses are testable. Furthermore, unlike everyday guesses, scientific hypotheses tend to be more systematic and frequently bear some relation to a scientific theory about a larger phenomenon. Ideally, scientific hypotheses tend to be verified, whereas everyday hypotheses may often lead to untested beliefs.

Although hypotheses that bear no particular relation to a theory are sometimes formulated and tested, most hypotheses are derived from a theory. In fact, hypotheses are the means by which theories are tested. A complex theory may give rise to a number of hypotheses, each of which is tested independently. If most of the hypotheses are verified with positive results, then the theory is said to have received experimental support.

Need for Hypothesis: Two Viewpoints

Whether or not hypotheses are considered essential in the conduct of meaningful empirical research depends upon the investigator's research style and philosophy. The statistical approach to research asserts that hypotheses are essential in empirical research (Kerlinger, 1973). It is argued that hypotheses give direction to research, since they are said to tell an investigator what to look for. It is believed that without a hypothesis, there may be nothing to investigate. It is also believed that hypothesis testing is the most important— if not the only—means of verifying scientific theories. Moreover, the hypothesis is said to be "the most powerful tool man has invented to achieve dependable knowledge" (Kerlinger, 1973, p. 25).

An alternative view on the usefulness of hypotheses has been suggested by the experimental analysis of behavior (Bachrach, 1969; Sidman, 1960;

Skinner, 1974). This viewpoint questions the need for, and the importance of, formal hypotheses in the conduct of research. The proponents of this view suggest that it is possible to investigate important research problems without the directive of formal hypotheses (Sidman, 1960; Skinner, 1950, 1956). One of the famous statements of Newton concerning the research process is "Hypotheses non fingo," which means that "I do not make hypotheses." Skinner has also stated that he has "never attacked a problem by constructing a Hypothesis" (1972, p. 112).

Hypotheses, as noted earlier, are proposed after a research question has been formulated. In this sense, a hypothesis is nothing but the prediction of results of a planned experiment. Skinner suggests that one can ask a question and immediately proceed to answer it through an experiment. He sees the intermediate step of hypothesis formulation as an unnecessary exercise. Whether predicted or not, a well-designed experiment may produce results that throw light on the relation between the variables investigated. Since the experimental results are the final test of a relation between variables, the need to predict those results beforehand is not clear. Because it is the evidence that stands, not necessarily the hypothesis, it is best to ask a question and produce results through experimentation. The results then help shape a valid statement of cause–effect relation.

There are other problems with the formulation of hypotheses prior to experimentation. If one insists that all meaningful research should start out with a well-formulated hypothesis, it is hard to imagine how unsuspected relations between variables could ever come to light. Hypothesis testing minimizes the importance of accidental discoveries. And yet, as we noted in Chapter 1, many important scientific discoveries were made accidentally. By nature, accidental discoveries are unsuspected and hence unformulated in terms of an a priori hypothesis. Often, accidental findings are noted during the course of researches designed to test formal hypotheses. The history of natural sciences is replete with examples of accidental discoveries that proved to be more important than some of the planned research during which such "accidents" occurred (Bachrach, 1969).

Another problem with formal hypotheses is that they can bias the investigator. A researcher who hypothesizes that A is the cause of B fully expects to support that hypothesis by the results of his or her experiment. If not, there would be no point in proposing that hypothesis. Theoretically, negative results should lead to a prompt rejection of the hypothesis. In practice, however, some investigators may show a tendency to explain away the results in an effort to breathe life into their troubled hypotheses. There is always the possibility that the hypothesis was true but was not supported by the results because of methodological problems, but in the absence of convincing reasons, the hypothesis must at least be temporarily rejected. This may not happen because of the researcher's belief in the hypothesis.

The biasing effects of formal hypotheses are recognized by those who support the use of formal hypotheses. Since the need for hypotheses is taken for granted, statisticians have offered a unique solution to the problem of bias: the null hypothesis (Fisher, 1956). The term *null* means zero, and a null hypothesis is a statement of no relation between two variables. It is also known as a statistical hypothesis. An investigator who believes that *A* is the cause of *B* would actually propose that *A* and *B* are unrelated. For example, an investigator who thinks that the parental punishment of dysfluencies in speech causes stuttering would actually state that the parental punishment and stuttering are unrelated. The investigator then hopes to show that this null hypothesis is not true and that parental punishment and stuttering are indeed causally related. When a hypothesis is stated in positive terms, the investigator expects to support it, and when it is stated in the null form, the investigator expects to reject it. Nonetheless, it is presumed that an investigator who proposes a null hypothesis *instead* of a positive one would not be biased in the interpretation of results.

It is highly questionable whether the null is an answer to the biasing effects of hypotheses. The null is no more than a surrogate for a positive hypothesis the investigator believes in. All knowledgeable readers of research papers know that a null hypothesis really means the opposite of what is stated. An investigator's efforts are directed toward *rejecting* a null hypothesis just as much as *supporting* a positive one. Therefore, when the results fail to reject a null, the investigator may try to explain the results away, since the null was not what was really believed in. The null is a facade, and a transparent one at that. It is hard to imagine how it can help remove or reduce the investigator's bias. For these reasons, those who do not believe in the use of formal hypotheses do not take the null seriously. Skinner has stated that in his research, "the null hypothesis finds itself in the null class" (1969, p. 81).

The biases of an investigator are a fundamental problem that cannot be eliminated by statistical devices and null hypotheses. It is possible that such biases exist even when investigators do not state a hypothesis, but simply proceed to experiment once the research question has been stated. Therefore, not stating a hypothesis is not suggested as a means of overcoming one's own biases regarding the outcome of research. On the other hand, an explicit statement of a hypothesis can amount to a public commitment to a certain position. It can thus create an additional pressure on the investigator to support the stated position. Typically, hypotheses are derived from already published theories for which the investigator may be well known. In such contexts, formation of hypotheses can have an especially biasing effects on the interpretation of results.

Objective interpretation of experimental results needs a certain degree of intellectual discipline. This discipline is a part of the scientist's disposition to value evidence higher than his or her opinions and expectations. Artificial devices such as the null do not even address the difficult problem of investigator bias. The problem is one of training objective scientists. Objectivity is a matter of a scientist's personal history, shaped mostly by education, training, and experience.

THEORIES AND SCIENTIFIC REASONING

It is common knowledge that scientists build theories. Probably it is no exaggeration to say that most people equate theory building with scientific research. Many philosophers of science believe that the aim of scientific research is to develop theories. Theories help us understand events around us. Undoubtedly, theories are the most valued products of scientific investigations. It is therefore necessary to understand the nature and types of theories and the scientific reasoning involved in their development.

A theory can be defined as a set of statements concerning a functional relation between a class of independent variables and a class of dependent variables. In simpler terms, a theory specifies a cause–effect relation between two or more events. Therefore, it can also be said that a theory *explains* an event. In the technical sense, a clearly specified functional relation between variables is the heart of a theory.

In a more general sense, a theory can be described as a systematic body of information concerning a phenomenon. A theory begins with a thorough description of the event or the effect to be explained. It states the conditions under which the occurrence of that event is probable. The properties of the event, such as the topography (form), frequency, magnitude, intensity, and levels of complexity are also specified. Variations in the properties and the conditions associated with specified variations are described.

After having described the event, the theory explains the event by specifying why it occurs. In other words, the causal variable or variables are specified. In essence, a theory states that Y exists because of X. Furthermore, the theory may also describe limitations of the discovered causal relation. It might specify any exceptions noted during the systematic, experimental observations. Finally, a good theory clearly specifies how it can be verified. In other words, a theory also specifies conditions under which the proposed cause–effect relations can be verified by other investigators.

A hypothesis can be contrasted with a theory. A theory is a more comprehensive description and explanation of a total phenomenon. A hypothesis, on the other hand, is concerned with a more specific prediction stemming from a theory. Hypotheses are testable propositions derived from a theory. It is possible, however, to propose certain hypotheses that are not a part of theories. In either case, the scope of a hypothesis is more limited than that of a theory. For example, a theory of language disorders might explain all kinds of language disorders found in all age groups, whereas a hypothesis might be concerned with the specific language problems of a particular group such as the mentally retarded.

Inductive and Deductive Reasoning

Logic and reasoning play an important role in designing and conducting research studies and in the formulation of theories. As a part of philosophy, logic describes formal rules of correct reasoning. Since incorrect reasoning may lead to faulty experiments as well as faulty interpretation of results, it is necessary to understand the logical basis of science and scientific experiments. The early development of the scientific method was due to philosophers' interest in logic and reasoning. In fact, many early scientists were also the philosophers, logicians, physicists, and psychologists of their times.

The philosophers have recognized two most important modes of logical reasoning: deductive and inductive. Deduction and induction are a part of everyday reasoning as well, but they are used in a more formal manner in scientific thinking. These modes of reasoning are especially involved in the process of constructing scientific theories. Therefore, theories themselves are often described as either inductive or deductive.

A common description of induction is that it is reasoning from the particular to the general. Inductive reasoning starts from an observation of particular instances of an event and eventually arrives at some general conclusions regarding the nature and causation of that event. Every time an event is observed, such factors as the precipitating conditions, intensity, magnitude, and so on are carefully recorded. Observations of this kind are made until several individual instances of the event have been observed and described.

The observed individual instances are categorized to see if some common patterns emerge. It may be determined that whenever the event occurred, certain common conditions were also present, and whenever the event failed to occur, the common conditions were absent. For example, a clinical researcher might observe that whenever some patients took a certain prescription drug, their hearing thresholds were temporarily elevated and whenever they were free from the drug, the thresholds were lower. It may also be observed that when certain conditions systematically vary across instances, the magnitude of the event also varies. In our example, whenever the dosage increased, the hearing thresholds were lower, and vice and versa. Such observations could result in a collection of reliable facts about the event.

The facts gathered through observation lead to certain conclusions regarding the nature and causation of the observed event. The scientist may conclude that the antecedent events that are reliably associated with the occurrence of the event are the causes of the event.

In the inductive reasoning used in modern science, observation is not limited to describing the observed event. Observation also includes experimentation, without which a valid theory cannot be built. Instead of waiting for the event to occur, a scientist may create it by manipulating what is believed to be the causal factor, and then withdraw the factor to see if the event disappears. The cause–effect relations receive their maximum support when such experimental manipulations are successfully carried out. When such experimenters are repeated with comparable outcome, a theory may emerge out of the data.

Inductive reasoning is the very method by which we draw conclusions based upon our personal experiences. We know that it is not prudent to draw conclusions based upon isolated experiences regarding an event or an individual. When similar experiences accumulate, certain conclusions may be considered more appropriate. For example, a person who knows nothing about the education of speech–language pathologists might come in contact with one of them and find out that the pathologist is a college graduate. The same person may later come in contact with another clinician who is also a college graduate. In this manner, the person may meet many clinicians, each with a college degree. That person may then conclude that all speech–language pathologists are college graduates. Inductive reasoning used in theory building is a more systematic use of this process with the added feature of controlled experimentation.

Deductive reasoning, on the other hand, starts with what are known as logical premises that are assumed to be valid. Premises are general statements, which suggest that given their validity, certain specific statements are also true. In other words, conclusions are *deduced* from valid propositions. A set of assumed and deduced statements is known as a *syllogism*, which is a logical device described by the ancient philosopher Aristotle. A syllogism starts with two general statements whose validity is assumed. For example, one may state that "All speech–language pathologists have a college degree"; and "Jane is a speech–language pathologist." These two statements will then serve as the basis for a *deduction*, or conclusion, which is that "Jane has a college degree." Syllogisms, as described by Aristotle, are used in modern deductive logic with very little modification. Thus, deductive reasoning begins with generalities and ends with relevant specific instances.

In building a deductive theory, a scientist first makes a series of proposals. Of course, these proposals are based on certain observations. Such observations lead the investigator to suggest the existence of certain cause–effect relations. In essence, a *theory* may be proposed on the basis of observations. From this theory, specific predictions may be derived. Predictions suggest that if the theory is valid, certain specific results must be observed. These predictions are then put to experimental test. If the results of the experiment confirm the prediction, the theory is said to have been supported. If repeated experiments confirm various predictions of the theory, then that theory is accepted as valid.

Deductive theories are more commonly proposed in physical sciences. In behavioral sciences, many have tried to develop such theories, but few if any have succeeded. This is because a large body of well-established facts is needed to attempt even a rudimentary deductive theory. Compared to behavioral sciences, physical sciences do have an impressive body of accepted facts and methods of observation. They have a longer tradition of experimentation that has produced more solid data base. Because of this, better deductive theories can be proposed in physical sciences than in behavioral sciences.

An investigator who uses the deductive method proposes a theory without having conducted certain crucial experiments. As such, the investigator takes a certain risk in proposing a deductive theory. The ensuing experiments may not support some or all of the predictions made by the theory. The investigator is then expected to revise the theory in light of the evidence gathered. Further predictions of the revised theory are then tested experimentally. Thus, continued experimentation may appropriately modify, and eventually validate, a deductive theory.

It is useful to compare inductive and deductive theories. Both types of theories start with certain systematic observations of a given phenomenon. Questions are then raised regarding such aspects as the nature, frequency, and magnitude of the phenomenon under investigation. The two approaches immediately diverge, however. The investigator using the deductive approach will propose a theory, whereas the one using the inductive method will proceed to experiment. In other words, within the deductive framework, questions lead to answers that need to be verified, whereas within the inductive method, questions lead to experiments, which may supply the answers. The deductive method is quick in providing an explanation but slow in verifying it. The inductive method is slow in offering an explanation, but the offered explanation tends to be based on better evidence. A considerable amount of experimental work lies *ahead* of a deductive theory but *behind* an inductive theory. The inductive theorist must resist the temptation to offer a theory without evidence, and a deductive theorist must resist the tendency to avoid the difficult course of experimentation after having proposed an explanation.

Most if not all of the differences between the two approaches lie in the *process* of theory construction, not necessarily in the final product, which is a validated theory in either case. Validated deductive theories are no different from inductive theories. Whether one builds a deductive or an inductive theory depends upon the state of the art of the scientist's subject matter and his or her personal dispositions shaped by the history of training, education, and experience.

By and large, the inductive method is relatively safe in disciplines that do not have widely accepted dependent variables, methods of observations and measurements, and a relatively long tradition of experimentation that has produced data of some generality. Communicative disorders is still such a discipline, and therefore the inductive approach may be the more desirable of the two strategies. Deductive theories in communicative disorders tend to be based on meager evidence and hence more speculative than they ought to be. Besides, it takes much time to verify a deductive theory, and in the meanwhile many persons may prematurely accept it as valid.

Other dangers are personal in nature. Some of those who propose deductive theories may find it harder to face negative evidence that refutes their well-known position. In such cases, instead of revising or rejecting the theory, some investigators may be more inclined to find faults with the data. A much worse situation arises when investigators propose deductive theories but fail to launch a program of research to verify their theories. This type of mistake is quite common in many fields, including communicative disorders. Some deductive theorists seem to imply that their theories are already validated, since some evidence suggested them. Such a tendency betrays a misunderstanding of the deductive process. The initial observations help develop a deductive theory, but they do not validate it. The theory is validated only when experimental tests of specific propositions deduced from that theory produce positive results. When this difficult validation process is neglected, the deductive approach becomes an excellent refuge for armchair theorists whose easy victims are their colleagues who lack a sophisticated understanding of logic and science.

THEORIES AND SCIENTIFIC LAWS

Validated theories allow scientists to move on to the next stage of scientific activity: formulation of scientific laws. Scientific laws are relatively brief statements of relations between events; they are mostly predictive in nature. Theories are broader in scope, whereas scientific laws may apply to a set of events defined more narrowly. Theories may still have portions that need to be verified or evidence that needs to be replicated. Scientific laws, on the other hand, are statements that have received maximum experimental support. Scientific laws are tersely written summaries of replicated evidence. Therefore, scientists are more confident of scientific laws than they are of theories.

It takes a long tradition of experimental research for a discipline to state some of its laws. Laws cannot be based upon controversial evidence, and therefore what is needed is agreement among scientists that similar observations lead to the same or similar results. Therefore, whether a set of statements (theories or laws) is accepted as valid depends largely upon the opinion of scientists in the field. Scientific evidence is always relative, since no scientist can claim that all possible observations of the phenomenon under investigation have been exhausted. Though the same cause of a given event may have been repeatedly observed by several scientists, there is no assurance that some other cause of the same event will not emerge in a later observation.

The relativity of scientific evidence also means that evidence suggests probabilities and not certainties. Observed cause–effect relations may be more or less probable. When the same empirical relations between certain events are observed repeatedly and by different investigators, the probability that the relations are valid is increased. In essence, continued accumulation of positive evidence increases the probability that a cause of the event investigated has been isolated. The continued efforts to gather more evidence may also help identify exceptions to the commonly observed relations. Special conditions under which the generally valid cause–effect relations do not hold may become evident. This will also help the scientist refine his or her statement of the cause–effect relations. When the evidence reaches a certain point of accumulation, scientists begin to think that a theory has been validated or that a more specific statement of a scientific law can be made.

DATA AND EVIDENCE

It is clear from our previous discussions that theories are validated by scientific evidence. At this point, it is necessary to consider the process of developing scientific evidence. The process typically starts with observation and collection of data. Data can be defined as the results of systematic observation. When a scientist observes an event and records some measured value of that event, data begin to accumulate. Scientific data are empirical in the sense that they are based upon actual happenings that resulted in some form of sensory contact. This then may lead to a more systematic measurement of the phenomenon. Such measured values constitute empirical data.

A phenomenon can be observed at different levels. As a result, the data generated by observations can differ in terms of their validity and power to support theories. At the first and the lowest level of observation, an event is witnessed and a description provided. This results in what is known as descriptive data, which are data in the minimal sense of the term. Descriptive data are useful in identifying the properties of an event, but not in supporting a theory. Generally speaking, descriptive data pertain to dependent variables. Although they might suggest potential independent variables, descriptive data cannot isolate such variables.

At the second level of observation, an event may be witnessed and thoroughly described, and some aspect of that event may be systematically measured. For example, one might *describe* and *measure* the frequency of stutterings, misarticulations, and so on. This level of observation provides the investigator with more than mere descriptive data. Included here are the quantitative data. This is an improvement over the first level of observation, but it still lacks the kind of evidence needed to explain the event and thus support a theory.

At the third level of observation, the event is not only described and measured but is also systematically manipulated. In other words, the event is brought under experimental control. To manipulate the event, the experimenter may select and apply a potential independent variable. This level of observation is comparable to clinical treatment in applied settings. A disorder, for example, is described, measured, and *treated* to modify it. However, such treatment or the manipulation of an independent variable may have been done without any *controls*. In other words, the experimenter may not have taken any steps to rule out other potential causes. In such cases, the resulting data may be suggestive of a cause–effect relation, but they still cannot support a theory. This is the level of uncontrolled experimentation, which yields *uncontrolled data*.

The fourth level of observation includes everything specified under the third level, plus adequate controls to rule out the influence of extraneous independent variables. For example, the investigator may show that a clinical group that received treatment improved while a second comparable group, untreated, showed no improvement. This level of controlled experimentation produces *controlled data*, which are essential for supporting a theory. Controlled data are capable of explaining an event since the cause of the event will have been isolated through controlled experimentation. In order for the scientific community to accept the theory, however, one still needs an additional set of observations.

The fifth and the last level of observation is probably the most time-consuming and complex because it seeks to establish the *generality* of controlled experimental data. Experimental data established in one setting (laboratory or clinic), with one set of subjects, by a given investigator, may or may not have generality. In other words, whether the same data can be obtained by other investigators in other settings with different subjects would not be known. A theory begins to gain a wider recognition only when its generality across settings, subjects, and investigators is established. *Replication* is the method of establishing generality of experimental findings that yields *controlled replicated data*. Replicated data are obtained at different stages. Therefore, at any one time, there may be a greater or lesser degree of replicated data supporting a theory. We shall consider procedures of, and issues relative to, replication in Chapter 9.

Scientific data obtained at any level of observation are objective in the sense that they are publicly verifiable. In order to establish the reliability of some data, different observers observing the same event must report similar values of measurement. Verified and replicated data are also known as scientific *evidence*. In essence, evidence, not mere observations, supports a theory.

18 Discuss the need for hypotheses in scientific research.

19 What is a null hypothesis? Why was it suggested?

20 Describe a theory. Find a theory in your reading of the scientific literature. Identify the elements of that theory.

21 Give your own examples of inductive and deductive reasoning in everyday life.

22 What is a syllogism? Give an example of your own.

23 How are inductive and deductive theories built?

24 Distinguish between theories and scientific laws.

25 Distinguish between data and evidence. Describe the different levels of observation that produce different kinds of data.

■ CHAPTER 4

Types of Research

■ Ex post facto research, 75

■ Normative research, 79

■ Standard-group comparisons, 84

■ Experimental research, 87

■ Clinical and applied research, 93

■ Sample surveys, 96

■ Evaluation research, 98

■ The relation between research types and questions, 99

■ Study guide, 101

In its everyday usage, the term *research* is used to describe a variety of activities. A student wishing to buy a computer may "research" the market, the hardware, the software, the service provided by different dealers, and so on. A couple planning to buy a house will research the housing market, interest rates, and lending institutions. The term *research* in these contexts refers to relatively well-planned and systematic activity.

Scientific research, on the other hand, may require more formal planning, and the questions addressed may be related to some publicly verifiable issue. Nevertheless, scientific research can also be more or less formal and may include a variety of activities designed to obtain different kinds of information or answer different kinds of questions. For example, a speech–language clinician may research the number of children with articulation disorders in a school district. A second clinician may research the typical language behaviors of a group of 5-year-old children. A third clinician may research the conditions under which stuttering began in a group of children. A fourth clinician may research the effects of a given treatment procedure on the speech and language behaviors of aphasic patients.

Each of the research activities just described has a different question behind it. Different research activities use different methodologies. The results across those activities will also be different in nature. They will have unique strengths and limitations. The kinds of conclusions to be drawn from the results will depend on those strengths and weaknesses. It is therefore necessary to understand different types of scientific research so that questions are researched with appropriate methods and the results are interpreted within the scope of those methods.

There are different ways of classifying research (Kerlinger, 1973), and several classic types are common across classifications. An overview of typical research activities in communicative disorders and related disciplines suggests the following system of classification: Ex post facto research, normative research, standard-group comparison, experimental research of both the basic and applied variety, clinical research including the descriptive and experimental subtypes, sample surveys, and evaluation research. In some respects, the research types described in this book are not categorical. There are research styles that combine different types or their elements.

EX POST FACTO RESEARCH

A considerable portion of research studies published in the field of communicative disorders is ex post facto. It is a type of research in which no independent variables are manipulated by the investigator. As the term suggests, it is an "after the fact" type of research in that the independent variables have occurred in the past and the investigator starts with the effect. Thus, a retrospective search of the causes of events under investigation is the essence of ex post facto research (Kerlinger, 1973).

Procedures of Ex Post Facto Research

The case history method used in clinical sciences is an excellent example of ex post facto research. Many disorders or diseases are initially researched through the ex post facto method. In fact, most human disorders and diseases are not experimentally manipulable to the extent required by experimental logic and philosophy. Some experimental research on certain diseases and disorders may be possible only at the subhuman level. However, the results of subhuman experiments may or may not be applicable to human beings. Therefore, much of the research in clinical fields, including medicine, remains ex post facto in nature.

In the case history method, the starting point of an investigation is a disease or a disorder. The investigator then proceeds to find out what may have caused that clinical condition. Evidently, the onset has occurred in the past. Therefore, the investigator cannot experimentally manipulate the potential causes of the condition. Therefore, the investigator begins by taking a detailed case history. The case history is a chronology of events that are relevant to the disorder under investigation. The client and other informants (such as parents) may be interviewed. Information that might help determine the conditions under which the disorder was first noted is gathered. If some set of events that may be potential causes of the disorder is reported to have occurred, the investigator may conclude that a potential cause–effect relation has been identified.

The retrospective search of causes is often guided by past research and theoretical expectations. The past research may have provided some clues to the causal factors of the phenomenon under study, and the investigator may search the history for evidence of those factors. The investigator may look for causes suggested by deductive theories. Should the case history provide evidence of events suggested by either past research or a theory, the investigator may conclude that the disorder is due to those events.

A number of currently accepted cause–effect relations are based only on ex post facto research at the human level. For example, the relation between smoking and lung cancer is based entirely upon ex post facto research. Repeatedly, studies using the case history method have shown that smokers have a higher chance of developing lung cancer than nonsmokers. A majority of people who have developed lung cancer report a history of smoking. On the basis of such observations, it has been concluded that smoking and lung cancer are causally related. Such conclusions have formed a basis for significant social policies such as those requiring warnings on cigarette packages.

In communicative disorders, extensive research by Johnson on the onset of stuttering in young children illustrates ex post facto research on a large scale (Johnson, 1955; Johnson and associates, 1959). In a series of studies, Johnson and his associates tried to determine the conditions under which stuttering was first noted by the parents of a large number of stuttering children. With the help of an extensive schedule of interview, the parents of stuttering children were questioned about such factors as the family conditions, the children's health, their speech and language development, amounts and types of dysfluencies, and so on. Similar interview data were gathered from parents of nonstuttering children as well.

Johnson made a comparative analysis of the interview information obtained from the parents of stuttering and nonstuttering children. The parents of stuttering children reported that their children exhibited such dysfluencies as repetitions, interjections, and prolongations, which prompted them to consider their children as stutterers. However, the parents of nonstuttering children also reported that the children had various kinds of dysfluencies in speech. Based on this information, Johnson concluded that *at the time of stuttering onset*, children who are thought to stutter speak no differently than those who are considered normal speakers. This became the well-known diagnosogenic theory of stuttering. Essentially, the theory stated that the origin of stuttering was the parental negative evaluation of normal nonfluencies and the mistaken diagnosis of stuttering. Of course, the negative evaluation and the unfavorable diagnosis would soon start the real problem: apprehension, anxiety, struggle, and avoidance reactions on the part of the children. For Johnson, dysfluencies themselves were not the major problems. The problems were the events that followed the diagnosis of stuttering based on normal nonfluencies.

Johnson's research and the resulting theory illustrate both the method and the problems of the ex post facto research. In terms of the method, it is clear that Johnson's was a retrospective study. The identified independent variable was the parental diagnosis of stuttering in the absence of stuttering. One can speculate whether Johnson had that assumption before he started his investigation or whether it was indeed a conclusion based on the interview data. It is clear, however, that the presumed independent variable had occurred in the past. He did not (of course, could not) observe the parental diagnosis that in his judgment caused stuttering. There was no experimental manipulation of an independent variable. Therefore, the cause–effect relation between the parental diagnosis and stuttering was based upon interview information, not upon experimental evidence. In other words, Johnson did not show that no other factor was responsible for stuttering.

Strengths and Weaknesses of Ex Post Facto Research

It is clear that ex post facto research (1) is not experimental in the sense of manipulating an independent variable and (2) lacks control in that extraneous independent variables are not ruled out. When the observations are ex post facto, the experimenter has no control over the independent variable. As a result, a direct relation between the presumed cause and effect cannot be established.

Carefully done case histories may reveal that language disordered children did not receive enough "language stimulation," or that they had limited intelligence, or that they experienced certain "emotional problems," or that they came from lower socioeconomic strata. Assuming that there are reliable and valid ways of measuring these variables, one can conclude that those variables were indeed observed and measured. However, whether they actually caused the language disorder is a different question. The ex post facto observations that documented the existence of those variables would not have done anything to show that they were the causes of the language disorder.

The documented observations within the ex post facto method cannot assert cause–effect relations for both empirical and logical reasons. As pointed out earlier, the empirical reasons are a lack of experimental manipulations and an absence of controls to rule out competing hypotheses. The logical reason is that both the effect and the presumed cause are measured at the same time. As a result, even the minimum requirement of a causal relation, which is that causes precede effects, is not fulfilled in ex post facto research, because in most cases, the prior existence of the presumed causal factor is not documented. The presumed causes and their effects are both studied simultaneously.

Statistical correlations are often used in the analysis of the results of ex post facto studies. The analysis might reveal significant correlations between events. However, such correlations do not necessarily suggest causation. Correlations suggest that events tend to coexist or covary, but the actual cause of one variable or both of the variables may be some other unobserved factor.

The often cited justification of ex post facto research is that it is the only possible type of research that can be implemented in many important areas of investigation (Kerlinger, 1973). Ethical restrictions prohibit experimental research on human diseases and disorders. The only way, then, is to explore the past history of patients with given diseases and disorders for possible causal factors. In such situations, however, one should be clear about the distinction between social and scientific implications of ex post facto research. From the standpoint of science, the impracticality of experimentation is beside the point. Weak scientific evidence does not become stronger because better evidence cannot be produced.

Similarly, from the standpoint of social policies designed to protect human lives, the limitations of scientific evidence may be recognized but considered unimportant. In such cases, each society makes an evaluation of the available evidence to support social policies that are best for its people. Scientists would support those policies as long as social versus scientific evaluations of research data are not confused. People may justifiably accept the social implications of weak scientific evidence because such a course of action serves their best interests. Relative to questions such as smoking and lung cancer, members of a society may be more willing to take the risk of being scientifically wrong than that of being prematurely dead.

The scientific evaluation of ex post facto research may be done independent of social policies. The main limitation of ex post facto studies is that it is not possible to explain an event on the basis of their results. The social or personal significance of the results is beside the point. Ideally, ex post facto research should lead to a suggestion of variables that may be verified through other means of investigation. In this sense, it is a desirable exploratory method of research. In practice, however, many investigators whose characteristic research method is ex post facto may not be inclined to find other means of verifying potential causal relations suggested by their method. Disregarding the limitations of the method, explanatory theories may be offered that might enjoy a certain degree of incongruous acceptance in the discipline.

It is possible that the inability to conduct better controlled research is somewhat exaggerated in many cases. Certainly, Johnson could not have asked parents of fluently speaking children to diagnose stuttering to see what happens. However, it is possible to think of large-scale preventive studies in which parents of high-risk children are asked not to diagnose stuttering and see if imminent stuttering is avoided. Or, selecting children in the very early stage of stuttering, one can modify the punitive parental behaviors to see what effects follow. With appropriate control measures (such as a control group whose parents are not asked to change their behaviors), it is possible to gather more convincing evidence than that produced by the ex post facto method. In the case of human diseases, similar preventive experimental studies are possible. For example, cholesterol intake of individuals may be differentially monitored and modified to see what health benefits and risks follow. Such naturalistic experiments have been conducted. In addition, when appropriate, animal experimental research might support ex post facto data.

NORMATIVE RESEARCH

Another extremely popular form of research in communicative disorders as well as in child psychology can be called normative research. Traditionally, it is not recognized as a separate type of research, but the enormous amount of efforts that go into this kind of research makes it necessary to consider it separately.

Normative research can be defined as a type of research in which the distribution of selected dependent variables across age groups is observed and recorded. Its purpose is to arrive at norms that are the averaged performance levels of presumably typical reference groups. Normative research seeks to establish behavioral differences across age groups. This type of research is often called developmental research or descriptive research. It tends to provide descriptive data on typical behaviors of different age groups.

It is generally believed that for clinical disciplines, norms are extremely important. It is argued that first norms tell us how children's behaviors change as they grow older and then such information will help us judge whether a given client's behavior is normal or disordered. It is further suggested that unless the clinician knows age-based norms, target behaviors for clinical intervention cannot be determined. For example, in order to determine whether a 4-year-old child is delayed in language, one needs to know the typical language behaviors of 4-year-olds. Also, once it is determined that the child is language delayed (because "the child's language approximates that of a 2-year-old"), norms are needed to establish the target behaviors for the clinical intervention program. Assuming that the child in our example has all the behaviors of average 2-year-old children, initial target behaviors may be that of average 3-year-olds and eventually that of 4-year-olds.

The bulk of research in the areas of morphology, syntax, phonology, semantics, and pragmatics is normative and theoretical. It is thought that a lack of norms in certain aspects of speech and language creates problems for making clinical judgments relative to evaluation and treatment. Therefore, it is considered a high-priority research.

Procedures of Normative Research

Normative research typically uses the subject and response sampling procedure to establish the statistically averaged response patterns across age groups. Theoretically, norms are established on *randomly selected* subjects who are representative of the population. Unless the sample is representative, conclusions cannot be extended to all the children in the population. Because the goal of normative research is to determine the typical behaviors of children in the population, not merely that of selected children, normative research must use adequate statistical sampling procedures.

In order to achieve an adequate statistical sampling, one must meet two conditions. The investigator must have access to the entire population, such as all school-age children with language disorders. Once this type of population has been identified, every member of that population must be willing to participate in the study. These two conditions are important because the random theory is based on the assumption that a representative sample of a population can be drawn only when the population is large and when every member had an equal chance of being selected into the sample. The sample size is related to the size of the population. The larger the population, the bigger the sample size required to represent that population. The sample is typically cross-sectional in that a certain number of subjects are drawn from each age level.

After having drawn a random representative sample of the population, the investigator proceeds to *sample the behaviors* of selected subjects. Speech, language, or auditory behaviors are sampled in a relatively short period of observation. Each subject may be administered a brief test designed to sample the behaviors of interest. Various tests of articulation, language, and hearing ability are used to sample behaviors in normative research.

The behaviors sampled across selected age levels are statistically analyzed. The mean performance levels of each age group are determined along with standard deviations. The mean scores may be statistically transformed into other types of scores to reduce variability across subjects and to facilitate comparisons among subjects. The means and other kinds of scores typical of the age group are considered the "norm" for that age group. Children in the population at large are expected to show the same kinds of behaviors as those of the sampled children at specific age levels. In evaluating individual clients, the clinician is expected to use such norms to judge whether a child is showing deviations from the expected (typical) performance levels. The presence of deviations suggests a clinical problem, whereas the degree of deviation determines the severity of the problem.

Strengths and Weaknesses of Normative Research

The strength of normative research is its logical appeal and not its empirical validity. The reasoning that we need to know the typical behaviors of subjects in different groups formed on the basis of age, sex, socioeconomic status, or occupational levels is logically consistent with the clinical demands of determining deviations and disorders based on such variables. It would be useful to know the typical language behaviors of children of different ages, of male and female subjects, and of people in different walks of life. The determination of the presence of a disorder or deviation would be a less demanding task with the availability of such knowledge.

It would also be useful to know how the dependent variables are distributed in the population. Science does start with the observation of some effects (dependent variables). Before other kinds of research manipulations can be achieved, one must be clear about the dependent variables. Therefore, a good description of speech, language, fluency, vocal, and auditory behaviors across variables that do make a difference in these behaviors would be essential for further empirical research and sound clinical practice.

Most of the serious problems of the normative research are empirical. The procedures and assumptions of this type of research seem to lack empirical validity, a problem that has received surprisingly little critical attention in communicative disorders.

The problems inherent to normative research are common to most research studies based upon the statistical theory of probability and random sampling from the population. These problems will be discussed in Chapters 7 and 9 and therefore will be mentioned only briefly here. The first empirical problem is that true random samples that permit the nationwide use of the resulting normative information are rarely drawn. Most normative studies draw local samples based upon varying degrees of randomization. Therefore, the behavior patterns found across age groups may or may not be representative of the children in the target population. As a result, the major goal of normative research is rarely achieved in practice.

The second empirical problem is also related to the sampling procedure. The normative researchers not only sample subjects but also sample responses under investigation. Since groups of subjects are examined at different age levels, most often the investigators are able to obtain only a brief sampling of responses. Whether it is language or articulation, the opportunities to produce specific behaviors are extremely limited. For example, children may be given two or three chances to produce a given phoneme or a grammatical morpheme. When age-based norms are derived from such limited sampling of responses, their reliability is doubtful. Unfortunately, the only kind of sampling the normative researcher typically thinks of is the subject sampling, which is done inadequately anyway.

The third empirical problem is a more serious one, and it involves a logical problem as well. It is known that any population is heterogeneous, not homogeneous. That means that when a large number of persons are studied, there is a tremendous degree of variability. This is nothing but the popular notion of individual differences and uniqueness. A good sample, therefore, must be as heterogeneous as the population it seeks to represent. Consequently, the more heterogeneous the sample, the more variable the subject performance. Unfortunately, the more variable the performance, the less meaningful the average (the "norm"). In other words, even when an investigator achieves a representative random sample, the resulting "norms" will be highly variable, a contradiction of terms. Therefore, it is quite possible that the notion of norms constitutes both a logical and empirical fallacy.

The fourth empirical problem is probably due to a misapplication of the statistical theory of probability and the random procedure to questions of individual performance. The theory and procedure are designed to extend the results from the sample to the population, and not from the sample to an individual. An average performance of a smaller group is supposed to help predict the average performance of the larger group. Within the theory, there is no empirical basis to predict an individual's performance based upon a sample study. Disregarding this, clinicians routinely assume that what is true of an averaged sample performance is also true of an individual client's specific (unaveraged) performance.

The fifth empirical problem of normative research is also a matter of practice. Normative research asks how the behaviors are distributed across certain arbitrarily selected variables such as age; it was never intended to answer the question why those behaviors are distributed the way they are. In other words, normative research can only describe the events observed; it cannot explain those events. Investigators do not exert any kind of control on potential independent variables. As such, no matter how extensive, normative research cannot support a theory. It seems that this limitation is also mostly ignored in practice, for most of the theories on how and why children acquire language, semantic notions, pragmatic rules, or phonological systems are based upon normative research.

Normative research assumes that the arbitrarily selected variables across which the behaviors seem to show different patterns are indeed the independent variables. For example, most investigators of language acquisition explicitly or implicitly assume that age is an independent variable. This commonly held assumption needs a careful look.

Age as an Independent Variable

Age is a measure of the passage of time relative to the beginnings of some living or nonliving entity. While time is impersonal and physical, age is personal and often biological. When it is observed that as age changed, certain behaviors changed, can we assume that age is the reason why such changes were observed? A positive answer is typically taken for granted, and it is an implicitly or explicitly offered explanation of any kind of behavioral "development" in most normative research.

It is hard to think that age, which is a personal measure of the passage of time, is an independent variable of anything. If it is, it is a discouraging variable for clinicians who wish to remediate disorders. The only course of action open to clinicians is to let the time pass in order for the communicatively handicapped child to show improvement. Of course, the disturbing question why the time that passed did not help the child would have to be stoically ignored. Fortunately, *in practice*, most clinicians do not believe that age is the independent variable of communicative behaviors. An observation of the actual clinical practice suggests that certain events are considered more important than the mere passage of time. The more familiar term *treatment* refers to these events. Treatment consists of controlling certain events to produce desirable effects on the client's communicative behaviors.

Age is a convenient term for known and unknown variables that influence observable behaviors. Some of these variables include biological changes that take place within organisms, and others are events in the environment. A better explanation of behaviors might emerge if manipulable independent variables are taken seriously. More importantly, a better technology of treatment would simultaneously become available. There is some evidence to show that "developmental milestones" of language are susceptible to environmental contingencies that can be experimentally manipulated (Capelli, 1985; De Cesari, 1985). In other words, experimental research on language acquisition is possible and it offers a more valid means of explaining the language learning process.

If normative research is applied strictly to observe and describe dependent variables, it can serve a meaningful purpose. However, in order to generate clinically useful data, the normative researchers may have to curtail the overuse of the cross-sectional method in which the individual behaviors are sampled inadequately. Repeated and more intensive observation of small numbers of children may produce data that are more applicable to individual cases (Brown, 1973). When behaviors are observed more intensively, patterns that may not become apparent under the cursory cross-sectional method may be observed. Such observations would still not explain the behavioral changes, but can possibly suggest potential independent variables for further experimental enquiry.

STANDARD-GROUP COMPARISON

Another type of research not traditionally recognized as a distinct variety can be called standard-group comparison. The method of standard-group comparison is a cross between the ex post facto and the normative types. Though it is not recognized as a separate type of research, it is necessary to consider it as such because of the sheer volume of this kind of research done in clinical sciences. In communicative disorders, standard-group comparisons are almost as popular as normative research.

Standard-group comparison is a type of research in which groups formed on the basis of one dependent variable are compared on the basis of the same or other dependent variables. An a priori dependent variable serves as an initial basis to form groups, and then the presence or the absence of selected dependent variables across the groups is measured. Typical group comparisons involve two groups that are different on the initial a priori variable. On the subsequent measured dependent variables, the group may or may not be different, though the expectation is that they will be. In many clinical disciplines, including communicative disorders, "clinical" groups are compared with "normal" groups on some measure of one or more dependent variables.

Standard-group comparisons are not the same as the two (or more) group experimental research. The latter type of research is experimental, and it is described in the next section. The type of experimental research that involves two or more groups is a more active research arrangement in which an independent variable is manipulated by the experimenter. In the standard-group comparison, there is no manipulation of an independent variable. Only the dependent variables are measured.

Procedures of the Standard-Group Comparison

For the most part, the standard-group comparison is an extension of the logic and methodology of normative research. After having discovered the distribution of certain dependent variables in certain general samples of subjects, some clinical researchers move on to find out if the distribution of those variables is in some way different across *selected* samples of subjects. The general sample is the "normal" group, and the special samples selected for comparison are the "clinical" groups.

The clinical groups are formed on the basis of a clinical diagnosis. For example, language disordered children, aphasic patients, or stutterers can be identified through clinical assessment. Once a clinical group has been formed, the researcher proceeds to form a normal group with no communicative problems. Certain screening procedures may be used to rule out the existence of communicative disorders. The two groups are then compared on selected dependent variables.

There are two strategies of comparing the two groups. In one strategy, the groups are compared further on the same criterion variable that separated the groups in the first place. In the second strategy, the groups are compared on variables that did not serve as explicit criteria for the initial separation of the groups.

The first strategy is illustrated by studies in which language disordered children are compared with normal children on the age at which they master selected grammatical morphemes. In fact, they may be compared on any or several of the many language measures: phonological, grammatical, semantic, or pragmatic variables. It must be noted that comparisons in such instances are made on the same criterion variable that separated the two groups. Language handicapped and normally speaking children may be compared on some specific measures of language. Phonologically disordered children may be compared with normally speaking children on certain phonological variables.

This kind of comparative analysis may lead to a description of further linguistic differences between the normal children and the language disordered or phonologically disordered children. For example, an investigator might find out that compared with normally speaking children, language disordered children are not able to use certain pragmatic structures or passive sentence forms. Similarly, the phonologically disabled children may be found to be deficient in acquiring certain phonological processes.

In the second strategy, the criterion and the comparison measures are different. For example, an investigator may wish to assess the difference between stutterers and nonstutterers on motor performance. The criterion variable in this case is stuttering, presumably speech dysfluencies and related behaviors. The frequency of those behaviors would be high in the stuttering group and low in the nonstuttering group. The variable on which they are compared, on the other hand, is entirely different. It is a measure of motor proficiency, which is not the same as speech dysfluencies. Later, stuttering and motor proficiency measures may be linked theoretically, but they are different kinds of responses. There are many examples of this kind of comparison. Aphasic and nonaphasic subjects, distinguished on the basis of some overt language measure, may be compared on the basis of memory skills or on a test of intelligence. The performance of phonologically disordered children on a motor proficiency test may be compared with that of normal children. A measure of intelligence of normal children may be compared with that of language disordered children.

In recent years, the standard-group comparison method has been used extensively in the study of neurophysiological differences between stutterers and nonstutterers. These two groups have been reported to be different on several neurophysiological variables. Many theoretical speculations have flourished on the basis of standard-group comparisons of this kind. Comparative analyses of phonatory reaction time alone have been made by numerous investigators. In a majority of studies, adult stutterers have been found to be slower than normal speakers in initiating and terminating phonation upon a signal. Other variables on which stutterers and nonstutterers have been compared include phonatory transition between voiced and voiceless sounds, laryngeal muscle activities, dichotic listening tests, and hemispheric processing of linguistic stimuli. Most of the studies on these and other variables have reported differences between stutterers and nonstutterers to varying degrees, with a remarkable extent of individual differences among both the groups.

Strengths and Weaknesses of Standard-Group Comparisons

The standard-group comparison can yield useful information regarding the differences between the normal and clinical populations. It is necessary to understand the differences between those who have a disorder of communication and those who do not. Furthermore, it is also necessary to understand the difference between particular disorder groups and the normal groups. The standard-group comparison studies can describe, for instance, the dependent variables on which the normal and stuttering groups or normal and language disordered groups differ. The method is useful in identifying and describing dependent variables. Since it is necessary to have clear descriptions of the dependent variables we study, the standard-group comparisons serve a useful purpose.

The standard-group comparison method poses no significant problems when it is used to identify and describe dependent variables across clinical and nonclinical groups. Problems arise when the method is misapplied, however. The problematic tendency on the part of many investigators is to *explain* the disorder on the basis of standard-group comparisons. For example, on the basis of standard-group comparisons, stuttering has been explained as a problem of inherent phonatory slowness. In other words, slow phonatory reaction time is treated as the cause of stuttering. However, in a standard-group comparison, there is no independent variable at all. As observed and measured in the studies, the slow phonatory reaction time is a dependent variable, not an independent variable. Therefore, there is no reason to suggest that phonatory slowness is the cause of stuttering. Of course, the cause of phonatory slowness is also not clear. In fact, no causal relation of any kind would be clear in a standard-group comparison, because it is not an experimental procedure. There is no assurance that an unidentified and unobserved variable is the cause of the effect under study. As such, standard-group comparison cannot support theories or explanations.

Some investigators designate the normal group as the control group and the clinical group as the experimental group in a standard-group comparison research. The use of this terminology is misleading, since the method is not experimental. Clinical groups are not to be automatically considered experimental groups. Unless a group receives a treatment variable, it cannot be considered an experimental group.

EXPERIMENTAL RESEARCH

The most powerful strategy available to discover functional relations among events is experimental research. This type of research shares many characteristics with other types. The formulation of a research question, the task of finding a suitable method, systematic observation of the phenomenon under investigation, and analysis and interpretation of data are all common across research types. The distinguishing feature of experimental research is the *experiment*. The normative, the ex post facto, and the standard-group comparison types of research do not involve an experiment. Therefore, the term *experiment* is not a synonym of research, although one can find such an inappropriate use of that term in the literature. An experiment is only a part of a series of technical operations in *some* research studies.

An experiment can be defined as a series of controlled conditions of dynamic arrangement in which one or more independent variables are manipulated and the effects of such manipulations on the dependent variable are measured. Alternatively, an experiment is a method of arranging conditions in such a way that a functional relation between events may be revealed. In an experiment, the investigator manipulates conditions to produce a dependent variable (effect) which is nonexistent, or to increase the magnitude when it is present at a small scale, reduce the magnitude when it is present at a larger scale, and in some cases eliminate the effect when it is present at some level. Logically, any one of those successful manipulations constitutes evidence of a functional relation between events, and a combination of such manipulations will further strengthen that evidence. Replications of those functional arrangements and comparable results will enhance the generality of the evidence.

Procedures of Experimental Research

The effect (or the "purpose") of an experiment is to reveal a functional relation between events in a reasonably unambiguous manner. In this sense, an experiment is more advanced than descriptive research, in which the investigator is asking a fundamental question relative to the existence and properties of events. An experiment, on the other hand, is designed to answer the question what events are functionally (causally) related to the phenomenon that is known to exist and whose descriptive properties are reasonably well understood. In other words, experimental research seeks to explain an event by discovering its causal variables. Therefore, this type of research is essential for constructing either deductive or inductive scientific theories.

There is no experiment without the manipulation of one or more independent variables. An experiment is the most active of the research arrangements because it seeks not only to observe a phenomenon, like many other types of research, but also to control that phenomenon. The term *control* in this context simply means that some change in the phenomenon has been effected. The experimenter, however, cannot exert a direct control over the phenomenon. The only means of affecting the event is to gain control over its independent variable(s). This is true of applied situations as well. A physician, for example, cannot directly manipulate a disease condition. The disease is brought under control only through treatment known to be effective. A speech–language pathologist cannot directly affect aphasia; it can be affected only through certain treatment techniques.

The manipulation of an independent variable constitutes a series of activities on the part of the experimenter. An independent variable is manipulated when it is introduced, increased or decreased in magnitude, withdrawn, or reintroduced. For example, in assessing the effect of white noise on stuttering, the experimenter may first establish the baseline of stuttering and then introduce noise through headphones while the stutterer is talking. The experimenter will continue to measure the rate of stuttering. The level of noise may be increased or decreased in appropriate experimental conditions. In subsequent conditions, the noise may be withdrawn to observe the effects on stuttering. Finally, the noise may be reintroduced to find out if the original effects can be recovered.

Two independent variables are manipulated when one of them is introduced and another is later added, which is subsequently subtracted, which is then added a second time, and so on. For example, in assessing the effects of providing both feedback on performance levels and verbal praise for correct articulation, one may start with giving only feedback to the subject. In the next experimental condition, verbal praise may be added to feedback. In the subsequent condition, the verbal praise may be withdrawn, leaving only the feedback as the independent variable. In a final condition, the verbal praise may be reintroduced. Throughout, the correct production of target phonemes is measured to assess the effects of the experimental manipulations. There are other and more complex manipulations of independent variables, but these help illustrate the basic strategy.

A critical aspect of experimental manipulations is that they must be done under controlled conditions. Experimental conditions are controlled when it is possible to rule out the influence of potential independent variables not under investigation. When this is done, the effects observed on the dependent variable can be attributed to the independent variable manipulated by the experimenter, since no other variables were present. In effect, under controlled conditions, the experimenter isolates a cause–effect relation.

In many respects, conditions are controlled to simplify the typically complicated empirical relations that exist in nature. Normally, multiple controlling variables may be simultaneously active, though not to the same extent. When different variables are allowed to exert their varying and as yet undetermined influence on the dependent variables, no specific empirical relation can be isolated.

Physically isolated and specially constructed laboratories are often used in creating controlled conditions. The need for such physical control measures vary across disciplines and with the nature of the problems under investigation. Generally speaking, a certain degree of control over the physical setup is necessary in all types of experimental research. But the setup can be more or less structured depending upon the nature and stage of research. For example, an experiment on auditory perception might need a highly controlled experimental setup (a soundproof booth). A clinical experiment in which a certain language treatment procedure is evaluated may also initially need a controlled physical setup. However, in the later stages in which generalization to the natural environment is evaluated, the setup must be more natural. In all cases, the extraneous independent variables must be controlled.

It is somewhat difficult to control independent variables in natural settings, but it can be done. Experiments on the effects of teaching methods evaluated in regular classrooms, or experiments on child social behaviors conducted in playgrounds, illustrate naturalistic experiments. Experiments conducted in naturalistic settings are sometimes called *field experiments*.

In addition to physical control measures, an experiment should also include control measures designed to minimize the influence of other variables related to the subjects themselves. An investigator must make sure that other events in the life of the subjects were not responsible for the changes observed in the dependent variable. In many cases, biological events such as those included under the term *maturation* must also be ruled out. For example, a clinician wishing to assess the effects of a language treatment program must make sure that no other treatment was simultaneously applied or that the maturational factors were not responsible for the eventual gains in language behaviors shown by the subjects. There are two basic approaches to rule out such extraneous variables: the between-groups strategy and the single-subjects strategy.

In the between-groups strategy, two comparable groups are formed on the basis of random selection and assignment. One of the groups, the experimental group, receives treatment, whereas the other group, the control group, does not. If the desirable changes are seen only in the experimental group, both the extraneous environmental and possible biological variables are ruled out. The only reason the experimental group showed changes is that its members received the clinician's treatment.

In the single-subjects strategy, the subjects are exposed to different conditions of the experiment, and the differences in their response rates under those different conditions are taken as evidence of the effect of the independent variable under study. Typically, there is no control group that does not receive treatment in a single-subjects strategy. These two strategies of designing experiments are described and evaluated in Chapters 6 through 9.

Basic and Applied Experimental Research

Experimental research has two varieties: basic and applied. It is sometimes assumed that experimental research is always basic and laboratory-oriented whereas applied research does not use experimental methods. This notion is strengthened by the viewpoint that basic research finds out answers to important questions and applied research simply exploits those answers in solving practical problems. This is certainly a mistaken notion. Both basic and applied research can use the same experimental methods. When related applied and basic research are equally experimental, a useful interaction results. Such an interaction can speed up the process of finding solutions to practical problems.

In some cases, it may take a long time for the basic researcher to give answers to applied questions. In other cases, there may be no basic science that would ask and answer the same questions that have to be answered by the applied scientist. To a certain extent, this seems to be the case with speech–language pathologists. In the area of language, speech–language pathologists have often looked to linguistics for a variety of answers. But by its very nature, linguistics is not likely to ask such questions as whether language treatment procedure A is more effective than procedure B. Fields such as linguistics may be able to describe potential dependent variables but may not give any clues as to what independent variables may be necessary to change those dependent variables. That is the task of speech–language pathologists.

A prudent applied or clinical scientist learns to do at least some of the basic research to take care of his or her own business. Contrary to popular notions, experiment is the most needed operation in an applied science. Based on whatever the information is made available by basic researchers, an applied scientist may begin to experiment to find out answers to practical questions. Interestingly enough, applied or clinical experimental research not only can help solve practical problems, but also can generate new knowledge that can influence basic sciences. In essence, an experiment is a method to answer certain types of questions, and those types of questions must be answered in applied sciences as well.

We shall return to the question of applied experimental research in the section on applied or clinical research.

Strengths and Weaknesses of Experimental Research

By way of pointing out weaknesses, it is sometimes argued that in behavioral sciences, experimental research is artificial, too mechanistic, and therefore inappropriate (Bannister, 1966; Gadlin and Ingle, 1975). Specially created and fully controlled experimental situations are so far removed from the social settings in which behaviors naturally occur that the results may not have much validity. The experimental investigator tends to isolate an independent variable responsible for the effect under study. However, under natural conditions, single variables may not be responsible for specific effects. For this and other reasons, the experimental results may not be relevant to the behavioral events taking place in the natural world.

The argument that experimental research is too mechanistic for human behavioral sciences is an old one. There is a long-held belief that the scientific approach may be appropriate for physical phenomena but not for human phenomena. It is further believed that the mechanistic approach of science will dehumanize the human species. The origin of such beliefs is in the ancient philosophical position that human beings are unique in the scheme of the universe. Although Darwin did much to dispel this cherished sense of self-importance, some of the prejudices against the science of human behavior have persisted and have appeared and reappeared in various disguises.

Another weakness of experimental research, according to some critics, is that the effects of independent variables manipulated in human experiments are very weak (Kerlinger, 1973). Many times, controlled experiments manage to demonstrate only small changes in the dependent variables, whereas the same variables in real life situations may produce very large effects. For example, "expansion" of children's utterances in a laboratory study may result in only small increases in language complexity, but the same variable in real life may produce larger effects.

None of those weaknesses of experimental research seem to be valid. The fact that independent variables are isolated is a strength, not a weakness of experimental research. It is only by isolating the effects of a variable that an experimenter can observe functional relations between variables. Real-life situations are typically confounded, and therefore, it is hard to determine specific cause-effect relations. That in natural situations variables are multitude and the relations complex is not contradicted by technical isolation of specific causes. The need to isolate and individually analyze the different causes of a complex event arises from logical as well as technological considerations. After having analyzed the isolated effects of major factors, the scientist proceeds to analyze the interactive effects of those multiple factors. Such analytical steps are taken to eventually obtain an integrated picture of the phenomenon under investigation. In this way, a better approximation of the reality is achieved through laboratory research.

The critics of the experimental method do not suggest an effective alternative to an analytical approach to determining functional relations. If isolated functional relations are unreal, then the complex, real, but hopelessly confounded relations do not permit any conclusions. In addition, many events cannot be "held" for observation in their totality. Often, there is no technological means of experimentally manipulating a multitudinal complex. Besides, some apparently complex situations may hold only a few causal factors while the rest of the multitude may be a collection of covariables with very little functional significance.

The objection that the experimental approach is too mechanistic may be consistent with certain scholastic traditions but is not consistent with any empirical evidence. Science neither glorifies nor degrades its subject matter. Human behavior will not be transformed into mechanical events because the methods of science have been used in studying it. For example, when we gain a better understanding of the language learning process through application of the experimental procedure, human language will not turn into machine language. Behaviors called *love* or *cooperation* will remain the same even after scientists have experimentally analyzed them.

The final criticism—that compared with situations in real life, experiments tend to produce relatively weak effects of independent variables—is probably true in the context of some research traditions. However, this problem is not inherent to the experimental approach itself. Experiments can and have produced large effects to be significant in natural settings, but the traditional statistical approaches to experimentation have asserted that large effects are not necessary to draw valid conclusions. Statistically "significant" small effects are considered sufficient to permit statements of cause-effect relations. The experimental tradition can be completely divorced from this statistical philosophy. There is nothing in the logic or the tactics of the experimental method that would prevent the production of larger effects of independent variables.

The strengths of experimental research are the strengths of science itself. It is the most appropriate method to isolate a cause–effect relation. Many other types of research can suggest possibilities of such relations, but only the experimental approach can confirm them. Therefore, in developing theories and testing empirical hypotheses, no other research type matches the power of experimental research. Since a theory is both a description and an explanation of some natural phenomenon, investigators need the experimental procedure to rule out alternative explanations and hypotheses. Types of research such as the ex post facto and the normative may suggest hypotheses and theories, but typically, the same piece of research may suggest several rival hypotheses without testing their relative validity. Only experimental research can examine alternative hypotheses and theories and support one while ruling out the others.

CLINICAL AND APPLIED RESEARCH

Clinical and applied research are often contrasted with basic or experimental research. Clinical and applied research are thought to be qualitatively different from experimental research. However, only a few contrasts are valid, since basic/experimental and applied/clinical research have much in common.

Clinical and applied research both address questions of immediate practical significance. They are designed to solve some pressing physical, social, or personal problems. While experimental research may yield data that may be used in the future to solve some practical problems, clinical and applied research seek solutions to current problems. Basic experimental research may be theoretical or may be designed to find order and uniformities in natural events. That type of research may seek to explain events, understand their causes, and predict their occurrences. Clinical and applied research, on the other hand, may seek to modify undesirable effects that have already taken place, improve certain existing conditions, or prevent certain unfavorable consequences. Research studies aimed at treating language disorders, improving an articulation treatment program, or researching a stuttering prevention program in a high-risk group illustrate these kinds of applied or clinical efforts.

The term *clinical research* is used here to describe research that is in some way connected with diseases and disorders of living organisms. Therefore, as in medicine, a considerable amount of research in communicative disorders should be clinical. Research aimed at understanding and treating various disorders of communication is necessarily clinical.

The distinction between applied and clinical research is not crucial except that in many cases applied research may be nonclinical as defined here. For example, research aimed at reducing energy conservation in homes is applied but not clinical. Similarly, research aimed at building better bridges or safer highways is applied without being clinical. However, both clinical and applied research try to solve problems, and in this sense, they are the same. Therefore, in this book, the terms *clinical* and *applied* will be used interchangeably and will be distinguished only when that is considered necessary.

Clinical research uses the same procedures as the other types of research. Its procedures are not necessarily unique. Depending upon the particular clinical study, the method may be descriptive or experimental. Therefore, we shall consider these two varieties of clinical research.

Descriptive and Experimental Clinical Research

Clinical research can be either descriptive or experimental. One of the popular misconceptions is that clinical research is always descriptive and therefore less exacting. However, clinical research is not necessarily less exacting than basic research. If, in practice, much of the clinical research is informal and less exacting, it is because of the belief of some researchers that that is the way it *must be*.

Generally speaking, nonexperimental research can be less demanding than experimental research. When clinicians begin to ask experimental questions, they will have to be as rigorous as the basic scientists. For example, if the research question is whether school teachers and speech–language pathologists differ in their attitudes toward stuttering, the method required to answer this question does not involve controlling operations. The researcher is interested in some existing differences in the two groups; he or she is not asking whether something can be done to change anything. On the other hand, if the question asked is whether articulation disorders are affected by treatment *A* or treatment *B* or with a combination of *A* and *B*, then the clinician needs the experimental method in which the disorders are changed. Since changes should be demonstrated under controlled conditions to rule out the influence of other potential independent variables, the method is as demanding as in any basic experimental research.

In the early stage of clinical research, the concern is to establish the dependent variables. In other words, we first need to know the effects well. This is often the stage of descriptive research. The behaviors or disorders, their form and frequency, and their variations over time or conditions are described. Once the dependent variables have been clearly established, the question of causes emerges. An answer to this question demands experimental analysis. In essence, after having clearly described the effects, the clinical scientist proceeds to find out their causes.

The clinical investigator may search for instigating or maintaining causes. In communicative disorders, experimental analysis typically involves maintaining causes, not instigating causes. An experimental analysis of stuttering or an articulation disorder, for example, would be concerned with potential independent variables that decrease those behaviors while increasing their counterparts: fluency and appropriate articulation. The brain damage that resulted in aphasia may be the original cause, but it is not accessible for experimental analysis, whereas that patient's verbal behavior is.

The Importance of Experimental-Clinical Research

In communicative disorders, experimental–clinical research is essential in three areas of investigation. First, it is essential in generating basic knowledge about the acquisition, production, and maintenance of various aspects of communication. We need to know the neurophysiological, genetic, environmental, and other factors that are functionally (causally) involved in the processes of speech. While other methods of research can suggest possibilities that remain speculative, the experimental method can produce more definitive evidence regarding the independent variables that may be responsible for normal speech, language, voice, and fluency behaviors. It is possible, however, that some kinds of independent variables are more easily investigated through experimental research than are other kinds. For example, environmental variables are more easily built into experimental designs than the genetic variables.

Second, the experimental method is essential in gaining an understanding of the factors that lead to disordered communication of various kinds. The method can isolate the factors involved in the production of disordered communication. Once again, the experimental method can be more effective in isolating environmental independent variables of disordered communication than genetic variables.

Third, experimental research is essential in evaluating the effects of various treatment programs designed to remediate disorders of communication. Even routine clinical treatment is more like an experimental research than normative research. Treatment, by definition, is an operation designed to change a clinical condition. By modifying an independent variable, the scientist modifies some effect, and by manipulating the treatment variable, the clinician also modifies the disorder or disease. The only difference between routine clinical treatment and experimental research is that the former may lack controls for extraneous variables. Such controls are considered essential in experimental research. However, when the question is whether or not a given treatment procedure is effective, we need the experimental methodology, which is no less exacting than that used in basic research.

Since determining the effects of treatment procedures used in clinical sciences is of paramount importance, it is distressing to find the meager amount of experimental research done in communicative disorders. It appears that compared with other types of research, controlled evaluation of treatment is of low priority. Ex post facto, normative, survey, standard-group comparisons, and speculatively theoretical research papers far exceed the number of experimental reports in most issues of journals in our field. Annually, very few experimental treatment evaluation studies are published in our professional and scientific journals. In language and phonology, most studies are either normatively descriptive or categorically theoretical. Categorically theoretical papers usually suggest various ways of categorizing the dependent variables (language or phonological classificatory schemes).

Clinical investigators justify nonexperimental research on the basis that first we need descriptive evidence. The belief is that one needs to prepare for experimental research. This justification is valid to a certain extent. However, from a technical standpoint, experimental research has been possible for a long time. Therefore, it appears as though communicative disorders is preparing itself endlessly for the much-needed experimental research.

Instead of experimentally demonstrating the effects of treatment programs, investigators who do not appreciate the experimental method often resort to offering speculative "recommendations" for treatment. When such recommendations are incorporated into existing therapeutic procedures, needless diversity of questionable treatment practices results. In such cases, clinicians do not know whether the incorporated recommendations contribute anything to therapeutic success. In this sense, experimental research is as crucial to a clinical science as it is to basic sciences.

When experimental data are lacking, theoretical speculations flourish. Such theoretical speculations create vigorous debates and controversies involving rational premises and subjective opinions. A desirable side effect of experimental–clinical research is a mitigation of such endless and useless debates and controversies. Experimental research may not settle all arguments, but at least it will force the debaters out of their armchairs and into the clinical laboratories so that instead of offering arguments, the specialists can collect data that matter.

SAMPLE SURVEYS

Surveys are designed to assess some characteristics of a group of people or a particular society. Like normative research, surveys try to determine the distribution of certain variables in the population. For example, a survey researcher might be interested in finding out the attitudes of teachers toward hearing impaired students in certain elementary schools. Another investigator might be interested in the most frequently used stuttering therapy procedure in university clinics. Yet another researcher may wish to assess the opinions of school administrators regarding the necessity of speech–language services in schools under their administration. Research concerns such as these require the survey method.

Technically, surveys try to find out how the variables such as attitudes, opinions, and certain social or personal practices are distributed in the population. However, rarely can a surveyor assess the entire population. The typical strategy is to draw a representative sample of the population and find out their reactions to a set of questions designed to evoke answers of interest. Therefore, scientific surveys are often called sample surveys.

Surveys are routinely used in assessing public opinions and attitudes of various kinds. Some of the well-known surveys include the Gallup polls, the Harris polls, and those that are conducted by television networks and national newspapers. Most of the attitudes and opinions assessed in these polls are related in some way to political, social, or economic issues. Predicting voter behavior, for example, is a regular form of survey research. Assessment of people's attitude toward contemplated legislations and economic policies is also done frequently. The need for such sample surveys is so great that many commercial firms specialize in them.

In academic and clinical fields, surveys might address questions regarding the distribution of certain variables either in the population at large or in specific groups. A professional organization may wish to find out how many people know about speech–language pathologists. In this case, knowledge, defined in some operational way, is the dependent variable whose distribution in the general population is measured in a survey. Similarly, when a speech–language pathologist wishes to determine the number of aphasic persons in a given town, the dependent variable is aphasia, whose distribution in the population is assessed.

The results of surveys are only as valid as the sampling technique used in them. Technically, a random sample is needed to assess the dependent variable accurately. A nonrepresentative sample will lead to invalid conclusions. The issues surrounding the random theory are discussed elsewhere in the book. It is sufficient to note here that all sampling techniques have a margin of error. Currently, the typical national sampling of citizens of voting age in the United States involves about 1,500 individuals. It may carry a sampling error of four to six percentage points. For example, assuming a 5 percent sampling error, when a survey reports that 34 percent of the voting-age population favor a tax reform package, the actual percentage in the population may be anywhere between 29 and 39 percent.

It is necessary to understand what surveys can and cannot do. Surveys can help formulate certain professional and social policies. They let us know what people are thinking on certain issues or what kind of actions the people think they might take in certain situations. For example, it may be important to know whether school administrators might support more speech–language pathology positions in the schools.

Surveys, however, cannot answer questions of causality because of a lack of experimental manipulation. For example, a survey might show that a certain procedure is widely used in the treatment of laryngectomies, but it cannot determine whether the technique is indeed effective. Such a survey reflects only a current practice, not its validity. As in normative research, when the question concerns the distribution of the dependent variables, surveys are useful, but when the questions concern functional relations between events, they are not.

The best surveys with adequate random samples can help predict group behaviors but not the behaviors of an individual. One might find out, for example, that a given stuttering treatment is used by a majority of clinicians. However, from this survey information, one cannot answer the question whether a given clinician is using the same technique in treating his or her stutterers. Similarly, the fact that an opinion survey shows that a given candidate is likely to be elected by a majority of voters is of no help in predicting the voting behavior of an individual citizen.

Another major limitation of surveys is that they tend to focus on "soft" dependent variables. Attitudes and opinions are the most frequently sampled dependent variables in a survey research. However, in most cases, attitudes and opinions themselves are of little interest to the survey researcher, who in fact tries to predict actions or behaviors of individuals in the populations. The researcher infers certain imminent actions on the part of the people to whom the conclusions of the sample survey are extended. Unfortunately, there is very little assurance that reflected attitudes and opinions always translate into actions. In some limited instances, opinions and attitudes may accurately reflect a group behavior. For example, just before the polls open, or during the polling hours, an accurate sampling of voters may reflect the actual voting behaviors. In such cases, a television network may be able to declare a winner a few minutes or a few hours ahead of the official announcement. Such accurate but competitive predictions may have commercial advantages, but their scientific utility is limited.

EVALUATION RESEARCH

Evaluation research is a relatively new form of social research that is designed to assess the effects of large-scale social, economic, and educational programs planned and supported by government agencies. Large-scale governmental programs such as those for the poor, the elderly, and the mentally and physically handicapped have created a need to develop procedures to assess the usefulness of such programs (Freeman, 1977; Patton, 1978).

Typically, agencies that support a program require evaluation research. For example, a state agency that has supported a program to reduce the number of drunk drivers on the streets during the holiday season may wish to know the answers to several questions, including whether the program was effective; if so, to what extent; and if not effective, how to improve the program. Evaluation research is often a tool for enhancing the public agency's accountability. Ideally, evaluation research is a means of making better political decisions. The criticism, however, has been that in practice, the outcome of evaluation research is rarely used by the politically controlled government agencies (Patton, 1978).

Three types of evaluation research have been described in the literature (Freeman, 1977): process evaluation, impact evaluation, and comprehensive evaluation. *Process evaluation* is designed to find out whether the program was implemented the way it was described, and whether the program served the specified target population. For example, a special educational program designed to serve communicatively handicapped children may be evaluated first to see if all of the children in need of services were served. It is possible that children with some specific disorder of communication were excluded because the clinicians or educators lacked professional interest or expertise. The next step in process evaluation is to examine the procedures that were used in the implementation of the program. Whether the procedures specified in the original plan were used; if not, what kinds of modifications were made; and what effects those modifications had on the target population would be analyzed.

In the actual evaluation of the program, the investigator may use a variety of techniques, including direct observation, interviews, and examination of the project records. The activities of the project staff members may be directly observed by the investigator. The staff may be interviewed to determine whether the procedures and targets were appropriate. The members of the target population may also be interviewed to determine whether the procedures were used as planned. Records kept by the staff may be examined to see if the procedures and results were accurately documented.

Impact evaluation is concerned with the effects of the program on the target population. The most important question here is whether the target group benefited as prescribed by the program. In some ways, an impact evaluation resembles experimental research. However, in practice, appropriate experimental methods are not used in impact evaluation. In most cases, the impact is assessed with the help of the data and documents provided by the project staff and the additional information gathered by the project team. The evaluative team cannot arrange controlled experimental conditions to assess the effects. Most social and educational programs are not set up as controlled experiments, and therefore the data they generate may be less reliable than the results of an experiment. By their very nature, large-scale social and educational programs are affected by numerous uncontrolled variables.

Comprehensive evaluation includes both an assessment of the process and the effects of the program under review. The process evaluation is completed in the initial step. If it is determined that appropriate procedures were used and the target population was served, then the investigator proceeds to evaluate the effects of the program. One might argue that this is the only useful type of evaluation research. The usefulness of mere process or impact evaluation is limited.

Evaluation research that yields a certain amount of useful information is possible only when the program is written clearly. The concepts and procedures must be specified in operational terms. The goals of the program must be stated unambiguously. The criteria for judging the success of the program must also be clear. Many government-supported programs, such as the special educational program, have broad guidelines. Broad guidelines encourage innovation at the local level, but they make a comprehensive national assessment of programs difficult.

THE RELATION BETWEEN RESEARCH TYPES AND QUESTIONS

We have discussed seven major types of research: ex post facto, normative, standard-group comparison, experimental, clinical, survey, and evaluation. It must be clear to the reader that each research type handles a unique type of research question. The nature of the question determines the type of method to be used.

Research types are not entirely matters of methods, however. They reflect both methodological and philosophical stances. As noted earlier, each type of research is capable of answering certain kinds of questions. Therefore, what kinds of methods one typically uses depends upon the kinds of questions one typically asks. As such, a researcher can use different methods to answer different kinds of questions. In practice, however, most researchers develop a typical tendency to investigate certain types of questions. A majority of those who are typically interested in normative research in language development, for example, may not be inclined to ask questions that require experimental analysis. Those who wish to determine the independent variables of their dependent variables rarely indulge in normative research.

Broadly speaking, the seven research types can be grouped into three categories. The first category contains the ex post facto and evaluation types of research, which can answer questions regarding potential relations between events that have passed. In ex post facto research, the investigator infers a cause of an effect from a knowledge of the past events. It may be noted that evaluation research is essentially ex post facto in that it tries to establish whether certain events took place (process) and whether certain other events followed (impact).

The second category contains the normative, standard-group comparisons, and survey types of research, which are capable of answering questions concerning "the way things are." All three types of research in the second category are concerned with the distribution of dependent variables in the population. There are philosophical and other differences between the three types within the category. Normative research is based on the philosophy of developmentalism and seeks to establish typical performances of defined groups. Standard-group comparisons are made to find differences between identified groups. Both normative and standard-group comparisons are thought to help determine boundaries of normal and disordered or deviant behaviors.

The third category contains experimental research of all varieties—laboratory, clinical, and nonclinical. Experimental research does not search for causal relations in the past, nor does it simply ask a question about the way things are. It creates conditions under which expected or unexpected things may happen. What happens when an independent variable is manipulated under controlled conditions is the concern of experimental research. Therefore, research questions about cause–effect relations in which the experimenter must have a reasonable degree of confidence dictate the use of the experimental method.

Many beginning researchers often wonder what type of research they should do. Instead, they should wonder about the types of questions they would like to investigate. Within their limitations, all types of research contribute something to the knowledge base. Some types of research, however, do more than others in helping us understand the events we study. The experimental method does the most in helping us both understand the events and gain control over those events. Understanding and controlling events are the essence of *science*, regardless of such qualifications as applied, clinical, and basic. ■

S T U D Y **G U I D E**

1 Define ex post facto research. Describe its procedures.

2 You are seeing a client with a sensorineural hearing loss. Design an ex post facto study to identify some of the potential causal variables. Describe possible independent variables and the procedures of uncovering them. Specify the limitations of this kind of study.

3 Justify the need for ex post facto studies in clinical disciplines.

4 What are the logic and the procedures of normative research?

5 Suppose you wish to establish the stages by which children learn to produce the regular and irregular plural forms with 80 percent accuracy. You also wish to have a local representative sample. Design a study to accomplish your objectives.

6 Summarize the strengths and limitations of normative research.

7 Is chronological age an independent variable? Why or why not?

8 Describe the method of standard-group comparison. It is similar to what other type of research?

9 Selecting a clinical group, design a standard-group comparison study. Describe fully the dependent variables, assigned variables, and measurement procedures.

10 Justify the statement that standard-group comparisons cannot establish cause–effect relations.

11 Define experimental research. Describe its procedures.

12 Suppose you wish to experimentally evaluate the effects of an articulation treatment procedure. Describe a hypothetical treatment procedure and design an experimental study to evaluate its effects.

13 Specify the criticisms of experimental research. How would you refute those criticisms?

(continued next page)

Study Guide *(continued)*

14 Distinguish between clinical and applied research.

15 Summarize the importance of experimental–clinical research.

16 What is the purpose of sample surveys? Write two research questions that can be answered by the survey research.

17 What are the limitations of survey research?

18 What is evaluation research? What are the different kinds of evaluation research?

19 Design a study to make a comprehensive evaluation of a communicative disorders program in a public school system.

20 Justify the statement that each research type handles a unique type of research question. Give examples.

■ C H A P T E R 5

Observation and Measurement

■ Observation and measurement, 104

■ Philosophies of measurement, 105

■ Traditional levels of measurement, 107

■ Some measures of communicative behaviors, 109

■ Client-assisted measurement, 117

■ Indirect measures, 118

■ Covert measurement, 119

■ The observer in the measurement process, 121

■ Mechanical aids to observation and measurement, 124

■ Reliability of measurement, 126

■ Study guide, 129

O bservation and measurement are two basic activities of science. The beginnings of observation are in the sensory experiences about some natural phenomena. When people see, hear, touch, and smell things and events, they may also wonder about their qualities and causes. They may then take a closer, more systematic look at the event. At the simplest level, looking at something and describing what is seen is observation. In fact, a systematic report of any kind of sensory experience is observation. In this sense, observation is an everyday activity.

Compared with everyday observation, scientific observation is more systematic, thorough, and objective. Scientific observation is systematic in the sense that it is relatively organized and the results of observations are recorded in some form. The observation is thorough in that the scientist attempts to observe as many aspects of a phenomenon as possible. It is objective because different observers try to achieve the same results of observation.

Scientific observation is rooted in empiricism. Normally, events that do not generate sensory consequences are not taken seriously by scientists. Exceptions emerge when the existence of a phenomenon is suggested by a variety of indirect evidence and theory in the absence of direct sensory stimulation. The existence of a phenomenon that cannot be measured may be *temporarily* postulated when many strong empirical reasons support it. In many cases, instruments mediate observation of events that do not generate sensory stimulation. I shall address the issue of mechanical aids to observation in a latter section.

OBSERVATION AND MEASUREMENT

Scientific observation is essential for measuring a phenomenon. Without systematic measurement, a scientist is often unable to go beyond observation. For example, the important task of experimentation requires that the event be measured before, during, and after the introduction of the independent variable. Changes in events are documented through measurement.

Measurement has been defined variously as "assignment of numbers to represent properties" (Campbell, 1952, p. 110), "assignment of numerals to objects or events according to rules" (Stevens, 1951, p.1), or as a "process involving quantification of observations with respect to a reference scale composed of and defined by units that are both absolute and standard" (Johnston & Pennypacker, 1980, p. 55). In essence, objects, events, and their properties are quantified in measurement. This is done according to a standard set of rules that define units of measurement.

Quantified observations are often called the measured value of an event, object, or its property. From a technical standpoint, what is measured is not the event, object, or its property, but some *dimensional quantity*. Frequency of an event, for example, is a *dimensional quantity* of an event. Standard number units can be assigned to that frequency. Other dimensional quantities of behavioral events include duration, latency, and interresponse time.

PHILOSOPHIES OF MEASUREMENT

As pointed out by Johnston and Pennypacker (1980), social and psychological sciences have evolved a philosophy of measurement that is different from that of natural sciences. Natural sciences have found that absolute and standard units of measurement are essential to objective quantification of observations. Johnston and Pennypacker (1980) have called this kind of measurement *idemnotic*, which they defined as "the type of measurement that incorporates absolute and standard units whose existence is established independently of variability in the phenomena being measured" (p. 71). Without idemnotic measurement, natural scientists would not have been able to achieve the level of precision and objectivity for which they are well known.

Social and psychological sciences, on the other hand, often do not measure the dimensional quantities of events in terms of absolute and standard units of measurements. Instead, they measure those quantities in terms of relative standards that are defined within the confines of the variability of the phenomenon under investigation. Johnston and Pennypacker have called this type of measurement *vaganotic*, which they defined as "the creation of scales and units of measurement on the basis of variation in a set of underlying observations" (1980, p. 64).

In vaganotic measurement, standards of measurement keep changing depending upon the amount of variability shown by the individual phenomenon of interest. For example, a rating scale developed to measure the severity of stuttering typically yields different values depending upon the amount of variability found in different groups of stutterers. Different rating scales designed to measure the same stuttering severity yield different values when used on the same clients. Similarly, rating scales developed to measure different disorders will result in vastly different values.

Social and psychological sciences often measure dimensional quantities indirectly. Instead of directly observing behaviors, social or psychological scientists may seek verbal statements by subjects or other people who are supposed to know. For example, a supervisor may fill out a questionnaire on the productivity of his or her employee. The investigator will use the questionnaire responses as though they were direct observational values of productive behaviors themselves. However, the investigator will not have directly observed and counted productive behavior with a standard and absolute system of numbers.

The proverbially derogative statement that "by taking a new job, he raised the IQ of the people he left and the people he joined" illustrates this philosophy of relative and indirect measurement defined in terms of the variability of the phenomenon being measured. Nobody's intelligence increased or decreased by a person's move, but because the variability changed, the assumption is that the measured value also changed. If one were to assume that a given individual student on a university campus is as intelligent as the "average student" on that campus, then that student's intelligence will continuously change depending upon which university he or she attends. Compared with a group of clinically anxious groups, I may have less anxiety, but compared with someone who is unusually calm, I may have more anxiety. But all along, my level of anxiety may not have changed, but the relative scale used to measure it assumes it has.

The history of vaganotic and idemnotic measurements has been traced by Johnston and Pennypacker (1980). In the 17th and 18th centuries, mathematicians and scientists were concerned with the variability in measured values of a given phenomenon. When a natural phenomenon is measured repeatedly, the values are typically not constant. The question, then, was what is the "true" value of the phenomenon? This concern eventually led to the development of modern statistics in the works of Adolphe Quetelet (1796–1874). Quetelet proposed that human characteristics such as height vary only because nature missed the ideal. What nature missed could be calculated by measuring the heights of many individuals. In effect, when repeated measures are plotted, the result is normal curve, which to many suggests the ideal in the form of a mean. Thus, the nonexistent average person, created to neutralize the measures of variability in people, gave not only a stable measure of persons but also the concept of an ideal person.

It was Francis Galton (1822–1911) who believed that mental abilities are also distributed normally and that the distribution of measured values across a vast number of subjects would suggest the ideal (the average). Tests of intelligence were soon developed by Binet (1857–1911) and Cattell (1860–1944), and the tradition of vaganotic measurement in terms of variability of the phenomenon measured became firmly established in psychology and social sciences. The tradition was strengthened by the developments of statistical techniques designed to infer the true value of a population from the measured sample values.

Although psychology and social sciences use indirect and relative system of measurement, the radical behaviorism of Skinner has shown that the use of absolute and standard units of measurement is possible in the study of human behavior. Skinner (1953) avoided indirect and statistically based measurement of behavior by defining his dependent variable as the *rate* (frequency) of observable and directly measurable responses of an organism. When the occurrence of a given response of a class of responses is counted, a direct and absolute number system is used. For example, when a clinician counts the number of times a child produced the regular plural morpheme /s/ in a segment of conversational speech, an absolute value of frequency is established. The value would not be relative to the variability found in the phenomenon of plural /s/ usage. On the other hand, the normative statement that "on the average 5-year-olds produce the plural /s/ with X percent accuracy" is relative to the variability found in that phenomenon.

The measurement philosophy and the nature of a subject matter interact in a curious manner. A measurement philosophy can influence the way a subject matter is conceptualized and researched. To a certain extent, intelligence and personality were conceptualized as they were because of the measurement philosophy and technique that were adopted by those interested in mental measurement. In turn, the way a phenomenon is conceptualized determines to some extent how it can be measured. If it is believed that the variability is intrinsic to the behaving organism, as does the statistical approach, then group designs and statistical methods of neutralizing variability are necessary techniques of research. On the other hand, if it is believed that variability is extrinsic to the behaving organism, it becomes a subject of experimental analysis. The measurement procedure adopted in this case would not be solely determined by the variability of behaviors.

TRADITIONAL LEVELS OF MEASUREMENT

Social and psychological scientists typically describe what are known as levels of measurement. These levels are an integral part of the indirect and relative measurement strategy. Some of the levels are closely related to statistical scaling techniques.

Typically, four levels of measurement are described: nominal, ordinal, interval, and ratio. In *nominal* measurement, a number assigned to an event or object has no mathematical meaning. Those numbers simply help distinguish one event or object from the other. As such, the numbers are much like proper names; hence, the term *nominal measurement*. Nominal measurement yields categorical data: 1 may stand for the female subject and 0 for the male subject. What is "measured" is simply given a parallel symbol system, which may consist of numbers without their arithmetic meanings. Questionnaires that evoke "yes" or "no" responses illustrate nominal measurement, as do telephone numbers and numbers assigned to football players. Diagnostic categories such as stuttering and aphasia are included under nominal measurement.

Nominal measurement is described as the crudest or the simplest of the measurement levels. It is probably no measurement at all. It does not measure a dimensional quantity, and it does not serve any purpose other than distinguishing one set of observations from another. It does not accomplish anything that a name would not, and naming a thing is not the same as measuring it.

Ordinal measurement assumes that the property being measured is continuous, not categorical. Relative concepts such as "greater than" and "less than" are involved in ordinal measurement. It is usually accomplished in terms of rank-ordering events, objects, or properties in terms of graded increases or decreases. For example, a school that graduates the most straight-A students may be assigned the rank number 1, and one that graduates the least number of straight-A students, the last rank. In rank-ordering students on the basis of their GRE scores, admission officers use the ordinal measurement. Ranks only tell that one student has scored more or less on the GRE in relation to students with higher or lower ranks. Ranked values do not tell how much more they scored, nor do they indicate an absence of the quality measured. In other words, there are no absolute numbers and there is no zero that indicates the total absence of the measured property.

The frequently used five-point Lickert type of rating scale consists of ordinal measurement. When a subject expresses *strong disagreement, disagreement, neutral, agreement,* or *strong agreement,* the opinion on some issue is said to have been measured on an ordinal scale. The categories of judgments can be given numbers to derive numerical values. However, such numbers and their corresponding categories do not have mathematical meaning. Also, the intervals between numbers or categories are unknown and probably not equal. For example, one cannot assume that *strong agreement* is twice as strong as *agreement.* Therefore, numbers assigned to ordinal categories cannot be added or subtracted.

Ordinal scales at best provide indirect and subjective measures of properties measured. They are greatly influenced by the uncontrolled, momentary, and subjective judgments of the observer. There is no standard unit of measurement. This type of measurement is commonly used in the assessment of such subjective and highly variable intervening variables as attitudes and opinions.

Interval measurement is an improvement over ordinal measurement in that the numerical distinctions of the scale do suggest similar distinctions in the measured property. That is, the difference between 1 and 2 on an interval scale would be the same as that between 3 and 4. As noted before, there is no such assurance in an ordinal scale. The interval scale has a zero, but it is arbitrary. The zero does not mean the absence of the measured property. Therefore, the scale values of an interval scale, though of known distance (intervals), cannot be added or subtracted.

Measurement of temperature and calendar time are examples of interval scales. On either the centigrade or Fahrenheit scales, zero does not mean an absence of temperature. The beginning of the Christian calendar is also arbitrary. If four clients' stuttering is measured on an interval scale, the client who is assigned a score of 4 stutters twice as severely as the client who receives a 2. Again, because of a lack of zero, the numbers are not additive or subtractive.

The final level of measurement is known as the *ratio*. It has all the properties of the earlier levels and also has a zero, which suggests an absence of the property being measured. Ratio measurement uses the number system in its mathematical sense. It is possible to count, add, and subtract the values of a ratio scale. Most measures in the natural sciences are on this scale; most of those in the social sciences are not. However, when the dependent variable is the frequency of discrete events, it is possible to use the ratio measurement. The frequency of a given discrete response can be measured with real numbers. A zero response rate does mean that the organism did not respond.

SOME MEASURES OF COMMUNICATIVE BEHAVIORS

Communicative behaviors can be observed, measured, and recorded in different ways. What kinds of measures are used would depend on the definition of the specific communicative behavior targeted for measurement. Some definitions allow direct measurement whereas others permit only indirect and inferential measurement. For example, language may be defined either as linguistic competence or as the production of various language responses. Linguistic competence cannot be measured directly; it is inferred from other kinds of data. The production of particular responses, on the other hand, is directly measurable. Generally speaking, a phenomenon can be measured more directly if it is defined operationally. Operational definitions are descriptions of procedures involved in measuring an event. For example, the term *articulatory proficiency* does not define anything operationally, but the production of /s/ in initial positions of ten words at 90 percent accuracy does.

I shall describe seven types of measures that are relevant for most clinical research in speech–language pathology: frequency, duration, interresponse time, latency, time sampling, momentary time sampling, and verbal interaction sampling.

Frequency Measures

The frequency with which a behavior is exhibited under specified stimulus conditions is one of the most useful, objective, and often used of the measured values of communicative behaviors.

Frequency measures can be used in counting the number of times a client produces language responses of particular classes, the number of sounds misarticulated, the number and types of dysfluencies, the number of pitch breaks, and other such communicative behaviors. To establish frequency measure of various speech and language behaviors, the observer often must also count the number of contextually correlated behaviors. These are typically the number of syllables or words spoken.

The measurement of the frequency of communicative behaviors poses a special problem. Communicative behaviors are discriminated. In other words, their production is not reflexive and automatic, but context-dependent. Therefore, in measuring the frequency of communicative behaviors, the investigator must first arrange the discriminative stimulus conditions that set the stage for the particular kinds of behaviors targeted for observation and measurement. Various kinds of stimulus pictures, objects, topic cards, and conversational devices help evoke communicative behaviors.

In establishing the frequency measure of specific speech–language behaviors, the investigator must take into consideration the number of opportunities afforded those behaviors in a given period of observation. For example, in the measurement of the frequency of grammatical features, the number of discriminated opportunities to produce those features must be considered. Brown (1973) has described such opportunities as obligatory contexts. They are the structural contexts of phrases and sentences in which the use of a particular grammatical feature is obligatory from the standpoint of the rules of a given language. For example, the regular plural inflection would be obligatory in the context of "I see two (noun) here." The concept of discriminated opportunities can be used in measuring semantic and pragmatic response classes as well.

The productions of specific sounds also have their discriminated opportunities. An omission is suggested when a child does not produce the /s/ in the word *soup* because of this discriminated opportunity for that production. The number of syllables or words spoken may be the discriminated opportunities for the production of dysfluencies. Speech itself is the discriminated opportunity for various voice qualities.

When the discriminated opportunities and the number of opportunities in which the behavior under observation appears are both measured, a percent correct response rate can be derived. This measure can be calculated for most of the communicative behaviors that can be measured in terms of frequency. The percentage of (correct) articulation of a given sound in a given word position and that of dysfluencies are among the commonly reported frequency-based measures in research studies. Studies on language have also frequently reported percent correct measures of productions of various grammatical features and vocabulary items.

Frequency measure, though simple, direct, and objective, may not be practical in measuring all kinds of communicative behaviors. Frequency measure is most appropriate for behaviors that are of relatively low rate and have a clear beginning and end. In other words, the behaviors must be discrete and should be a part of other behaviors. Many speech and language behaviors fulfill these two criteria. Grammatical features, for example, are used in the context of other behaviors and are therefore of relatively low rate. They are also discrete behaviors in the sense that their onset and termination can be easily determined.

Some nondiscrete communicative behaviors of high rate are not appropriately measured by frequency count. For example, some of the voice qualities, such as hoarseness or harshness, may not be most efficiently counted according to their rate. A pervasive hoarseness of voice (high rate) that does not have a discernible beginning or end (except for speech/silence dichotomy) must be measured some other way.

Another limitation of frequency count is that it may not be a comprehensive measure of certain behaviors. In other words, mere frequency count may miss other equally significant dimensional quantities of a behavior. For example, the duration of certain behaviors may be an important dimensional quantity that may be missed in the frequency count. For instance, a frequency measure of dysfluencies may not necessarily reflect their durational quantity. Theoretically, dysfluencies of low frequency may be of relatively long duration, and those of high frequency may be of short duration. This theoretical possibility has not been observed in a majority of stutterers, however. In most cases, low frequency of dysfluencies is associated with relatively shorter duration, and vice versa. But in those exceptional cases where frequency and duration are unrelated or opposite to each other, both the measures must be obtained.

Procedures of counting the frequency of a behavior can be simple or complex. Many speech–language behaviors can be counted with the help of various kinds of counters. In most clinical sessions, behavioral frequency can be counted with certain kinds of marks on a piece of paper. Speech–language behaviors, because of their transitory nature, require some form of recording before they can be reliably counted. Audio or video recordings are often necessary to count speech–language behaviors. In most cases, the recorded behaviors must be reviewed repeatedly to obtain accurate measures. Other mechanical devices can help count behaviors, and in some cases they may do most of the counting.

Durational Measures

The duration over which a specified behavior is sustained can be a useful measure. It is especially useful in the case of continuous behaviors. The total number of seconds or minutes for which the behavior is sustained is usually measured and compared against the total duration of time for which the observation was made. For example, the duration for which an inappropriately high pitch is maintained by a client within a 30-minute conversational speech can be recorded. In this case, the percentage of time spent exhibiting the appropriate pitch can also be calculated.

Duration, being a temporal measure of behavior, gives a different kind of information than does the frequency. While the frequency specifies the number of times a behavior is exhibited, it gives no clues to the length of each behavioral episode. As pointed out earlier, duration of dysfluencies is an important dimensional quantity, and a direct measure of it can be of both empirical and theoretical significance in a research study. In communicative disorders, most vocal qualities are better measured in terms of duration. If talking behavior (a global measure of language use) is the subject of experimental manipulation, the time spent talking, instead of specific language behaviors, may be a more appropriate measure.

The durational measure can be impractical with many behaviors. Apparently, duration is a valid measure of behaviors that have an appreciable temporal dimension. It is true that all behaviors have a temporal dimension, but depending upon the purposes of a study, measurement of duration may or may not be essential or practical. For example, in the measurement of grammatical features or semantic notions, the interest may be in frequency and not duration. How many times a child produces the present progressive /ing/ in a conversational sample may be of greater interest than the duration of /ing/ productions.

In clinical research, duration measures are less frequently used than frequency measures because extremely brief durations of behaviors are hard to measure without sophisticated instrumentation. The duration must be noticeable in order for it to be used in routine clinical research. For example, sound or silent prolongations of stutterers have a noticeable durational dimension, whereas the schwa interjections do not. Therefore, measurement of duration is relatively easy in the case of prolongations and difficult in the case of interjections.

In clinical research, durations that can be measured with a stopwatch may be reported more frequently than those that require complex instrumentation. Clinical target responses of extremely brief durations are better measured for their frequency. Generally speaking, without instrumentation, duration measures are harder to record than are frequency measures.

Whenever possible, duration measures must be combined with frequency measures. Together, they give a better measure of behaviors. In some cases, a pure duration measure can be meaningless unless the frequency measure is also reported. For example, it may be misleading to report merely that a stutterer's mean duration of sound prolongations was 3 minutes. For this observation to be meaningful, the frequency of such prolongations must also be reported.

Interresponse Time Measures

Another time-based measure of behaviors is the duration that lapses between any two discrete responses or other events. Interresponse time can be a useful measure in some kinds of research. In clinical studies that are concerned with too sparse response rates, the clinician might be interested in decreasing the interresponse time.

Clinically, interresponse time may be a function of the rate at which the clinician presents the training stimuli. For example, a clinician may present language or articulation stimulus cards at a relatively fast or slow rate, generating a shorter or longer interresponse time. When the rate of stimulus presentation is changed, the interresponse time may also change. Other treatment variables may affect interresponse time. One can investigate such variables with a view to increasing the response rate and decrease the time spent in not giving the target response.

It is obvious that interresponse time is closely related to the frequency of responses. A high response frequency is likely to be associated with short interresponse durations; a low frequency is likely to generate relatively long interresponse durations. Therefore, it is meaningful to report the frequency measure along with the interresponse durations.

Latency Measures

Latency, or reaction time, is also a temporal measure of behavior. It differs from the duration measure in that it is not a measure of time for which a response was sustained. Latency is the time that lapses between the termination of an environmental event (often a stimulus) and the onset of a response. The time it takes for an organism to respond after stimulation is sometimes taken as a reflection of learning: the faster the reaction time, the stronger the learning. Whether this is valid or not, reaction time can be an indirect measure of frequency: other things being equal, the greater the latency, the lower the frequency of responses per unit of time.

Latency is an important aspect of communicative behavior. In conversational speech, the listener and the speaker switch their roles alternatingly. Each provides certain verbal as well as nonverbal signals to the other person or persons to switch the role (initiate or terminate responses). Therefore, latency measures may be necessary in an analysis of conversational speech. In clinical research, a client's response latency can be a useful dependent variable in that shorter latencies are often one of the targets of treatment. A delayed response may be as good as no response, and often it is scored as such. Decreasing the latency, then, becomes a primary target of treatment.

A few seconds of reaction time is considered typical in clinical situations. Most clinicians probably allow a few seconds, perhaps up to 5 seconds, for the client to respond. If the response latency is too long, the clinician tends to shape progressively shorter latencies.

Latency has been a dependent variable in several studies concerned with stutterers' vocal behaviors. Two latency measures have been researched extensively: the voice initiation time (VIT) and the voice termination time (VTT). Several kinds of stimuli can be used to get a vocal response initiated or terminated although auditory stimuli have been used most frequently. In using an auditory tone as the stimulus, the experimenter may instruct the subject to initiate a vocal response such as /ah/ as soon as the tone is heard and terminate the response as soon as the tone ceases. The actual time that elapses between the onset of the tone and the onset of the vocal response is the VIT. The time that elapses between the termination of the tone and that of the response is the VTT. Studies of this kind have generally shown that stutterers' reaction time is somewhat slower than that of nonstutterers and that it tends to improve with practice (Bloodstein, 1980).

Time Sampling Measures

Time sampling is a measure of behaviors observed and recorded during selected time periods. It is not to be confused with the response duration measure, which is also based on time. The *time* in time sampling refers to periods during which the occurrence of a behavior is observed and recorded, whereas in duration measurement, the length of a response is recorded.

In time sampling, the investigator observes a behavior during selected intervals of time. The intervals may be of short durations: a few seconds to few minutes. An entire treatment session of 45 minutes may be subdivided into 5-minute blocks. During each block, whether or not a specified behavior occurred is recorded. During the observational interval, multiple occurrences of the same behavior are not distinguished; the behavior is scored only once during the interval. The duration of the response is also ignored.

The observational periods may be consecutive or may be interspersed with nonobservational periods. This method requires intensive observation, because during the interval or period of observation, the investigator must pay continuous attention to the subject being observed. For example, a special education specialist might observe a child for 10 minutes, divided into 10-second intervals. During the interval, it is noted whether the child is exhibiting a given target behavior such as quiet sitting or reading. At the end of the interval the presence or the absence of the behavior is recorded. Similarly, in an assessment of mother–child interactions, an investigator may use time sampling to observe specific communicative behaviors during specified intervals.

Time sampling, because it generates categorical data (presence or absence), may not accurately reflect the frequency of measured behaviors. The results of time sampling are analyzed in terms of the number of intervals during which the behavior occurred as against the number of intervals in which the behavior was absent.

Momentary Time Sampling

When it is known that a behavior is relatively constant or of high frequency, continuous observation and measurement may not be necessary. It may be sufficient to observe the behavior periodically and record its occurrence. This method is known as *momentary time sampling* or *spot checking*.

In momentary time sampling of behaviors, the investigator first predetermines the times at which the behavior will be checked. Some kind of signaling device, such as a timer or a wrist-alarm, may set the occasion to observe the behavior. As soon as the timer goes off, the investigator looks at the subject and determines whether or not the subject is exhibiting the target behavior. The behavior is scored as present or absent *at the moment of observation*. A percentage is then calculated by dividing the number of momentary samples during which the behavior was present with the total number of samples and multiplying the quotient by 100. For example, at 30-minute intervals that are set off by a wrist-alarm, a special education specialist may observe a child to see if he or she is sitting quietly. Assuming that over a few days, the specialist had 38 total spot checks and the behavior was scored as present in 24 of them, the percentage of time sampled values would be 63 (24/38 × 100 = 63).

One advantage of momentary time sampling is that it does not require continuous observation of the target behavior. Clinicians and classroom teachers working with groups are not able to observe a particular client or child constantly. And yet, clinicians and teachers need to measure and monitor various behaviors of the individuals in the group. In such cases, momentary sampling can be useful. Momentary time sampling can be appropriate to measure various noncooperative behaviors of specific children in a group therapy session. At predetermined times, the clinician can check a particular client to see if the client is exhibiting nonattending, off-seat, or any other undesirable behavior.

VERBAL INTERACTION SAMPLING

Most of the measures considered so far are suitable for measuring behaviors that are relatively independent, discrete, and exhibited by one or a few individuals. The various language productions of one or a few individuals may be measured for their frequency, duration, and interresponse time. Many of these measures may be obtained through either time sampling or momentary time sampling. However, verbal behavior presents a need for another kind of measure, which has been used only in recent years. It is the measure of *verbal interaction* between individuals.

Ethologists and animal psychologists have observed social interactions between members of groups of animals either in natural habitats or laboratories. In this method of observation, sometimes called *sequence sampling*, a sequence of behaviors of multiple individuals is recorded (Altman, 1974). In some respects, the problem faced by the speech-language pathologist is similar to that of the ethologist and the animal psychologist interested in patterns of social behaviors. Communicative behaviors are essentially social interactions. Studied in natural settings, communicative behaviors involve an interaction in which multiple sequences of verbal behaviors can be simultaneously active.

The term *dyadic interaction* is often used to describe the kind of behavior that is sampled in what I have called here verbal interaction. In many cases, verbal interaction is dyadic. Much of the current research in normal and disordered communication is concerned with interaction between two individuals, often a child and his or her mother or other caregiver. Nonetheless, verbal behaviors are not always dyadic. An analysis of verbal interaction between three or more individuals has barely begun, but it can be expected to be an important part of language analysis. Therefore, the term *verbal interaction sampling* may be more suitable to describe a method of observation designed to measure interactive verbal behaviors of multiple individuals. The term does not restrict, on a priori grounds, the number of individuals involved in verbal interactions.

In verbal interaction sampling, two or more individuals' verbal behaviors are sampled. Interactions are usually arranged for the specific purpose of observation, and in this sense they may not be as naturalistic as everyday conversations. However, every attempt is made to make the interaction as natural as possible. A mother and a child, for example, may be asked to talk to each other in a normal manner. A variety of play materials, pictures, and other stimulus items may be provided to stimulate verbal interaction. This kind of observation may be made at the subjects' home or in a research laboratory.

The actual measures obtained through verbal interaction sampling depend upon the research questions and theoretical orientations of the researcher. For the most part, the frequency of a variety of *types* of verbal responses is noted. For example, the number of requests, comments, and topic initiations made by the child and the mother may be observed and recorded. In addition, the development of conversational skills, including of turn-taking, has been studied by verbal interaction sampling (Brinton & Fujuki, 1984; Hurtig, 1977; Martlew, 1980; Snow & Ferguson, 1977; Wanaska & Bedrosian, 1985).

The verbal interaction sampling has been used mostly to study the patterns of interactions between the child and the mother. These studies have been typically nonexperimental (nonmanipulative), and in this sense they are comparable to ethological studies of animal behaviors in natural habitats. The purpose has been to document the dependent variables in the form of interdependent speech of mothers and children. Potential independent variables of those interactive behaviors have rarely been addressed in research studies.

The method of verbal interaction sampling can be equally useful in studies designed to manipulate the potential independent variables of the interdependent speech of multiple speakers. The frequency of various interactive verbal behaviors under conditions of experimental observations and manipulations can be measured and analyzed. In the case of mother–

child dyadic interactions, one might systematically alter some aspect of the mother's speech to her child to see what effects follow. For example, what happens when mothers are trained to reinforce certain kinds of utterances produced at a low level by their children? Or, what happens when mothers are trained to expand their children's limited utterances into grammatically or semantically more complex utterances? Such experimental studies have been few, but they generate heuristic as well as clinically relevant data (Goldstein, 1984; Scherer & Olswang, 1984). Unlike observational studies, experimental studies can identify the independent variables of verbal interactions.

The frequency, duration, interresponse time, latency, time sampling, momentary time sampling, and verbal interaction sampling measures all require direct observation of the behavior to be measured. When necessary, the conditions of behavioral occurrence must be carefully arranged and the observer or a mechanical device must be present to record the dimensional quantity of the measured behavior. Any of these measures can be obtained in experimental or nonexperimental research conducted in naturalistic settings or laboratories.

Measures obtained by investigators are preferable to those obtained by subjects themselves. However, in clinical research, it is sometimes necessary to obtain the measures of behaviors in the client's natural environment in the absence of the clinical investigator. In such cases, client-assisted measurement may be used.

CLIENT-ASSISTED MEASUREMENT

In client-assisted measurement, some important task necessary to document the occurrence of the behavior of interest is performed by the client himself or herself. The clinical investigator is not present while the behavior of interest is naturally occurring. The client can record his or her own behavior with audio or video recording devices and submit the records for the clinician's review. It is the clinician who measures the frequency or other dimensional quantity of the target behavior.

This kind of measurement is especially important in establishing a reliable frequency of the target behaviors in the natural environment before, during, and after treatment. It is possible that no amount of direct measurement in the clinic or laboratory will fully and accurately reflect the communicative behaviors of clients in the home, school, office, and supermarket. When the concern is the assessment of treatment effects sustained in such natural environments, client-assisted measurement can be useful.

Client-assisted measures may be preferred even when the clinical investigator can be present in a client's everyday situation to measure the target behaviors, because the presence of the clinician may affect the frequency of measured behaviors. Usually, the effect is positive; the clinician is a discriminative stimulus for the treated behaviors. Since the clinician is not a permanent part of the client's natural environment, a more valid measure of the target behavior can be recorded only in the absence of the clinician.

The client must be trained to record his or her behavior in natural settings. In many cases, clients may have to be trained in the correct use of a tape recorder or a video recording machine. In communicative disorders, clients are often asked to record their conversational speech at home or in other situations. They must be given detailed instructions on how to arrange the conversational situations. The conversational speech must be natural (habitual) and must be long enough to permit reliable measures of the dependent variables targeted for treatment. Possibly, the conversations with different individuals may have to be recorded at different times of the day. Typically, repeated recordings are also needed.

When both are obtained, direct and client-assisted measures can give a more comprehensive and reliable picture of the dependent variables. However, some investigators may also use another kind of measurement in which the dependent variable is neither observed as it occurs nor measured through client-submitted recordings. This is the indirect measurement of behaviors.

INDIRECT MEASURES: SELF-REPORTS

Indirect measures are obtained without the experimenter coming into contact with the dependent variable in vivo or after the fact. Instead of directly observing or scoring recorded behaviors, the investigator asks clients to describe their behaviors. The subject can report orally or in writing, and the format of the report may be more or less standardized. These are the methods of self-reports.

The most commonly used self-reports are questionnaires of various kinds. Questionnaires of personality, attitudes, interests, fear, anxiety, and avoidance reactions are frequently used in clinical research. Most of these questionnaires are used by clinical psychologists and psychiatrists in the assessment of behavior disorders. In communicative disorders, attitudinal scales to measure stutterers' reaction to various speech situations are used by some researchers and clinicians. Also available are various rating scales that seek information from stutterers regarding their fluency and dysfluency levels in many speaking situations. Other questionnaires may measure attitudes and reactions of parents, teachers, or employers toward various speech–language disorders. Speech and hearing centers may seek the reaction of its patrons regarding the services offered.

The validity of questionnaire measures depends upon the correspondence between what the subjects report and the actual behavior that is being reported upon. If there is a good correspondence, self-reports may be valid. However, the approach assumes that the subjects themselves are reliable and keen observers of their own behaviors, a questionable assumption at best.

A distinction must be made between those self-reports that seek information from the client on specific behaviors exhibited in situations that are not easily accessible to direct observation and those that seek to assess internal states such as attitudes and personality traits. A stutterer, for example, may be asked to compare the extent of his or her dysfluencies in home and at work. When a stutterer reports less dysfluency at home than at work, one might take it as a reasonably valid statement. However, if the investigator then assumes that the stutterer has a negative attitude toward the work place, he or she is going beyond reported observations. Therefore, self-reports that simply supply additional information on behaviors exhibited in extra-clinical situations are more useful than those that seek to measure internal states or inferred entities.

Accepting even those self-reports that simply describe behaviors exhibited in extraclinical situations can be problematic, however. One cannot be sure that a subject's reports are reliable. Therefore, self-reports of clients are an inadequate substitute for direct observation. When practical, subject-assisted observation is preferable to self-reports.

Self-reports are an indispensable method in the case of some dependent variables, however. When an investigator is concerned with what the client thinks and feels, verbal or written reports are the only means of assessing them. For example, in assessing an obsessive patient, the clinician has to ask the patient to describe his or her obsessive thoughts and feelings. In communicative disorders, it is possible that a clinician is interested in the feelings and thoughts associated with a speech or language disorder. In such cases, self-reports provide the only means of assessment. The clinician then should exercise caution in interpreting self-reports because the dependent variables may not have been quantified objectively.

COVERT MEASUREMENT

Whether direct or not, most of the measurement techniques described so far are overt in the sense that the fact of measurement is not hidden from subjects. Even when it is direct, most subjects may not fully understand all aspects of the measurement. They may not understand what specific target behaviors are measured by what methods. Nonetheless, most subjects know that some of their behaviors are observed and measured by the investigator.

There are reasons, however, to measure behaviors without the knowledge of the subjects. In unobtrusive or covert measurement, the subjects are unaware that their behavior is being observed and measured. Covert measurement may be necessary for at least two reasons. First, reactive behaviors may be better measured covertly. When subjects do not know that their behavior is being measured, the behavior cannot change simply because it is being measured.

Thus, in the measurement of attitudes, opinions, and other such reactive dependent variables, covert measurement is useful.

Second, in clinical situations, covert measurement (assessment) may be necessary to avoid the influence of discriminated responding. Discriminated responding means that the treated clients are more likely to exhibit the target behaviors in the presence of the clinician, in the clinic, when the treatment technique is in force, and in the presence of persons or stimuli that are associated with the treatment. Since these stimuli are typically absent in the client's natural environment, the treated target behavior may not be produced there. Nevertheless, when the clinician observes the client in one of the natural settings, the behavior may be produced, giving the invalid impression that the behavior is present in such settings. In essence, an accurate measurement of the target behavior in the client's natural environment requires that the clinician or other stimuli associated with treatment not be present during measurement.

Covert measurement requires the cooperation of individuals who are not associated with the treatment process. Those individuals must also be part of the client's everyday situations. A clinician working in a school may request the teacher to observe a child's language and report to the clinician on the production of specific target behaviors. The teacher does this under routine classroom situations and therefore the child may be unaware that his or her speech or language behaviors are being measured. Another clinician may request a stutterer's work supervisor to report on the number of dysfluencies in conversations. The spouse of an aphasic client may be requested to note the number of verbal responses produced at dinner time.

On occasion, certain individuals may be hired to measure the target behaviors. For example, salespersons or pollsters may be hired to make telephone calls to treated clients and report on specific aspects of speech–language behaviors to the clinical investigator.

To be more reliable, the person doing the covert measurement must submit tape-recorded samples of speech to the clinician. The clinician can then score the presence of grammatical features, correct production of phonemes, dysfluencies, and so on. Tape recording without the permission of the client, however, may violate ethical principles, and may also be illegal. In such cases, the covert observer must be trained by the investigator to observe and record behaviors covertly and instantaneously, a task that can be prohibitively expensive in most situations. Even without the permanent records of the behavior being observed, covert measurement raises ethical issues. Obviously, when covert measurement is made, the client will not have given his or her informed consent. Clients who are *debriefed* (see Chapter 15) may still express objections to the procedure and consider it an invasion of their privacy. See Chapter 15 for a detailed discussion of ethical issues in research.

When covert measurement is planned, human subjects committees (see Chapter 15) may or may not approve the procedure. In order to increase the chances of approval, a modified covert procedure may be proposed. The investigator may seek the permission of the client for covert measurement but not inform the client when and where covert assessment will be made and who will make it. In communicative disorders, covert measurement of stuttering has been researched by Ingham (1984) and Howie, Woods, and Andrews (1982).

THE OBSERVER IN THE MEASUREMENT PROCESS

The process of observation has two important components: the phenomenon being observed and the individual who observes it. The scientist-observer is supposed to record the events impartially and without injecting his or her own prejudices and biases. Sometimes the mere fact of observation may change the phenomenon. However, the reactivity of dependent variables is not as major a problem in communicative disorders as it is in such fields as social psychology.

Two issues are often raised in the discussion of the human observer: observer bias and the training of the observer. The first, *observer bias*, refers to a potential tendency on the part of the observer to produce data that might support his or her preconceived ideas about the phenomenon being observed. Subtle changes in the method, duration, and intensity of observation can distort data. For example, if a child is known to talk more at home but less at school, the investigator who spends more time observing the behavior at home may introduce subtle biases into the data. The short-term effects of treatment may be more impressive than the long-term effects, and an observation may be terminated before the data show a decline. The percentage of dysfluencies calculated on the basis of the number of syllables spoken may give a different picture than that based on the number of words spoken.

Faulty analysis of results and improper conclusions drawn from data may also be due to observer biases. However, this is not a significant problem when the data resulting from the observations are clearly separated from the inferences and conclusions. It is only when the observer records inferences instead of the dimensional quantities of events that this problem becomes serious. For example, when a clinician records that "the client was aggressive on five occasions during the treatment session," independent observers have no data to judge the client behaviors. On the other hand, if the clinician records the observable actions (five times the client hit another person) instead of inferring what the actions meant, then the independent observers can come to their own conclusions.

Observer bias is not a problem restricted to the person observing. It is also a matter of the way the dependent variables are conceptualized. Biases are inevitable when the dependent variables are poorly conceptualized and methods of observing them must of necessity be indirect. In essence, indirect measurements and vague dependent variables create opportunities for observer bias. When discrete responses are dependent variables, observer bias can be minimal or at the least, when it does occur, external observers can rectify it.

The second issue, *observer training*, is much more important because proper training can help generate reliable and valid data with minimum or no observer bias. As pointed out by Johnston and Pennypacker (1980), observation is a response of the scientist and objective (bias-free) observation is strictly under the control of the event being observed, not the preconceived ideas of the investigator. Like any other complex response, the act of observation is a learned skill and improves with experience.

In communicative disorders, the training of observers has received little systematic attention. Many investigators hire research assistants who may be only minimally trained in observational skills. Some of these assistants are graduate students who at best receive some instructions on what to look for and how to record what is being measured. Graduate students may consider themselves "experienced" if they have had an opportunity to watch a senior investigator make some scientific observations.

To make scientific observations, the observer (1) must be clear about the topographical aspects of the event, (2) must know the dimensional quantity selected for observation, (3) should be aware of the rough limits of variability of the phenomenon, (4) should have observed and recorded along with an experienced (reliable) observer before working on his or her own, (5) must have mastered the technical aspects of observing and measuring, and (6) must have the disposition of a scientist. These conditions will not guarantee reliable and objective observations, but in their absence, measurement is almost always questionable.

First, the observer must have a thorough knowledge of the form of the response targeted for observation. The observer should know what the behavior looks and sounds like. A person who is unsure of the topography of the response under observation is not likely to record its occurrence consistently, if at all. For example, a student who is not sure of the structure of a verb phrase will not be able to observe and record its occurrence in a language sample. Observers who do not know the form of various dysfluencies cannot be expected to count their frequency. Students who do not know how a vocal fry sounds like will not be able indicate its presence or frequency.

One can be relatively sure of the response topography when it is conceptualized directly and defined operationally. In the self-or-other training process, dependent variables that are unobservable internal events ("cognitive reorganization," for example) are often inferred, not directly observed. Inference is not observation, and if the act of observation itself requires inference, then training objective observational skills is especially difficult.

Second, a clear understanding of the dimensional quantity selected for observation is essential, and observer training must be specific to that. What aspect of the event must be observed and measured? Is it the duration, the frequency, or some other dimensional quantity? Are there multiple dimensions, such as duration *and* frequency, that must be measured simultaneously? How to record the repetitions of the same response topography? For example, when a stutterer says "I stu-stu-stu-stutter," the same response topography is repeated three times. Is this scored as one instance of syllable repetition or three? (Most researchers would count this as one instance of part-word repetition.)

Third, the observer should have some idea about the limits within which the phenomenon under observation can vary. Repeated events do show some variability in their topography. Sound prolongations may be relatively long or short, or they may be produced with greater or less muscular effort (force). But they are all still counted as sound prolongations only. The same morphological feature may be used in inflecting a word, or it may be a part of a phrase or a sentence. The hypernasality of a client may be more pronounced on certain speech sounds and less on others. But such variations may not be considered significant in measurement of the *presence* of hypernasality.

Fourth, an observer must first observe and record the same event along with an experienced observer. This is probably the most important aspect of actual training in observation. It is not sufficient for the awestruck student to merely watch the senior scientist's smooth observational skills. The student observer must observe and record the behavior along with the more experienced observer. The two (or more) persons must measure the same event simultaneously but independently of each other.

Contingent feedback is an essential part of this phase of training. The student and the scientist must compare their measured values and discuss the differences. It is often necessary to talk about the differences as soon as an instance of observational act is completed. This is more efficient when *recorded* behaviors are observed. While measuring behaviors from audio- or videotapes, the scientist and the student observer can "stop" the event to discuss the behavior and its dimensional quantity being measured. The student in this process must receive contingent feedback on all aspects of measurement.

Fifth, when instruments are used in observing and measuring a behavior, the observer must have the necessary technical skills. The use of relatively simple instruments such as tape recorders needs some training and skill. Complex instruments require much more training time, and the student observer must be sure of operating them correctly. The observer should also be able to recognize malfunctions of instruments.

Sixth, the observer must have the behavioral disposition of a scientist. The observer must separate observations from opinions, data from inferences. During the act of observation, the observer should not be interpreting the phenomenon. The sole purpose during observation and measurement is to record the selected dimensional quantity of the event under study.

Interpretations and inferences come later. They are offered in such clear distinction with measured values that other observers can make their own interpretations and inferences.

The training of observers is difficult and tedious, but it is the first step in the training of scientists. I have been involved in training undergraduate and graduate students in the measurement of stuttering, defined in terms of specific dysfluencies whose measured dimensional quantity is frequency. Instructors who have done this know that teaching students to observe and measure behaviors reliably takes several sessions. Accurate observational behavior must be shaped with contingent feedback in a series of small steps.

MECHANICAL AIDS TO OBSERVATION AND MEASUREMENT

Mechanical devices can extend, sharpen, or otherwise enhance the power of human sensory observation. Objects or events that are too small can be enlarged so that they can be seen, measured, and recorded. Objects or events that are too far away to be seen may be visually brought closer for more detailed observation. Events or processes that do not normally generate sensory consequences can also be tracked and recorded by machines or instruments. Instruments can also magnify processes that are too subtle to be measured by human observers. All of these instruments are valuable tools in scientific observation and measurement.

Mechanical instruments can be simple or complex. A hand-held counter may be useful in recording the frequency of many communicative behaviors. A tape recorder or a video recording machine can give scientists a relatively permanent record of fleeting and temporary behavioral processes. Such records can be used to observe a phenomenon repeatedly in training observers and obtaining more accurate measures. Various electronic response monitoring devices, such as operant programming devices, can help record responses mechanically and deliver response consequences contingently and automatically.

A variety of mechanical devices simply give the scientist access to what must be measured. For example, a fiber scope can be used to view the laryngeal area directly; it does not measure or record any of the laryngeal behaviors. However, a fiber scope can be a part of a video recording system in which case the video camera and the recording and monitoring system can make it possible to see the generally inaccessible laryngeal mechanism and record different laryngeal behaviors under different conditions of stimulation and experimentation.

Several other instruments help measure various neurobehavioral processes. Electromyography, for example, measures electrical activity in muscles. It can be used in basic research designed to analyze muscle activities in speech production. Electromyography can also be used in evaluating the effects of treatments on the muscles of speech with corresponding changes in some perceived aspect of speech. They are useful in biofeedfack research with stutterers, cerebral palsied, and people with voice disorders. A kymograph measures specific muscle activity (nonelectrical) involved in breathing.

Various instruments directly track the electrical impulses of muscles and nerves. With suitable recording devices, one can obtain a permanent recording of the electrical activities of different neuromuscular systems. Electroencephalography measures the electrical activity of the brain, picked up by surface electrodes placed on the scalp. Different patterns of discharge are indicative of different kinds of neurobehavioral activity, including linguistic and nonlinguistic activities. Equipment to measure the galvanic skin reflex or response (GSR) can help measure the resistance the skin normally offers to the electrical conductance. This resistance is reduced under conditions of emotional arousal. Therefore, GSR is typically taken as a physiological measure of emotion.

Cineradiography is one of the techniques used in recent years to measure various parameters of the movement-related variables involved in speech production. The technique helps measure the movements of the muscles of the jaw, tongue, and larynx in the production of speech. Such movements cannot be measured precisely without cineradiography, which films the entire sequence of action with x-rays.

The parameters of airflow involved in speech production can be measured by a pneumotachograph. Oscilloscopes make speech visible by displaying various wave patterns associated with differential speech forms on a television-like screen.

A variety of other instruments are available for the researcher in speech–language pathology. Recent advances in computer technology have provided additional mechanical capabalities in the measurement, monitoring, and modification of speech–language behaviors that cannot otherwise be measured precisely. This section is not intended as an introduction to instrumentation in speech and speech pathology. When a particular research investigation requires the mechanical tracking of an independent variable, the investigator must use the instrument that will permit an accurate and reliable measurement of the variable (Curtis and Schultz, 1986). The main point to be made here is that mechanical devices are aids to systematic observation and measurement of dependent variables targeted for scientific investigation.

Instruments are devices that help observe and record phenomena. However, in most cases, the human observer should also exercise his or her judgment in the use of instruments and in the evaluation of observations recorded by instruments. An adequate level of technical training in the use of instruments is necessary. The instruments themselves must be reliable so that they are not a source of internal invalidity of research data.

RELIABILITY OF MEASUREMENT

The results of measurement are subjected to certain kinds of evaluations. Measured values are useful only to the extent that they are adequate for the purposes of a scientific investigation. Measured values of phenomena are evaluated mainly for their reliability and validity. This section is concerned with the concept and procedures of reliability.

The concept of reliability can be understood in different ways. In everyday language, a person is said to be reliable if his or her behavior is consistent across situations and time. The term *stability* also means reliability: if a person's behavior is unstable, it is not reliable. In a restricted sense, predictability also suggests reliability: you can predict an event if it is known to be reliable. Unpredictable events are also unreliable. Dependability is yet another term that implies reliability: dependable phenomena are stable, predictable, and reliable.

Reliability refers to consistency among repeated observations of the same phenomenon. When the measurement of an event is repeated, the measured values should be comparable. If they differ widely, then the measurement is not reliable. When events are measured repeatedly, values are not likely to be the same. Chance fluctuations in the phenomenon and subtle variations in the measurement procedures can cause different values. Nevertheless, to be considered reliable, the divergence in the values of repeated measures must be within certain limits. These limits are usually arbitrarily defined.

The term *reliability* should not be confused with *accuracy*. While reliability refers to the degree of consistency between two or more observations of the same event, accuracy refers to the extent to which the measured values reflect the event being measured. For example, if the measurement of language behaviors in a group of children reflects the "true" performance of those children, one can say that the measurement was accurate. An unreliable measurement may still be accurate in the sense that it reflects the truly fluctuating response of some subjects. A reliable measure may not be accurate in that its repeated values are comparable but the values do not reflect the actual performance of the subjects studied.

Repeated observation is the key to establishing reliability. The same event is observed more than once either by the same individual or by different individuals. We have a measure of *intraobserver* reliability when the same person measures the same phenomenon repeatedly, and a measure of *interobserver* reliability when the same phenomenon is measured by different observers.

In most cases, intraobserver reliability does not pose serious problems. Generally speaking, an observer, even while not measuring something accurately, can be consistent with himself or herself. The same constant mistakes made in the measurement process can result in acceptable reliability of measures. Therefore, intraobserver reliability is typically not reported in research studies. However, it is often required in theses and dissertations. When the research question itself concerns the reliability of measurement of some specific phenomenon, both kinds of reliability may be important. This has been the case in the measurement of stuttering (Bloodstein, 1980).

Interobserver reliability is a crucial element of scientific measurement. Without an acceptable level of interobserver reliability, the results of a study cannot be accepted. Interobserver reliability is one means of convincing the audience that the data are objective. Objectivity in science is realized only by an agreement among different observers regarding the measured values (not opinions) of a given phenomenon. Therefore, interobserver reliability is one of the criteria used in the evaluation of scientific data.

Assessing Interobserver Reliability

There are three general methods of estimating the reliability of research data. In the first method, sometimes referred to as the *unit-by-unit agreement ratio,* two observers must agree on the individual instances of the response being measured. For example, if two observers measure the frequency of the correct production of /s/ in a language sample, they both must agree on the particular instance of /s/ production in order to score agreement. This is a stringent method of scoring agreement.

The procedure for estimating the unit-by-unit agreement ratio is as follows. First, the number of measured units (responses, events, and so on) on which both the observers agreed is determined (A). Next, the total number of units on which the observers disagreed is obtained (D). Finally, the following formula is applied to obtain the agreement index. It is usually expressed in percentages:

$$\text{unit-by-unit agreement index} = \frac{A}{A + D} \times 100$$

Suppose the two observers scored 37 responses as correct and 22 responses as incorrect. The agreement index in this case would be 62 percent ($37 + 22 = 59$; $37/59 \times 100 = 62$ percent). This index has been used extensively in clinical research involving various kinds of communicative behaviors.

The unit-by-unit agreement index is most useful when responses are scored on discrete trials or time intervals. In the measurement of stuttering, Young's work (1969a, 1969b, 1975) has pointed out the importance of the unit-by-unit analysis. He has also developed the following formula to calculate the unit-by-unit agreement index when three or more observers are involved:

$$\text{agreement index} = [1/(n - 1)] [(T/Td) - 1]$$

Where

n = number of observers
T = total number of words marked as stuttered
Td = total number of different words marked as stuttered

Young's (1975) formula has been frequently used in assessing interobserver agreement involving more than two observers. It is especially useful in assessing the effects of technical training programs designed to enhance reliable measurement skills in student clinicians (Gittleman-Foster, 1983).

Statistical correlations provide a second method of calculating interobserver agreement. A correlation, such as the Pearson product–moment coefficient, indicates the degree of covariation between any two sets of measures. In calculating interobserver reliability with this method, scores or measures of one observer are correlated with those of another observer. In calculating correlation coefficients of reliability, each observer must supply several measures. That is, each observer must observe the responses on different occasions, trials, sessions, and so on. For example, the observers may score the correct productions of /s/ in a total of seven sessions. Each observer supplies a *total* score for each session. This yields seven pairs of scores. These pairs can be correlated to obtain a measure of reliability.

The method of scoring unit-by-unit agreement ratio can be contrasted with the correlational method of scoring agreement. The correlational method gives only a global notion of reliability. In this method, the two observers may score comparable numbers of correctly produced /s/, but they may have disagreed on many individual instances. In other words, there may have been many /s/ productions scored as wrong by one observer and correct as another observer, but since both scored about the same total number of correct and incorrect responses, the resulting reliability index may be spuriously high. Generally speaking, a high correlation results as long as the total scores of the two observers are not too divergent. Such high correlations can mask the fact that the two observers agreed only on very few individual instances of responses. It is known that the unit-by-unit method of scoring agreement is a more accurate method of estimating reliability than the correlational method.

A third method, infrequently used, is called a frequency ratio. In this method, the smaller of the two observations is divided by the larger and the resulting quotient is multiplied by 100 to express the ratio in percentages. Each observer's total number of observations is used in this calculation. Suppose that one observer scored 22 correct productions of /s/ and the other observer scored 16. The frequency ratio for this would be 72 percent (16/22 × 100 = 72 percent). Because of its global nature of assessment of reliability, the method is less preferable to the unit-by-unit procedure.

If desired, the original unit-by-unit interobserver agreement formula can be used to calculate the intraobserver agreement as well. In this case, the units (response instances) on which the investigator agreed on both the occasions of measurement are first determined. Then the instances on which the two measurements of the investigator disagreed are determined. The same formula is then applied to derive the intraobserver agreement index. The Young formula should not be used to measure intraobserver agreement because it is meant for two or more observers only.

Reliability of Tests Versus That of Research Data

The reliability of a standardized test must be distinguished from that of research data. Different procedural details are involved in establishing the reliability of standardized tests. These procedures will not be discussed here and the student is referred to other sources (Kerlinger, 1973; Peterson & Marquardt, 1981; Ventry & Schiavetti, 1980).

The reliability of a standardized test may show that when the original sample of subjects is tested and retested, the scores are comparable. This is generally taken to mean that any time the test is used to measure other individual's behaviors, the resulting measures are automatically reliable. This is one of the most questionable assumptions associated with the popular practice of using standardized tests to measure behaviors. From the standpoint of scientific data, reliability is established for the particular measures; it is not inferred from the reliability established elsewhere, by someone else, and in measuring other individuals' behaviors.

The reliability in research is data-specific whereas the reliability of standardized tests is instrument-specific. Like a well-calibrated audiometer, the test may be said to be reliable. But the reliability of hearing thresholds reported in a research study may be questionable. That is, even when an audiometer is reliable, certain measured hearing thresholds may not be. Therefore, in scientific research, regardless of the previously demonstrated reliability of measuring instruments, the reliability of specific observations across the experimental conditions must be evaluated and reported. ■

S T U D Y **G U I D E**

1 As described in this chapter, what are the two basic activities of science?

2 Describe the characteristics of scientific observation.

3 Describe the relation between empiricism and observation.

4 How did Campbell define measurement? How did Johnston and Pennypacker define it?

5 What is another name for quantified observations?

6 Describe briefly the idemnotic and vaganotic measurement philosophies. Compare and contrast them.

(continued next page)

Study Guide *(continued)*

7 A clinician rates the severity of speech–language disorders on a three-point scale as follows: mild, moderate, and severe. Is this idemnotic or vaganotic measurement? Why?

8 In his study of behavior, what is the absolute and standard unit of measurement adopted by B. F. Skinner?

9 Are the "norms" of speech–language behaviors based on absolute or relative measurement? Why?

10 A research clinician assigns a number to each of the ten aphasic subjects in an experiment. What kind of measurement is this (nominal, ordinal, interval, or ratio)?

11 Roger Brown has rank-ordered 14 grammatical morphemes according to the order in which the children he studied mastered them. What kind of measurement is this?

12 A researcher sent out a questionnaire to measure the attitudes of stutterers toward speaking situations. The questionnaire asked stutterers to respond to items such as "my wife (or husband) makes telephone calls on my behalf" with such response options as "always, usually, infrequently, rarely, or never". What kind of measurement is this? What are its limitations?

13 In what sense is the interval measurement an improvement over the ordinal measurement?

14 Give an example of a frequency measure in speech, language, or hearing. Describe how you obtain the measure.

15 Taking the example of dysfluencies in conversational speech, show how a given measure of dysfluencies can be converted into a percentage value.

16 What are some of the difficulties faced in obtaining reliable and valid frequency measures of most communicative behaviors?

17 What are the general limitations of the frequency measure?

18 Define a durational measure and give an example. What kinds of behaviors are best measured with this procedure?

19 In routine clinical sessions, how would you measure hypernasality in conversational speech? What kind of scores or values would you derive from your measurement procedure?

20 When would you use the interresponse time measure in clinical research? Give an example.?

21 What are latency measures? In one of the *Asha* journals, find a study that measured a latency of a particular behavior. How was it done?

22 How would you use time sampling in measuring specified language responses produced in conversational speech?

23 How do you score the multiple occurrences of "nonattending" behavior of a child within blocks of time scheduled to measure that behavior? Are they counted once or as many times as the behavior occurs?

24 Give an example to illustrate the statement that time sampling generates categorical data.

25 Describe the momentary time sampling technique. Is this procedure suitable for high- or low-frequency behavior? Give an example from a group therapy situation.

26 Describe the potential of verbal interaction sampling procedure in conducting experimental studies of mother-child interaction and interaction between three or more individuals.

27 Specify the need for, and the importance of, client-assisted measurement in clinical research.

28 What are indirect measures? What are some of the frequently used indirect measurement tools?

29 What are the indirect measurement tools that focus on internal states? What are some of the problems associated with them?

30 Describe covert measurement and point out the need for it. What ethical concerns does this procedure raise? How do you handle those concerns?

31 What are some of the sources of observer bias?

32 What are the requirements of objective scientific observation? Summarize the six conditions that were described in the text.

33 What is the function of mechanical aids to observation? Do they negate the need for human observation and judgment? Justify your answer.

34 How is cineradiography used in research involving speech production? Find a published study that used cineradiography.

35 What is the instrument used to measure the parameters of airflow?

36 Define reliability. Distinguish it from accuracy of measurement.

(continued next page)

Study Guide *(continued)*

37 Describe interobserver and intraobserver reliability. Which one is generally more important in research?

38 What is the unit-by-unit agreement index? Why is it better than a global measure of reliability?

39 Two clinicians, measuring the number of correct and incorrect articulations of selected phonemes by a child, have scored the following: 63 correct, 45 incorrect. Calculate the unit-by-unit interobserver agreement index for these scores.

40 Specify Young's formula for calculating the agreement index when three or more observers are involved.

41 Describe how a statistical correlation can be used to assess reliability. What is its most significant limitation? Illustrate your answer with an example.

42 What is the difference between the reliability of standardized tests and that of research data?

■ P A R T **T W O**

Clinical Research Designs

■ CHAPTER   6

Research Designs: An Introduction

■ What are research designs?, 135

■ The structure and logic of experimental designs, 136

■ Variability: some philosophic considerations, 137

■ Intrinsic variability, 138

■ Extrinsic variability, 140

■ Experimental designs: means of controlling variability, 141

■ Validity of experimental operations, 143

■ Internal validity, 144

■ Generality (External Validity), 151

■ Concluding remarks, 159

■ Study guide, 161

A n investigator's knowledge of research designs is a crucial element in the successful implementation of research studies. Whether the investigator will produce reliable and valid data on the researched question will depend mostly on the design used in the study. Therefore, this chapter is about definitions and descriptions of research designs along with why they are needed and what purposes they serve.

WHAT ARE RESEARCH DESIGNS?

Research designs can be described in general as well as technical terms. Generally speaking, a research design is the overall plan of an investigation. The plan should describe the research question or questions, the methods of observation and measurement, the different conditions of observation and manipulation, procedures of collecting data under different experimental arrangements, and the method of data analysis. In essence, a research design refers to the methods and procedures of an investigation. Many investigators use the term *design* in this general sense. In this sense, all types of research studies have a design.

A technical definition of a research design is that it is a structure of temporospatial arrangements within which the selected variables are controlled, manipulated, and measured. In this sense, design refers to certain technical operations performed by the investigator under specified conditions or arrangements of an experiment. In this technical sense, a research design can be found only in experimental research.

It is useful to consider the various elements of our technical definition of a research design. A design is basically a *structure* within which certain operations are performed to see what happens. It is an arrangement of conditions for observation, manipulation, and measurement. For example, a design structure may arrange conditions of pretest or baselines, experimental manipulations, withdrawal of those manipulations, and posttests or probes of the dependent variables. Thus, each arrangement within the structure serves a particular purpose while making it possible to observe and measure the dependent variable. This is what is meant by the structure or the arrangement of conditions of a study.

A design structure is more or less flexible depending upon the philosophy on which it is based. Some research designs are less flexible; once selected, design changes during the implementation of the study are considered undesirable. Other research designs allow changes in the course of a study if warranted by data. Typically, group designs of research, described in Chapter 7, have more rigid structures than the single-subject designs described in Chapter 8.

The arrangements of a design allow the researcher to control variables. As we noted in Chapter 4, controlling the variables is a significant part of any experimental research. Variables must be controlled when a researcher wishes to establish a functional (cause-effect) relation between events. The researcher must make sure that the independent variables not under observation do not influence the dependent variable. A good research design makes it possible for the experimenter to rule out the influence of such "extraneous" variables. This is generally what is meant by controlling the variables.

A design is also a framework within which to manipulate the independent variable selected for the study. An independent variable is manipulated when it is introduced, withheld, varied in magnitude, withdrawn, or reintroduced to see if corresponding changes occur in the dependent variable. For example, in the initial stage of a study, the independent variable is typically not introduced to measure the dependent variable's typical frequency. In the next condition, the independent variable, say a new form of treatment for a speech disorder, is introduced. There may be a group of subjects who do not receive treatment. Alternatively, the same subjects who receive treatment in one condition may be observed in a no-treatment condition. Such manipulations can demonstrate the effects of an independent variable on a dependent variable.

Finally, a design is a condition that allows systematic observation and measurement of the variables of interest. In most research studies, the focus is on the dependent variable, though the measurement of the independent variable is also important. The variables are typically measured in terms of their frequency, magnitude, and intensity. For example, the number of times an independent variable such as a reinforcer is delivered in a treatment condition may be measured. In a drug evaluation experiment, the dosage and its frequency are measured throughout the study. Dependent variables such as the production of a plural morpheme in sentences may be measured in terms of frequency and complexity (the number of syllables or words per utterance). Dysfluencies or correct production of selected phonemes may also be measured in terms of frequency.

THE STRUCTURE AND LOGIC OF EXPERIMENTAL DESIGNS

An adequate understanding of experimental designs involves a full consideration of the logic and the empirical processes of science and research. As we noted in Chapter 2, the scientist's task is to find order in, and functional relations between, natural phenomena. However, order and causal relations are more often concealed than revealed in nature. Therefore, science is a search for something that is not so readily seen. Nature is a complex flux of multitudinous events that are in a constant state of change, variability, and transformation. Events in nature may be independent, correlated, causally related, or interactive.

Science seeks to determine whether certain events are independent or related, and if related, what exactly is the type of relation. Two events may coexist but still be independent of each other, with no causal or any other relation between the two. Two events may also be correlated in the sense that both increase or decrease at the same time, but they may be doing this because fluctuations in an unobserved third factor, responsible for both are the cause of the observed changes in the two events, giving an illusion of causality. The events may indeed be causally related in that one is the effect of the other. Finally, several events may produce the same effect, all of them may be simultaneously present, and they may interact with each other to produce an effect that is larger than the effect produced by any one of those events. This is called an interactive relation between events.

A scientist who discovers that certain events are independent, correlated, causally related, or interactive is said to have found order in nature. Order may be discovered in a small part of nature, but no part of nature is insignificant. The process of such a discovery is called an experiment, and how that experiment is temporospatially arranged is its design.

An experimental design must be arranged in such a way that if there is a relation between the two events, it will be revealed relatively clearly, since such a relation is anything but clear in the natural flux. In fact, the typically concealing nature can also be misleading, suggesting relations that are not real. Of course, nature does nothing of this, but it can certainly have such effects on those studying natural phenomena. An experimental design is the scientist's method of uncovering relations against a background of events that vary. The challenge the scientist faces is that a systematic relation lies in the process of what may appear to be chaotic and confusing variability. In some cases, the logic and the structure of a design permit the scientist to observe a relation between events in spite of their variability and the variability of surrounding and correlated events. In other cases, designs make it possible to reduce the variability and thus see the effects of manipulated independent variables on selected dependent variables. In this sense, variability and how to control it are important aspects of experiments and their designs. Therefore, we should take a closer look at the issue of variability and how it is handled in experimental designs.

VARIABILITY: SOME PHILOSOPHICAL CONSIDERATIONS

Both scientists and lay persons know that variability characterizes practically everything we experience. Physical and chemical events vary constantly, and natural scientists have always tried to analyze the sources of this variability. When biological events began to be studied more closely with the methods of science, the same variability seen in physical and chemical phenomena became apparent. Eventually, it became evident that animal and human behaviors are also highly variable under natural conditions.

The fact of variability, however, is not purely a scientific discovery. Philosophers, poets, and theologians as well as ordinary persons have been aware of variability in physical, biological, and behavioral phenomena. While the statement that all natural phenomena, including biological and behavioral phenomena, are variable has never been especially controversial, how to explain it and handle it from a technical standpoint has always been controversial. The controversy, however, has been more intense with respect to human behavioral variability. The variability of physical events may create philosophical as well as methodological problems for the scientist, but it does not seem to raise many philosophical concerns in people who are not natural scientists. It may be viewed more as a technical problem to be handled by physical scientists. However, the fact of human behavioral variability has been a matter of philosophical, theological, and scientific controversy.

Historically, there have been two distinct approaches to the question of variability in general, and human behavior in particular. (Barlow & Hersen, 1984; Johnston & Pennypacker, 1980; Sidman, 1960). One viewpoint, the older of the two, holds that variability is intrinsic to the events that vary. In other words, the variability seen in human behavior, including speech and language behaviors, is a part of "human nature" and therefore cannot be controlled. The other, more recent viewpoint is that behavioral variability is due to external factors that can be controlled.

INTRINSIC VARIABILITY

The assumptions of intrinsic variability have played an important role in the extrascientific understanding of human behavior. Traditional philosophies and theological thinking have asserted that behavior springs from within the individual and therefore is not controlled by external events. Internal causes have taken many shapes, the most famous of which is probably the concept of free will. Behaviors vary across time, situations, and individuals. A given individual's behavior also varies across time and across situations as well as as within them. Traditionally, this is explained by pointing out that people behave differently because of their free will. The notion of free will, so popular even today, is based on the assumption that physical events may have external causes, but an extension of such a concept to human behavior would violate the notion of freedom of action. In essence, behavioral variability has unique sources and therefore is not the same as the variability of physical phenomena.

Unfortunately, the concept of intrinsic variability has played a significant role in the purportedly scientific study of human behavior as well. In this context, mind has been an important internal source of behavior. It is proposed that people behave differently because each person has his or her own mind. Some speculative neurological theorizing has also buttressed this notion. Such theories have replaced mind with brain as the intrinsic source of action and behavior. Psychoanalysis and other kinds of psychological theories are also full of intrinsic causes of behavior and its variability. Unconscious forces of motivation, such as the id, ego, superego, self-image, self-confidence, have been considered intrinsic sources of behavior. It has been hypothesized that the acquisition of language has been made possible by innate ideas and innate knowledge of universal grammar.

The question of variability and the hypothesis of intrinsic causes of behavior may seem separate, but they are closely related. The assumption of intrinsic variability of behavior becomes inevitable when the presumed sources of behavioral control are inaccessible. Most hypothesized intrinsic causes of behavior are indeed inaccessible. It is believed that inaccessible entities such as the mind, soul, free will, unconscious forces, and innate knowledge that are thought to cause behaviors should also be responsible for the variability of those behaviors.

The concepts of intrinsic causes and intrinsic variability of behavior converge to produce a significant effect on the experimental strategy. Obviously, variability that is intrinsic to the behaving organisms cannot be controlled. Therefore, experimental attempts at reducing or eliminating variability would be futile. Consequently, the experimenter has no choice but to accept variability as inevitable and uncontrollable. Nonetheless, the scientist must reduce variability in order to find out cause–effect relations between variables. It is hard to identify the causes of events that vary randomly. Therefore, when the assumption of uncontrollable intrinsic variability is made, researchers must find ways of working around it.

The traditional answer to the problem of behavioral variability in social and behavioral research has been to use large numbers of subjects and determine the average performance of the group. Statisticians recommend that the greater the variability, the larger the number of subjects needed to show the effect of an independent variable. Obviously, the mean performance of a large number of subjects does not fluctuate, simply because it is a single measure. It is the behavior of individuals in the group that fluctuates, but a mean is no reflection of this fact. When this mean is used as the primary measure of the dependent variable in the inferential statistical analysis, it is supposed that somehow the problem of variability has been handled satisfactorily.

The amount of deviation from the mean shown by individuals (standard deviation) does affect the eventual inferential statistical analysis of the data. However, when a large sample is drawn to overcome the problem of variability, one is also sampling a larger amount of variability. The statistical answer to this problem is to require only a greatly reduced magnitude of the effect of the independent variable before the investigator can conclude that the cause manipulated in an experiment had an effect over and beyond chance.

In essence, the traditional research strategies based on the theory of probability and inferential statistics handle variability by ignoring it. Individual variability is minimized post hoc by the averaging method and by accepting only small effects of the independent variables. Typically, such effects are wrested by complex statistical analyses.

It is a common practice in social and psychological sciences to think of variability (the more frequently used term is variance) as random fluctuations that the investigator can handle only through statistical methods of averaging group performance data and inferential techniques (Christensen, 1980; Kerlinger, 1973). For the purposes of statistical analyses, variability of subjects within a group is considered *error variance*, which typically includes unexplained (and uninteresting!) individual differences, fluctuations in the behaviors introduced by random variables, and errors of measurement. The kind of variability introduced by the independent variable is called *systematic variance*. Yet another kind of variance is described as *extraneous variance*, which is the amount of variability introduced by independent variables that are not being manipulated or measured by the investigator. Within this framework, an experimental design is expected to enhance systematic variance, minimize error variance, and control extraneous variance. These recommendations are not controversial except for the way the basic variability of behaviors is handled.

EXTRINSIC VARIABILITY

The second philosophical position holds that behavioral variability is extrinsic to the behaving organisms (Barlow and Hersen, 1984; Johnston and Pennypacker, 1980; Sidman, 1960). Much behavioral variability is not a property of either the behavior or the organism but is imposed from external factors. Behavior varies because the factors responsible for it vary, and many of those factors are in the environment. Evidently, this viewpoint of variability seriously questions the traditional assumption that free will, soul, mind, and other such intrinsic entities are the causes of behaviors. According to the philosophy of extrinsic variability, behavior is a function of the individual's past history and the present environmental events to which he or she is exposed. Therefore, behavioral variability is not unique; it is just a part of the scheme of natural events.

Extrinsic variability does not imply that variables within the organism exert no influence on behaviors. Internal physiological states (such as thirst and hunger) and changes over time ("development") have certain effects on behaviors. The integrity of neuromuscular systems is also an internal factor that influences behaviors. Similarly, genetic factors set limits on the behavioral variability imposed by natural or experimentally created environmental events. Nevertheless, the assumption of extrinsic variability suggests that most of those sources of variability, when studied appropriately, lead to a better understanding of behaviors than the assumption that variability is a property of behavior itself.

It is clear that the two viewpoints of intrinsic and extrinsic variability have profound but contradictory philosophic implications. From the standpoint of experimental methodology, the ultimate truth or falsity of the two assumptions is not of immediate concern. Whether behavioral variability is intrinsic or extrinsic is an empirical question, a complete answer to which will require lengthy experimental research. However, whether systematic attempts to produce that answer will be made at all depends upon the assumption of extrinsic, not intrinsic variability. This is not one of those situations in which contradictory viewpoints are both testable, and either viewpoint has the same chance of producing a valid answer.

If all scientists took the position that behavioral variability is intrinsic, then there would be no reason to design experiments in which such variability is experimentally analyzed, for the assumption is inconsistent with such experimentation. In other words, the assumption of intrinsic variability precludes experimental analysis of the sources of behavioral variability. As Johnston and Pennypacker have observed, "it appears that intrinsic variability (analogous to indeterminancy) is an *a priori* assumption that thereafter guides experimentation and methodological development in the manner of a self-fulfilling prophecy" (1980, p. 205). After having placed (intrinsic) variability outside the scope of experimental analysis, researchers will continue to use statistical means of handling it.

A position most valid from an empirical standpoint is to treat all variability as extrinsic, at least tentatively, so that experimental analysis of variability is a possibility. It is reasonable to expect that sustained experimental analysis will reduce the territory held by variability supposed to be intrinsic. Every time a source of behavioral variability is identified, a chance to control it presents itself. As Sidman has pointed out, "each time such control is achieved, intrinsic variability loses another prop" (1960, p. 143).

Such an approach to variability has a chance of showing that it is not possible to control some sources of variability. This may be a result of the limitations of experimental techniques the improvements in which will change the situation. Or, the approach may show the limits beyond which individual variability cannot be controlled. In either case, it is only the assumption of extrinsic variability that can lead us in the direction of self-corrective data. As such, the assumption of extrinsic variability has a chance of disproving itself, whereas the assumption of intrinsic variability offers no such opportunity.

EXPERIMENTAL DESIGNS: MEANS OF CONTROLLING VARIABILITY

The two philosophical positions on variability are indeed associated with two kinds of experimental designs: between-groups design and single-subject design. But it must be noted that both the approaches to designing experiments recognize the need to control variability; they differ only in terms of what kinds of variability must be controlled and in what manner.

Group designs, even with the assumption of intrinsic variability, include mechanisms to control and isolate the variability produced by independent variables. This approach recognizes the need to control variability produced by factors not under observation (extraneous variability). There is no significant conceptual difference between the group and the single-subject designs on these issues, although there are some methodological differences which will be addressed in later chapters. The difference between the two approaches lies mostly in how the background variability created by differences in the individual response rates is handled and also in how the variability produced by the experimental variable is analyzed.

The effects of all experiments are analyzed against a certain amount of background variability. Suppose, for example, that an investigator wishes to evaluate the effect of a new stuttering treatment program. If the basic two-group design is selected, the investigator forms an experimental and a control group of stutterers using the random procedure. After taking pretest measures of stuttering in both groups, treatment is given only to the experimental group. At the completion of the treatment program, the two groups are given a posttest. To find out if the treatment was effective, the pre- and post test measures of the two groups are analyzed statistically.

The control group helps rule out the influence of extraneous independent variables. If the mean performance of the control group of stutterers did not change significantly from the pretest to the posttest, but the mean performance of the experimental group did show such changes, then it is concluded that extraneous variables were controlled. However, this evaluation of the effect of the treatment variable is made, of necessity, against the background of random (hence, uncontrolled) variability. The larger the individual differences within the groups, the greater the background variability in a group design. As noted before, much of this variability is handled statistically with the help of the arithmetic mean.

The effect of the treatment is also handled statistically. The difference in the performance of the two groups is evaluated on the basis of the mean, which ignores individual differences in response to treatment. Thus, in a group design, both the background and the systematic variability are evaluated nonexperimentally.

On the other hand, the investigator who selects a single-subject design to evaluate the same stuttering treatment program will not try to draw a random sample of subjects. Available stutterers will be used in the study, but each subject will be described in detail. The stuttering behaviors will be baserated until some criterion of stability is reached. The baseline helps reduce the intrasubject variability before the introduction of treatment. The treatment is then introduced and continued until it produces an effect. Subsequently, the treatment may be withdrawn to return the rate of stuttering to its baseline. Finally, the treatment may be reapplied to replicate the treatment effects. In this procedure, no effort is made to average individual performances to show some kind of stability before, during, or after treatment. Variability is handled on an individual basis. As long as the behavior continues to be variable, baselines are extended. It is generally found that when conditions are controlled, sooner or later the behavior stabilizes. Obviously, this approach to pretreatment variability is very different from that found in group designs in which a single pretest measure (arithmetic mean) represents stability.

The treatment effect within a single-subject design is not evaluated by statistical means. The assumption is that when the effects are large enough to be evaluated by visual inspection, there is no need for statistical analysis, which typically tries to identify relatively small effects against a background of uncontrolled variability. Such large effects of the treatment variable neutralize the issue of intersubject variability found in group designs.

Within the single-subject approach, when individual behaviors vary tremendously, either during baselines or during treatment, the experimenter may then proceed to find out why (Sidman, 1960). In other words, the variability itself becomes an object of experimental enquiry. Investigators may be willing to postpone their study of the original problem and begin the new task of tracking the intrasubject variability. It may be found, for example, that the variability found in the amount of stuttering exhibited by a stutterer during baseline sessions is due to the stutterer's participation in rather traumatic staff meetings held every other day. Many clients' variable response rates in treatment sessions may be a reaction to various uncontrolled factors that the clinicians dump under "a good day" and "a bad day."

Regardless of philosophical and methodological differences on the issue of variability, it is clear that experimental designs must handle them, for a design is a way of controlling some kind of variability while creating another kind of variability. It must control the variability found within and across individuals, and it must produce a large enough variability that can be attributed to the effect of the independent variable. In other words, a change in the behavior when treatment is introduced is also variability, but it is the type of variability the experimenter hopes to see and takes every step to create.

VALIDITY OF EXPERIMENTAL OPERATIONS

By allowing the researcher to control and create variability, experimental designs make it possible to identify functional relations between variables. The task of an experimental design is to isolate a cause–effect relation between events. Therefore, we must now consider issues relative to this task.

In human clinical and nonclinical research, the demonstration of a cause–effect relation is made with the help of selected individuals, whether in a few individuals, as in a single-subject design, or in groups of subjects, as in a group design. This raises two closely related questions. The first question is whether in the individuals who served as subjects in a given experiment, the cause–effect relation was demonstrated convincingly. This is the question of *internal validity.* The second question is whether the demonstrated cause–effect relations can be generalized to individuals who have not participated in the experiment. This is the question of *external validity* or *generality* of findings.

The validity of experimental operations refers to the confidence with which the experimenter's claim of a cause–effect relation can be accepted by other scientists. In nontechnical terms, the results of an experiment are valid when the observed cause of an event is not mistaken. When the results are not valid, conclusions drawn from the study may not apply to the individuals who served in the experiment as well as to those who did not. In other words, there is neither internal nor external validity.

The validity of *experimental operations* must be distinguished from the validity of *measured values* of the dependent variables. The validity of measured values is the degree to which the measurement of the dependent variable is indeed the best possible reflection of the true value of that variable. The validity of the experimental operations, on the other hand, is concerned with the overall experimental arrangements, manipulations, and control procedures. As such, the validity of measured values has a narrower scope than the validity of experimental operations.

Internal Validity

In order to achieve internal validity, the investigator must make sure that during the experimental operations, only the independent variable selected for the study was present and any of the other potential independent variables were not. In other words, when the selected independent variable produces acceptable changes in the dependent variable in the absence of other potential variables that could have produced the same results, the data are said to have internal validity. Therefore, the major concern is to make sure that the variables other than the one selected for study were appropriately controlled for in the design.

In some individual subjects, variables that affect the dependent variable may require special analysis. Historically, though, several common factors that affect internal validity across experiments have been recognized. These factors are also described as *threats* to internal validity or *sources* of internal *invalidity.*

Most of the sources of internal invalidity can be found in poor research designs. In fully understanding our discussion of the factors that affect internal invalidity in the following section, it is necessary to keep in perspective a prototype of a poor design in which those factors can easily come to play. Such a design is illustrated in the traditional case studies used frequently in clinical research. For example, a clinician may measure "language disorder" (the dependent variable) in a group of children (pretest) and then subject them to a new treatment program whose effect is being evaluated. After several months of therapy, the children's language behaviors may be evaluated again.

This posttest may show that the children's language behaviors have changed significantly. The investigator may then conclude that the new treatment program was responsible for the changes observed in the dependent variable. As discussed in the next section, a study such as this may contain several factors that affect internal validity.

Factors That Affect Internal Validity

1. HISTORY. History refers to the subjects' life events that may be totally or partially responsible for the changes recorded in the dependent variable subsequent to the introduction of the independent variable. A design that does not rule out the influence of those events cannot demonstrate that the treatment variable had an effect on the dependent variable. In other words, history is a source of internal invalidity in such a design.

In our prototypic example of language treatment research, it is possible that the treatment was totally or partially ineffective. A variety of extraneous factors not monitored by the clinician may have produced the results or may have created a significant portion of the effect. For example, the classroom teacher may have started a language stimulation program for the same children receiving treatment from the clinician, and this program may have been responsible for the improvement in children's language. Or, the parents, after having discussed their children's language problem with the clinician, may have begun to talk more to their children or read more stories to them at bedtime. Such changes in the parents' behavior may have caused improvement in the children's language. The clinician then is not able to conclude that there was a functional relation between the treatment variable and the changes in the language of the children.

It may be noted that the term *history*, though used to describe the effects of extraneous variables, may not be the most appropriate term. It does not refer to the events that have taken place in the past but to events that are contemporaneous with the experimental manipulations.

In the group design strategy, the influence of history is controlled by showing that those who do not receive treatment do not show significant changes in the dependent variable. When a control group, which is also exposed to factors of history, does not show changes, then history is ruled out as a potential variable responsible for changes shown by the experimental group. In the single-subject strategy, after exposing the subjects to treatment, the experimenter may withdraw treatment and reintroduce it later. When the behavior changes under treatment, but returns to the baseline when it is withdrawn, and changes again when it is reintroduced, the investigator is able to conclude that the factors of history were not responsible for the observed changes.

2. MATURATION. When experiments take a considerable amount of time, changes taking place within the subjects themselves may produce some effect on the dependent variable. In some cases, such changes may account for the entire effect supposedly produced by the independent variable manipulated by the experimenter.

Maturation refers to biological and other kinds of unidentified changes that take place in the subjects simply as a result of the passage of time. However, to what extent mere passage of time can produce effects on behaviors is not always clear. Obviously, maturation is indexed by the age of the subjects. In our discussion of normative research in Chapter 4, we took note of the issue of age as an independent variable. In evaluating maturation as a potential independent variable, we must consider all the problems that were identified in that discussion. It is quite possible that maturation and history are not as distinct as they are generally thought to be. Possibly, events in the life of the subjects while they are supposed to be maturing may be responsible for the changes, but such changes may be simply attributed to maturation.

In our prototypical example of research, during the time required to complete the experimental language treatment, maturational changes can be expected to have taken place. Those changes may have been responsible for the improved language in the children.

In both the single-subject and group design strategies, the problem of maturation is handled in the same way as the problem of history. Either a control group or a no-treatment condition that follows treatment can rule out the influence of maturation. It can be expected that the members of the control group who do not change over time experience the same amount of maturation as the members of the experimental group. Similarly, the subjects who change once when the treatment is introduced but change again when it is withdrawn indicate that maturation is not responsible for the changes in the dependent variable. The logic is that when maturation is given a chance, it fails to show its effects, and the only effect seen is that of the independent variable manipulated by the experimenter.

3. TESTING. When a dependent variable changes simply because it has been measured more than once, we have the effect of testing. Pre- and posttests may be sufficient to introduce some change in the dependent variable. In such cases, the experimenter's conclusion that the treatment variable of the study was responsible for the changes recorded on the posttest may be erroneous.

Some behaviors are known to change somewhat when repeatedly tested or measured. Measures of behaviors that change as a function of repeated testing are known as reactive measures. Scores obtained through questionnaires designed to measure attitudes, opinions, feeling states, personal "adjustment," and "personality" are known to be notoriously reactive. People answering a questionnaire on their attitudes toward racial minorities, for example, may show significant changes when retested in the absence of an independent variable manipulated by the investigator.

Because most experiments involve repeated measurement of the dependent variable, one must make sure that testing is not a source of control exerted on the behavior. One way of handling the problem of testing is not to use reactive measures at all, as measures of behaviors, opinions, attitudes, and personality are weak and inferential at best. Whenever possible, it is better to measure behaviors directly. For example, one may either ask a person to fill out a questionnaire on movie-going behavior, or measure the frequency with which that person goes to the movies. Obviously, the latter measure is difficult to obtain, but the more easily accomplished score on the questionnaire may be useless. Also, the actual behavioral measure is less reactive than the questionnaire measure. An employer who has never hired a member of a minority group is not likely to suddenly hire one simply because his or her "attitudes" showed reactive changes on an attitude scale.

Reactive measures are not as bothersome in single-subject designs as in group designs. Single-subject designs do involve repeated measures; in fact, more so than the group designs. For the most part, single-subject designs avoid the use of indirect and reactive measures of behaviors. Group designs have a method of handling testing effects by adding an additional group that does not receive pretests while receiving only the post test. This design, known as the Soloman four-group design, is described in Chapter 7.

4. INSTRUMENTATION. Potential problems associated with measuring instruments can negatively affect internal validity. This factor includes not only mechanical instruments that might deteriorate or improve between pre- and posttests, but also the changes that may take place in human beings who serve as judges, raters, and observers. In much social and psychological research, persons with varying degrees of expertise observe, score, and measure behaviors. Of course, human observation and measurement is basic to all sciences, but the experimenters' reliance on others to make measurements for them is more extensive in social and psychological research.

An instrument that was in normal working condition at the beginning of the study may develop problems by the time the posttest is made. Or, an instrument that already had some problem from the beginning may have been corrected just before the posttest. In cases such as these, the pre- and posttests would not reflect the actual effects of the experimental manipulations. Suppose that in a study of the effects of some medical or surgical intervention procedure designed to improve a certain type of hearing loss, the audiologist used a defective audiometer to establish the initial thresholds of the subjects. Possibly, because of the mechanical defect, all subjects' thresholds were 10dB higher than their actual level of hearing. Also suppose that as a matter of routine maintenance procedures, the audiometer was serviced and calibrated just before the posttests. Unaware of the history of the instrument, the audiologist may measure the hearing in the subjects after the completion of the medical or surgical treatment. Thresholds on this posttest are likely to show at least a 10dB improvement over the pretest, but this finding is entirely invalid. In the same study, an audiometer that was working normally but had deteriorated by the posttest would have led to an opposite finding, also equally invalid.

Judges who observe and score behaviors may induce invalidity of findings in several ways. When a group of speech pathologists is used to rate the severity of stuttering before and after some form of experimental treatment, the persons in the group may change their idea as to what constitutes different levels of severity between the pre- and post-tests. The criteria used by individual judges may become more or less stringent. The observers may get bored during the posttest. The judges also can become more experienced in measuring stuttering, so they may now score more stutterings that were missed during the pretest observations.

As a clinical supervisor, I have seen beginning clinicians who scored more and more stuttering behaviors as therapy progressed during the first few weeks. At one time, a very disconcerted student clinician came to my office and showed me this kind of data. This first-time clinician had her worst fears confirmed: her therapy was making the client stutter more and more although the client's fluency seemed to have improved. Her measurement procedures were then analyzed, and it was found that gradually she was becoming more and more deft at observing and measuring silent pauses, interjections, and more subtle forms of all other types of dysfluencies that she was not measuring at all in the beginning.

5. STATISTICAL REGRESSION. In clinical research, it is not uncommon to have subjects who happen to seek clinical services at the time of the study. However, it is known that many clients seek clinical services at a time when their speech problem is at its worst. This is more likely to happen with those disorders that vary across time and situations and hence are somewhat cyclic. Stuttering, for example, can be such a cyclic speech disorder. This means that stuttering may have a worst time but it is not likely to stay that way for long. It will soon return to its less severe and more common level. Such a return from an extreme point to an average level is known as statistical regression, or regression to the mean.

Regression can pose serious problems for internal validity if the stuttering clients selected for a study are at the peak of their problem at the beginning of the experiment, but as the experiment progresses dysfluencies begin to return to their average level. Such an improvement in stuttering can give the impression that the treatment is effective. Such an erroneous conclusion would not have internal validity.

Statistical regression does not mean that every client will improve without treatment. It is simply a change in the extreme scores of a group of subjects, and when such changes are confused with the treatment effects, a problem of internal invalidity exists.

Theoretically, our prototypical example of language treatment research study does not rule out statistical regression. Whether language disordered children show statistical regression is a different question, however. The problem of regression to the mean is controlled for in the group design by random selection and assignment of subjects to an experimental and a control group. The amount of regression would then be the same in the two groups. Unfortunately, the random procedure is impractical where it is needed the most. In clinical research, finding a population of clients with a given disorder from which a sample can be randomly selected is not practical. In single-subject designs, regression is handled by repeated measurement taken over the entire duration of the experiment. Since treatment typically follows a period of no treatment or treatment applied to some competing behavior, the regression phenomenon can be ruled out.

6. SUBJECT SELECTION BIASES. As is evident in our discussion so far, how the subjects are selected for a study can cause problems, but selection biases can create problems of their own. Whenever two groups of subjects are used in experimental studies, it is possible that the groups were different to begin with, and therefore any differences found on the posttest may not be due to the treatment at all.

The typical answer to the problem of subject selection biases is to use randomly selected and assigned groups or groups that have carefully matched subjects. As already noted, random sampling of clinical subjects is not always practical. In matching, one must find pairs of subjects who are similar on important variables, but clinically, this procedure is about as impractical as the random procedure.

In single-subject designs, subject selection bias is not a major problem because the conclusions are not based upon group comparisons. Whether or not the treatment is effective in individual clients whose characteristics are well described is the question for analysis. Therefore, there is no need to make sure that the subjects are similar, even when several subjects are used in a single-subject design.

7. ATTRITION. Also known as subject mortality, attrition is the problem of losing subjects in the course of an experiment, which in turn has an effect on the final results as interpreted by the investigator. Attrition of subjects is not as uncommon as most investigators hope it to be. Graduate students, who generally secure subjects for their theses and dissertations with great difficulty, dread this problem the most. Current ethical guidelines appropriately guarantee the subject's right to withdraw from a research with no consequences (see Chapter 12), and some subjects exercise this right freely and in the middle of a study.

Attrition can be a serious source of internal invalidity in group designs. Analysis of results based on group averages can be affected markedly by differential attrition of subjects. If in our prototypical study on language treatment, children with more severe language disorder were to drop out during the course of treatment, the mean of the posttest of language behaviors would be higher (better) than that of the pretest. This might then suggest a feigned treatment effect leading to invalid conclusions. When two groups are used, *differential* subject drop out in the experimental and control groups can create a problem of greater magnitude. More severely affected subjects may drop out from the experimental group whereas less severely affected subjects may drop out of the control group. This would create major differences in the pre- and post-tests of the two groups even when the treatment is totally ineffective.

Attrition is a problem only when statistical analysis based on group means is used. In the analysis of results, an investigator may take into consideration the subject attrition, and also describe individual data. However, these may not be practical when the groups are large. Unfortunately, even when it is possible, such individual-specific discriminated analysis is not a typical part of the *practice* of group design strategy.

In single-subject designs, attrition is not a factor affecting internal validity. Whenever possible, the subjects who drop out are replaced by others. A lack of statistical comparison of groups of subjects avoids the problems created by differential attrition. However, the single-subject researcher may face another problem relative to attrition: the study may have to be simply postponed to a later date when one or more subjects become available. In the case of subject attrition, the group design strategist runs the risk of drawing invalid conclusions, whereas the single-subject strategist runs the risk of not having a study at all.

8. DIFFUSION OF TREATMENT. A factor that affects the internal validity of some single-subject designs has been called diffusion of treatment (Kazdin, 1982). In most single-subject designs, the treatment is introduced once and then withdrawn to show corresponding changes in the behaviors. However, when the treatment is withdrawn, the behaviors may sometimes continue because they have come under the influence of other or even the same independent variables administered by other persons. Parents or spouses who have observed experimental therapy in which an aphasic person's language responses were reinforced may begin to reinforce those behaviors at home at a time when the investigator is trying to reduce the target behaviors to its original baseline.

Some single-subject designs involve two or more treatments whose relative (not interactive) effects are evaluated. Such designs may also have the problem of diffusion of treatment affecting internal validity. The two or more treatment conditions may not be clearly discriminated. In such cases, the effect of one treatment may influence the effect of another treatment, but such influences may remain obscured.

Diffusion of treatment is not a problem in most group designs of research. Because the subjects who receive treatment and those who do not are in different groups, the question of treatment diffusion from one condition or treatment to the other does not arise.

The eight sources of internal invalidity discussed so far are used in the evaluation of most research designs. It must be noted, though, that designs are not perfect and that they control for these sources with varying degrees of efficiency. Therefore, most designs are likely to have some control problems to varying extents, but these problems should not be serious enough to invalidate the study. A study appearing to have a single potential source of internal invalidity that may or may not have operated is judged differently from the one with multiple sources, each posing a definite and serious threat to internal validity.

Generality (External Validity)

Unlike internal validity, external validity (generality) is not always a matter of the experimental design itself. Generality is a matter of the extent to which the investigator can go beyond the particular study. Therefore, one may have internal validity but may not be sure of generality. In other words, the investigator may be confident that external variables have been ruled out and that the demonstrated relation between the dependent variable and the independent variable is therefore valid within the confines of the study. However, the extent to which the results can be generalized, which is of course the question of external validity, may not be clear.

In many books and articles, discussions of external validity, generality, or both can be confusing. Three sources have contributed to an elaboration of these concepts. One of the traditional sources of discussion on external validity is the group design strategy, with its emphasis on statistical inference. The second source of information is the single-subject design strategy. The third source is applied behavioral research, with its explicit clinical concerns. As a result of these converging approaches and sources, various terms and concepts are associated with the discussion of external validity. An attempt is made here to provide an integrated view of this important concept.

The statistical approach to research designs has classified external validity into two major categories of variables that affect it: population validity and ecological validity (Bracht and Glass, 1968). The major concern of this approach to external validity has been the extent to which the results of a study based on a sample of subjects can be extended to the population from which the sample was drawn.

The single-subject design strategy has faced the problem of external validity from a different standpoint. Because the strategy does not draw a sample of subjects from a population, extending the results of a particular study to a population is not of immediate concern. However, the strategy has faced a different kind of problem: extending the results from a single subject or a few subjects to other similar individuals. When the single-subject strategy began to be used more frequently in applied research, additional concerns emerged. For example, if a behavioral technique is demonstrated to be effective in the treatment of some problem behavior, can the technique be effective with other problem behaviors? Will the technique be equally effective in other clinical or professional settings? Answers to such clinical questions have helped identify additional sources of external validity.

The single-subject strategy with its applied emphasis has preferred the term *generality* to *external validity*. The concept of generality is more relevant to an understanding of clinical issues relative to external validity, and therefore we shall continue to use that term. What follows is a description of some of the major types of generality and the factors that affect them. It includes most of the factors of external validity identified in the group design strategy as well.

1. INFERENTIAL GENERALITY. Inferential generality refers to the extension of the conclusions of a study from a sample of subjects to the population from which it was drawn. A population is any defined group in research studies. For example, all citizens of voting age, all stutterers, all children in the 7th grade, and all children with unrepaired cleft, illustrate populations. A sample is a smaller number of subjects who represent a specific population. The sample must be randomly selected from the population and then randomly divided into two or more groups that participate in an experiment. Typically, one group receives treatment and one other does not. It is assumed that a random sample of a population is as heterogeneous as the population and that it is therefore representative of that population. Therefore, in order to have conclusions about a phenomenon found in the population, one need not study the entire population, which would be almost impossible. When it is shown that two events are causally related in a representative sample of subjects, it may be concluded that the events are so related in the entire population. The concept of inferential generality is illustrated in Figure 6-1.

Inferential generality is based on inferential techniques of statistics, such as analysis of variance. These techniques are so named because they help *infer* the values of the dependent variables in the population. Because the population is not tested, generality is a matter of making a valid inference as supported by the theory and technique of statistics. The random procedure is crucial to inferential generality. Unless the investigator has drawn a random sample of the population, there can be no assurance of inferential generality of findings.

Two major problems affect inferential generality: lack of random selection of subjects, and potential interaction between subject characteristics and treatment that is masked in group averages. Random sampling is very difficult to accomplish, especially in clinical sciences concerned with the experimental evaluation of treatment procedures. The population of children with articulation disorders, language handicapped persons, or aphasic persons is typically not available for the researcher. Therefore, when clients who seek help are selected for a study, there is no assurance that the results can be generalized to those who do not. Therefore, a serious threat to inferential generality is the lack of random sampling that is so typical of clinical research.

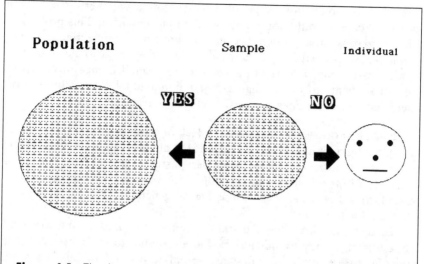

Figure 6-1. The direction of inferential generality: from a random sample to the population. It does not permit generalization from the sample to an individual.

A randomly drawn sample must also be assigned to the experimental and control groups to make sure that the two groups are equal. This, as we noted earlier, is a matter of internal validity. The critical factor for inferential generality is the original sampling of the subjects from the population.

The other factor that affects inferential generality, the interaction between subject characteristics and treatment, is related to the method of data analysis. Most group designs average the performance of individual subjects to make inferential statistical analyses. Therefore, one cannot determine whether all of the subjects behaved the same under the treatment condition or whether individuals with certain characteristics behaved one way and those with other characteristics behaved another way. For example, an experimental study may have demonstrated that a certain treatment is effective, on the average, with a sample of children with articulation disorders. However, it is possible that only those children with mild articulation disorders or high levels of intelligence benefited from the treatment, whereas those with other characteristics may not have shown any improvement. In other words, the interaction between subject characteristics and treatment effects is usually masked in the group performance analyses. Therefore, whether there was an interaction, and if so of what type, is usually unknown.

The problem of unknown but possible differential response to treatment by different subjects in an experimental group can pose a significant problem for the clinician who wishes to determine whether the results can be extended to individual clients with specific characteristics. The clinician can conclude only that *on the average*, particular sets of clients seem to improve under treatment. It would not be possible to determine whether or not given individual clients would not improve under that treatment. This problem is inherent to most group designs because the direction of inferential generality is from the sample to the population and not from the sample to the individual. In most cases, clinicians try to generalize from small groups of clients or individual clients to other small groups or individual clients. In essence, inferential generality does not serve a clinical science very well.

2. LOGICAL GENERALITY. Because of a lack of random samples, the results of single-subject designs cannot be extended to the population. In other words, the results of particular single-subject design studies do not have inferential generality. However, single-subject designs do not seek inferential generality. Instead, they seek what is known as logical generality (Barlow & Hersen, 1984; Eddington, 1967).

Logical generality is based on the assumption that it is possible to extend the results of a study to individuals who are similar to the subjects of that study. Because single-subject designs use only a few individuals at a time, the investigator is able to give a thorough description of each of the subjects. It should then be possible to tentatively conclude that persons who are similar to those who have served in the study may react to the experimental treatment in the same way as the subjects. The concept of logical generality is illustrated in Figure 6-2, which also contrasts it with inferential generality.

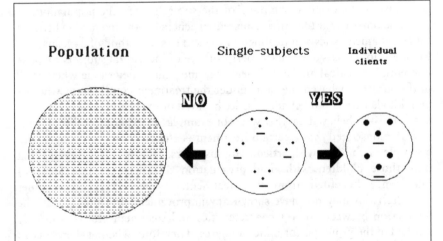

Figure 6-2. The direction of logical generality: from single subjects of a study to similar individual clients. It does not permit generalization from the subjects to the population.

Logical generality proceeds from a set of selected individuals to a single individual or a few individuals. It is generality from either a homogeneous or a heterogeneous set of experimental subjects to a similar set of individuals who have not been tested yet. For example, an experiment involving a new treatment for dysarthric persons may be conducted on five individuals whose specific characteristics are described in detail. Practically, five separate experiments, each involving a single subject, is conducted. However, the conditions of the experiment across the subjects are the same: baseline, treatment, withdrawal of treatment, and reinstatement of treatment. In making a report on the study, each dysarthric client's personal and behavioral characteristics are fully described. Their behaviors under the conditions of the study are presented and analyzed separately. A clinician reading such a report will be able to conclude that as long as the individual dysarthric client he or she is working with is like one of those in the experiment, the treatment tested may be applicable. Of course, any conclusion regarding how the population of dysarthric clients would react to the same treatment would be inappropriate.

Logical generality can eventually achieve the presumed power of inferential generality through various kinds of replications. If different experiments are performed by different clinicians in a variety of settings involving varied clients with the same disorder, the treatment in question will have been tested across different conditions of generality.

3. **GENERALITY ACROSS SUBJECTS.** Generality across subjects is an important factor in all human research, and especially so in clinical research. If a language treatment is known to be effective with 4-year-old children who do not produce morphological features, will the treatment be equally effective in the treatment of 10-year-old children with similar language problems? It is possible that the treatment would not be effective with older or younger children. When clients differ from subjects in an experiment, the results may not be generalized to those clients.

It may appear that inferential generality and generality across subjects address the same problem. However, they refer to two related but separate problems. In inferential generality, whether there was an interaction between subject characteristics and the treatment variable may be *unknown*, and therefore it may not be possible to generalize from the sample to individual subjects. The concern here is the direction of generality: from the sample to the population, and not from the sample to the individual. In generality across subjects, the concern is whether the results of an experiment performed on subjects whose characteristics are *well-known* can be generalized to subjects who have other, but equally well-known, characteristics. The individual subject characteristics are unknown in inferential generality; therefore, the concept permits the extension of conclusion only to the population. It is not critical to determine the characteristics of individual subjects in the population.

In generality across subjects, the investigator wishes to generalize from one set of known subject characteristics to a different set of known characteristics. For instance, the investigator may have determined that a given treatment is effective with dysarthric clients whose characteristics are well described in the study. Other clinicians can surmise that the treatment may be effective with individuals with the same or similar characteristics. (Even this supposition is not possible in inferential generality.) However, they would not know whether the treatment would be effective with dysarthric clients who are different from those in the original study. If there is no such generality, then the treatment must be limited to clients of certain characteristics only.

4. GENERALITY ACROSS SETTINGS. It is important to establish that the findings of a study conducted in one setting are valid in other settings as well. Of necessity, most research studies are conducted in a particular setting. The results may have excellent internal validity. However, it may not be clear that the same results would be obtained if the experiment were to be repeated in other settings. For the clinician, this is an important type of generality.

The extent to which a physical setting itself affects the generality of research findings is not always clear. Often, the reason why the results of a study are not replicated in another setting is a failure to use the procedure in its original form. In any case, if there is no setting generality, additional experimental analyses should be made to determine why. Such analyses may suggest ways of improving the procedure so that it can produce relatively uniform results in different settings.

5. GENERALITY ACROSS EXPERIMENTERS. Sometimes an effect demonstrated by one experimenter may not be obtained by another investigator. The results then do not have generality across experimenters. In clinical research, dramatic effects of certain treatment programs administered by some clinicians may not be replicated by other clinicians.

It is possible that special characteristics, training, and skills of the experimenter contribute to the effects of independent variables manipulated in experiments. However, when such factors are involved, the problem may not be one of experimental design, but of who implemented it and in what manner. In other words, designs cannot be blamed if they are used with varying degrees of efficiency and accuracy by different investigators or clinicians. Regardless, the effect on generality is negative.

Discussions on research in social sciences often include a reference to the Rosenthal effect: the effect of the experimenter on the dependent variable, much of which is due to the personal characteristics of the experimenter. The physical appearance, race, sex, "personality," and such other variables associated with the investigator as a person may play some role in changing the dependent variable under investigation.

It is also possible that experimenter effects are more troublesome when the independent variable manipulated in a study is relatively weak, and the dependent variable measured in the study is not a stable and nonreactive behavior. When the procedures are clear, variables are strong and nonreactive, and the experimenter is well trained in the methods of the study, these effects should not pose significant problems for experimenter generality.

6. **GENERALITY ACROSS RESPONSE CLASSES.** In human and clinical research, a certain independent variable may be demonstrated to have an effect on certain responses. The responses manipulated may belong to a single class, for example, the production of the present progressive *ing* in sentences. The results may demonstrate that the treatment program was effective in teaching the production of *ing*. A clinician then may wonder whether the same treatment technique may be used in teaching plural morphemes, passive forms of sentences, or sign language. Each of these clinical targets belongs to a separate class. This is the question of generality across response classes. One may ask whether the treatment will be effective in treating similar or very different responses—whether, for example, the technique known to be effective in teaching language behaviors can be used to train mathematical or musical skills.

Generality across response classes is important in clinical research and treatment. Clinicians sometimes assume that an independent variable demonstrated to be successful in the treatment of one disorder of communication may not be effective in the treatment of another disorder. However, clinical evidence shows a considerable degree of generality of treatment variables (Hegde, 1985). It is important to establish such generality through systematic research because it reduces unnecessary, often only an apparent, diversity in therapeutic practices.

7. **PRETEST AND POSTTEST SENSITIZATION TO TREATMENT.** The pretest, or the initial assessment of the dependent variable, may sensitize subjects to the treatment in such a way as to enhance the effect of the treatment variable. For example, smokers may become sensitized to the magnitude of their problem when the number of cigarettes smoked is measured prior to implementation of a treatment program. The treatment may have a larger effect in these subjects compared with subjects who were not pretested and thus were not sensitized. Therefore, the results may not be generalized to subjects who will not be given the same or a similar pretest.

In some research studies, the posttest may also act as a sensitizer of treatment variables. While the pretest may sensitize subjects to treatment, the posttest may help demonstrate the effect that would otherwise not have appeared. This can happen because the posttest can help recall the information presented in the treatment sessions. For example, questionnaires and interviews designed to find out the effects of a film on attitude change can help the subjects simply recall some of the information presented in the film, which may be interpreted as an effect of the film. The posttest of an academic teaching program may have similar effects on the dependent variable.

Sensitization is a more serious problem with reactive variables such as attitudes and opinions. After they are measured, they tend to become more sensitive to techniques designed to change them. The reactive variables then show additional changes simply as a function of the posttest. Rates of actual responses, on the other hand, are less reactive than a subject's verbal statements about those responses.

Sensitization to treatment that limits external validity should not be confused with testing that affects internal validity. When testing directly changes (to whatever the extent) the dependent variable, that is a threat to internal validity. In this case, the independent variable may not be responsible for some or all of the changes observed on the posttest. Sensitization, on the other hand, affects the external validity or generality of findings by making the results less relevant to the subjects who are not given a pretest. Testing can directly affect the dependent variable, whereas sensitization can make the subjects react more favorably to the treatment. What is common to both factors is the reactive dependent variable.

8. HAWTHORNE EFFECT. In social and behavioral research, the knowledge on the part of the subjects that they are participating in an experiment may produce an effect in addition to that of the independent variable. The results then may not be extended to subjects who do not have such a knowledge. The subjects may be aware of the purposes of an experiment, and besides, may know what kinds of responses are expected of them under the different conditions of the study. As a result, they may be more inclined to respond in expected directions. Furthermore, experimental subjects may be apprehensive about being evaluated in some way. Such apprehension may also affect the results either positively or negatively. Influences of this kind that limit the generality of research findings are grouped under the Hawthorne effect.

The well-known *placebo* effect is part of the Hawthorne effect. This effect is evident when subjects react to a treatment favorably simply because it is presented as a treatment by experts. The treatment may be totally ineffective, but the subjects may report otherwise. In drug evaluation experiments, a placebo, which looks like the drug being tested but is actually an inert material, is routinely used to rule out this effect. An effective drug should produce effects over and beyond the placebo effect. This effect can also be a troublesome source in behavioral treatment programs. When self-report data on the effects of treatments are sought, the clients may report a magnitude of improvement that is greater than the actual.

9. MULTIPLE TREATMENT INTERFERENCE: In most research studies, the effects of a single independent variable is assessed. However, in some experiments,

the effects of multiple independent variables may be investigated. Clinical research of this kind is especially valuable. For example, a clinician may wish to find out if immediate feedback on the accuracy of a client's response is more effective than delayed feedback in the treatment of articulation disorders. The two different methods of providing the feedback would constitute the two treatment variables in the study. When such experiments are conducted, a potential problem is that of multiple treatment interference.

When two or more treatments are applied in sequence to the same subjects, the effects of the second treatment may be confounded by those of the first. Also, the overall effect observed in the subjects may be at least partly determined by the order in which the multiple treatments were applied. If the same treatments are applied in a different order, the same results may or may not be obtained. This affects the generality of findings. The results may be valid only in terms of the sequence in which the treatments were administered. The generality of the findings with regard to individual treatments would also be unknown.

Multiple treatment interference is a serious problem when the same subjects are exposed to different treatments within a single design. Therefore, it is a problem with certain single-subject and within-subjects designs. However, this problem can exist within the group design strategy when the same subjects are repeatedly used in several experiments. It is known that often the same college students are repeatedly used in multiple experiments. The clients of speech and hearing centers may also be repeatedly used in certain experiments, including treatment evaluations. In such cases, the subjects' performance on subsequent experiments may be partly determined by their participation in earlier experiments. Therefore, the results of subsequent studies may not have much relevance to subjects who have not participated in a number of experiments.

Multiple treatment interference is further discussed in Chapters 7 and 8.

CONCLUDING REMARKS

Internal and external validity are factors that an experimenter, as well as those who evaluate a study, must be concerned with. Whether the demonstrated relation between variables is valid and whether the same relation would hold in other circumstances are the two most important judgments both investigators and consumers of research must make.

Although researchers may be able to control for some of the factors that threaten external validity in a study, it must be realized that no single study can be said to have all kinds of generality. Generality of research findings is a matter of replication. Unless studies are repeated by other experimenters in different settings using new subjects, the eventual generality of experimental findings is not established. There are different procedures of establishing the generality of research data, and I shall describe them in Chapter 9.

Before we conclude this chapter, a note on the distinction between *generality* and *generalization* is in order. Some investigators use the terms interchangeably. However, this practice is confusing because they are not the same. Our discussion so far makes it clear that *generality* refers to the applicability of research data to subjects, responses, settings, experimenters and so on that were not involved in the original study. It is achieved by the process of repeating the experiments under varied conditions. Generality, therefore, is a result of certain actions, but it is not in itself a behavioral process in the sense that generalization is. *Generalization* refers to a temporary response rate when the process of conditioning is discontinued and the response is allowed to be made. On the other hand, generality does not refer to any response rate; it refers to functional relations between events under new conditions of experimentation.

The *act* of establishing generality of research findings is a behavioral process, but that is true of the original experiment as well. In this sense, all research activity is behavior, as we noted in Chapter 3. There is one sense in which generality and generalization are similar, however. When experiments are repeated and the same functional relation is seen again and again, the scientists are said to have demonstrated generality. It means that as long as the same functional relation is encountered, scientists behave as though the differences in settings, conditions, subjects, and other such factors do not matter. The scientists' behavior, then, shows the same properties that characterize generalization. In essence, we can view generality as a functional relation that repeats itself in nature and generalization (in this particular context) as the behavior of scientists toward generality. A scientist would generalize only when the generality of findings has been demonstrated. ■

S T U D Y G U I D E

1 What is a general description of research designs?

2 What is the technical description of research designs?

3 What is meant by the manipulation of an independent variable?

4 Why is the concept of variability especially controversial in the study of human behavior?

5 How does the concept of free will relate to variability of behavior?

6 What is intrinsic variability? What are some of the sources of intrinsic variability of human behavior, including language?

7 How do the concepts of intrinsic variability and intrinsic causes of behavior converge to produce a significant effect on experimental strategy?

8 Which one is experimentally more controllable: intrinsic or extrinsic variability?

9 What is the name for the variability induced by the independent variable?

10 What is extraneous variance? Give an example.

11 What is error variance?

12 What is the traditional answer to the problem of behavioral variability in social and behavioral sciences?

13 Define extrinsic variability. What is its relevance to experimental research?

14 Does the concept of extrinsic variability rule out the influence of variables within an organism?

15 What are some of the variables within the organism that influence behavior?

16 A clinician wishes to find out why stutterers seem to exhibit varying amounts of stuttering on different occasion. How would you try to answer this question on the basis of (1) intrinsic variability and (2) extrinsic variability. What kinds of research will these two assumptions lead to?

17 Which assumption is self-corrective: intrinsic or extrinsic variability?

(continued next page)

Study Guide *(continued)*

18 How is variability handled in the group design and the single-subject design strategies?

19 Can variability itself be the object of scientific investigation? Which design strategy is more likely to investigate the causes of variability?

20 Distinguish between internal and external validity.

21 What is the other name for external validity?

22 What kind of validity is demonstrated by a clinician who convincingly demonstrates that a particular treatment procedure was indeed responsible for changes in his or client's communicative behaviors?

23 How is internal validity achieved?

24 What are the factors that adversely affect internal validity?

25 How is maturation controlled for in the group design and the single-subject design strategy?

26 What are reactive measures? What kinds of dependent variables are most likely to be reactive?

27 What is statistical regression? What kinds of disorders are likely to show this phenomenon?

28 A clinical investigator had ten subjects in each of two groups (experimental and control). The 20 subjects had a disorder of articulation whose severity varied across individuals. With this example, show how differential subject attrition could invalidate the conclusions based on the group means.

29 Is external validity strictly and always a matter of research designs themselves? Why or why not?

30 Describe the relation between internal and external validity. Can you have one without the other?

31 Distinguish between inferential and logical generality.

32 Specify the relevance of logical generality to clinical research.

33 Why is inferential generality not achieved in most group design studies?

34 What kinds of generalities are not demonstrated even by an ideal group design study? Why?

35 What is pretest–posttest sensitization to treatment? What kind of validity is affected by this?

36 How is "testing" different from pretest–posttest sensitization?

37 Define the Hawthorne effect.

38 The placebo effect in clinical research is a part of what effect?

39 What research strategy is especially vulnerable to multiple treatment interference?

40 How is generality different from generalization?

■ CHAPTER 7

The Group Design Strategy

■ Basic terminology and characteristics of group designs, 165

■ Preexperimental designs, 167

■ True experimental designs, 171

■ Designs to evaluate multiple treatments, 179

■ Factorial designs, 181

■ Quasi-experimental designs, 186

■ Time–series designs, 190

■ Counterbalanced within-subjects designs, 196

■ Correlational analysis design, 206

■ Group designs in clinical research, 207

■ Chapter summary, 209

■ Study guide, 213

It was noted in the previous chapter that there are two basic approaches to designing experiments: the group design and the single-subject design. I shall describe the group design strategy in this chapter and the single-subject strategy in the next chapter. Together, the two chapters will summarize a variety of designs that are used in investigating research questions.

The group design strategy is the more established and hence more traditional of the two strategies. Several excellent books on this strategy are available (Campbell & Stanley, 1966; Edwards, 1960; Huck, Cormier, & Bounds, 1974; Kerlinger, 1973; Shaughnessy & Zechmeister, 1985). Clinicians planning to use the group strategy must consult one or more of these books.

The group design strategy was greatly influenced by the development of statistics. As a result, statistics is often equated with research designs. In fact, many books that purportedly deal with research designs do not describe experimental designs to any significant extent. Instead, they describe statistical analyses of data generated by group designs. One must remember that statistics is neither research nor research design, but a method of analyzing certain kinds of data. This point was cogently made as early as 1923 by McCall, who stated that "there are excellent books and courses of instruction dealing with the statistical manipulation of experimental data, but there is little help to be found on *the methods of securing adequate and proper data to which to apply statistical procedures*" (italics added) (p. 23). Designs are methods of collecting adequate data, and statistics are but one method of analyzing them.

An entirely statistical approach to designs is illustrated by the work of Fisher (1925, 1942, 1956) whose writings are a classic within this philosophy of research. His methods of data analysis were originally developed in the context of agricultural research and were later extended to social and psychological research. The approach taken in this chapter, however, is based on another classic in the field of experimental designs: Campbell and Stanley's *Experimental and Quasi-Experimental Designs for Research*. This slim volume has had an enormous impact on research methods used in psychology and education. It has helped standardize the thinking on various design strategies, terminologies, and overall schemes of describing them. The approach taken by Campbell and Stanley (1966) is explicitly not that of Fisher: they emphasize experimental manipulations that reveal cause-effect relations between events. Although most of the designs discussed by Campbell and Stanley need statistical analyses, the book makes a clear distinction between designs as conditions of experimental manipulations and statistics as methods of analyzing data generated by such manipulations.

BASIC TERMINOLOGY AND CHARACTERISTICS OF GROUP DESIGNS

The group design strategy is also known as the between-groups strategy. The basic method used in this strategy is to compare the performance of two or more groups on one or more dependent variables. For the sake of this comparison, the performances of the individuals within a group in any one condition are averaged to form a single composite score.

The strategy requires the formation of groups on the basis of randomization. The investigator first identifies a population of subjects, all of whom are accessible and willing to participate in the study. The required number of subjects is then randomly drawn from the population—meaning that each subject had an equal chance of being selected into the study. Once the subjects are randomly selected, they are then randomly assigned to the different groups of the study.

The logic of the group design requires that the groups formed for the study be equal on all relevant variables at the beginning of an experiment. This is sometimes referred to as the *sampling equivalence* of groups. Then the treatment is applied to the experimental group and withheld from the control group. If, as a result of this experimental operation, the groups differ in their performance, the difference is attributed to the independent variable, since that was presumably the only difference between the groups.

Well-controlled group designs have at least two equivalent groups: the experimental and the control groups. However, a poor design may have only one group that receives treatment. Some advanced and complex designs can have more than two groups, and a "control" group can receive treatment.

A majority of group designs often involve measurement of the dependent variable only on two occasions: once before the independent variable is introduced (pretest) and once after (posttest).

Group designs that have representative samples attempt to establish inferential generality. Whether this is justified is somewhat controversial, and we will address this issue in a later section. In any case, group designs are not expected to help extend the conclusions from a random sample to a single or a few specific individuals. In other words, they do not have logical generality.

Since the publication of Campbell and Stanley (1966), it is customary to use diagrams with abbreviations to represent group research designs. For the sake of consistency and clarity, the same system will be used in this chapter in representing various group designs. In these diagrams, the experimental and control groups are represented with E and C, respectively. The measurement of the dependent variable is represented by O, which stands for observation. Pre- and posttests may be indicated by O_1 and O_2, assuming that there were only those two measures in a study. The treatment variable is indicated by X, and the random subject selection by R. In some books, the dependent variable may be represented by Y. In science and mathematics, X is the cause and Y is the effect. The Y is said to be a function of X.

It is also an accepted practice to describe group designs as preexperimental designs, true experimental designs, quasi-experimental designs, and correlational designs. In different books and articles, however, the reader will find differing and sometimes confusing terms in the description of the same research designs. When appropriate, multiple names of the same design will be pointed out throughout the chapter.

PREEXPERIMENTAL DESIGNS

Preexperimental designs are commonly used in clinical, educational, social, and psychological research. Although they have serious limitations, it is necessary to understand these designs mostly because we must evaluate the vast amount of published research that uses such designs.

The One-Shot Case Study

The one-shot case study is used frequently in clinical and educational research. In an effort to find out the effects a language treatment procedure, a clinician may select some children who have been diagnosed to have a language disorder and apply the selected treatment procedure. The clinician in this case does not have pretest results and simply assumes that the diagnosis of a language disorder provides a sufficient basis to evaluate the results of treatment. Also missing is a control group. The design is shown in Figure 7–1.

The posttest may contain some measure of the children's language obtained either through a standardized test or a language sample. If no evidence appears of a language disorder in the group, the treatment may be considered to have been effective.

The greatest weakness of this design is its total lack of control. The absence of a control group makes it difficult to rule out the influence of factors other than the treatment. There is no valid basis to evaluate the changes documented by the posttest because there was no pretest. Whether the children prior to the treatment were indeed not able to produce the language behaviors that were measured on the posttest remains speculative. In fact, the absence of a pretest makes it impossible to say whether there were any changes due to treatment at all. The clinician comes to some sort of conclusion because of the "common knowledge" that language disordered children do not produce certain language behaviors and therefore, if they do after treatment, the treatment must have been effective.

X	**O**
Treatment	**Posttest**

Figure 7-1. The one-shot case study.

The one-shot case study is not useful in making valid judgments regarding the effectiveness of the treatment variable. In spite of the logical appeal of the treatment program and thoroughness of the posttest, investigators are not be able to demonstrate a functional relation between the treatment and the target behaviors. Of the factors that affect internal validity, history, maturation, and statistical regression typically invalidate the results of one-shot case studies. Depending on the particular study, other sources of internal invalidity may also be involved.

The One-Group Pretest–Posttest Design

The one-group pretest–posttest design is similar to the one-shot case study in that there is no control group. A single group is used in the study. Typical case studies in clinical sciences follow this design format. Unlike the previous design, this one includes a pretest of the dependent variables. The treatment is introduced after the pretest, and a posttest is conducted to evaluate the effects of the treatment. The difference between the pre- and posttest scores is attributed to the effects of the independent variable. The design is illustrated in Figure 7–2.

To continue with our hypothetical example of language treatment research discussed under the previous design, the clinician using the one-group pretest–posttest design would have an opportunity to measure the language behaviors of children serving as subjects in the study both before and after the treatment.

The results of the one-group pretest–posttest design can be analyzed through statistical methods. The most frequently used technique is the parametric t test for correlated samples. Nonparametric tests may also be used in analyzing the results. Two such tests are the sign test and the Wilcoxon matched-pairs signed-ranks test.

Although the design is an improvement over the one-shot case study, it is still not able to generate data that can support a functional relation between the changes in the dependent variable and the independent variable. The clinician in our example can be reasonably sure that the language behaviors of children studied did (or did not) change over the course of the experiment. However, he or she will not be able to conclude that the observed changes

$$O_1 \qquad\qquad X \qquad\qquad O_2$$
Pretest   **Treatment**   **Posttest**

Figure 7-2. The one-group pretest–posttest design.

(the differences between O_1 and O_2) are due to the language treatment program. The design is not able to rule out the influence of history, maturation, testing, instrumentation, statistical regression, and differential subject attrition. In essence, the design lacks internal validity.

There is no assurance that a change in the parents' behavior or a new language stimulation program started by the classroom teacher, or an unspecified biological change taking place within the children, was not responsible for improved language in children. Similarly, the pretest itself may have introduced some changes in the language behaviors, or the testing instruments may have been unreliable. Although statistical regression may not be a problem with language disorders, the design itself is not capable of ruling it out. Differential subject attrition can certainly be an additional problem. The posttest scores may be better than the pretest scores simply because more severely affected children may have dropped out during the course of the experiment. However, because the design uses only one group, subject selection bias is not a factor.

The Static-Group Comparison

Another frequently used preexperimental design is known as the static-group comparison. This design uses two existing groups: one that has already received treatment and another that has not. Because the design does not require the formation of new groups, it is called the static-group comparison method. However, the design does not have pretests of the dependent variables. The design is diagramed in Figure 7–3. The difference in the dependent variable between the group that has received treatment and the group that has not is attributed to the treatment. For example, a clinician may evaluate a stuttering treatment program offered by a large clinic. The stutterers who just completed the treatment program may be compared with those who are yet to receive the same treatment. No pretest measures are obtained for the "control" group because none are available for the experimental group which has already received the treatment. The static-group comparison is also involved when the academic performance of students who have gone to junior

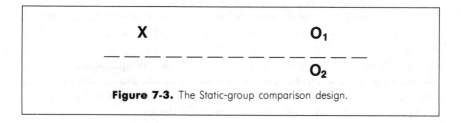

Figure 7-3. The Static-group comparison design.

colleges is compared with the performance of those who started at a four-year college. Similarly, children with repaired cleft palate who have had speech therapy may be compared with those who did not on some measure of speech intelligibility. Then the better speech intelligibility found in the "experimental" group may be attributed to their past speech therapy.

The results of the static-group comparison are analyzed through a parametric *t* test or a nonparametric test such as the Mann-Whitney U test or the median test. A chi-square test may also be used. In static-group comparisons, the group that does not receive treatment does not help control extraneous variables. The major problem of internal validity faced by this design is that of subject selection bias. The design does not require random selection or assignment of subjects into the two groups. Therefore, there is no evidence of the equivalence of the two groups before the treatment. For example, stutterers who were very mildly affected may have gone through the treatment program, whereas those in the "control" group may have been more severe stutterers. The "experimental" group of children with repaired cleft may have had good speech intelligibility all along. The second major problem is that of differential subject attrition. Even when the two groups are identical to begin with, they may become different not because of treatment but because of subject attrition. As such, the static-group comparison is not able to rule out the influence of extraneous variables and therefore cannot help establish functional relations between variables.

Summary and Summative Evaluation of Preexperimental Designs

Preexperimental designs are those that do not have adequate controls to rule out extraneous independent variables. Consequently, they lack internal validity. The one-shot case study, the one-group pretest–posttest design, and the static-group comparison are three commonly used preexperimental designs.

Generally speaking, studies that use one of the preexperimental designs are retrospective. The designs are frequently used in clinical sciences. The preexperimental designs are often justified on the basis of their practicality and clinical relevance. Studies that use these designs are typically considered to be exploratory. They can help identify potential causal relations. In clinical sciences, case studies and one-group pretest–postest designs are useful in generating suggestions for studies involving more rigorous designs. Investigators using one of the preexperimental designs must exercise caution in interpreting their results. The investigators must point out that any hint of causation is just that: only a hint that must be confirmed by more powerful designs. Readers of studies based on preexperimental designs should exercise similar caution in their evaluation of those studies. The readers must be especially careful not to accept an author's conclusions when they seem to disregard the limitations of a preexperimental design.

TRUE EXPERIMENTAL DESIGNS

As noted in Chapter 6, an experimental design must be able to establish a functional relation between an independent and a dependent variable. Within the philosophy of the group designs, true experimental designs are able to do this by ruling out many of the potential extraneous variables. Therefore, true experimental designs are those that reveal a reasonably clear cause-effect relation between the manipulated independent variable and the measured dependent variable. Therefore, the designs have internal validity within the theoretical and methodological limitations of the approach. Most investigators who do not consider alternatives to the group design strategy also make a claim that a single study with a true experimental group design can also have external validity. Such a claim is questionable because of the nature of generality and the limits of the probability theory. We shall return to this controversial claim in a later section.

The Formation of Control Groups

True experimental designs within the group strategy rule out the influence of extraneous variables, mainly through the use of control groups. Therefore, before we consider the designs themselves, it is necessary to understand the various ways of forming control (as well as experimental) groups.

Randomization

There are different methods by which two or more groups can be formed. The purpose, of course, is to have two or more groups that are equivalent at the beginning of an experiment. As noted before, of all the available methods, randomization is considered the best. According to the probability theory, an unbiased sample drawn from a population is representative of that population. As such, a sample, which is a smaller number of individuals, is drawn from a population, which is a large group with defined characteristics. All language disordered school-age children can be considered a population, for example.

Representativeness is achieved when the individuals in the same sample have the same variety of characteristics as the population. A population is heterogeneous in the sense that the individuals in it differ in terms of all those characteristics that make differences in people: health, intelligence, socioeconomic status, education, family background, and so on. Therefore, only a sample that is as heterogeneous as the population from which it was drawn can be considered representative. Such samples can be drawn only when the investigator does not let his or her biases influence the selection of subjects.

There are different methods of drawing a random sample. When a list of all names of individuals in a population is available, the investigator can simply select every second, fifth, or thirteenth person. Smaller samples can be drawn by the lottery method or by tossing a coin. But the method considered by many to be the best is to use the random table, which is a list of mechanically generated numbers. The investigator simply reads the numbers off the table and selects individuals on this basis.

When the required number of subjects has been selected randomly, the investigator must assign them to the experimental and control groups. This is also done randomly to avoid investigator bias in determining who receives treatment and who does not. The groups can then be considered equivalent on all the variables that could affect the results of the investigation.

The random procedure is thought to assure the equivalence of the groups because the selection and assignment are left to chance. In this case, each subject is said to have the same chance of being selected to the study and then being assigned to either of the two (or more) groups.

Random selection and assignment serve different purposes. Random selection assures that the sample is representative of the population. Therefore, the investigator can extend the conclusions to the population. Random assignment, on the other hand, assures that the two or more groups of a study were equal to begin with. Therefore, the investigator can conclude that any changes observed in the experimental group must be due to the independent variable that was absent in the control group.

Matching

An alternative to randomization is called matching. When it is not possible to gain access to a large population of subjects all of whom are willing to participate, the investigator may try to achieve sampling equivalence by one of several methods of matching subjects.

Matching *pairs of subjects* is one such method. In this method, the investigator matches pairs of subjects on known (relevant) variables and then randomly assigns one of the pair to the experimental group and the other to the control group. For example, suppose that an investigator knows that in the treatment of articulation disorders, the severity of misarticulations is a significant variable influencing the treatment outcome. In this case, the investigator may find pairs of subjects who are equal in severity of misarticulation. A member of each pair will be assigned to the control group and the other to the experimental group. Matched pairs can be created on multiple variables. For example, pairs of subjects can be matched on age, sex, and severity of the disorder under study.

Another method of matching subjects is to achieve *equivalent frequency distribution* of relevant variables in the two groups. For example, if age, severity, and intelligence of subjects are considered relevant variables in a particular investigation, a comparable distribution of these variables in the two groups may be obtained. The distribution of the variables is considered comparable when the mean and the standard distribution of the measured values of those variables are comparable. This technique of matching is less precise than the paired-subjects procedure, but it is more practical. Individuals are not matched one-to-one, but the groups are matched on a statistical basis.

The most serious limitation of matching is that under the best possible circumstances, it can create two groups that are comparable on *known* variables only. The groups may still differ on variables that have an effect but were unknown and hence were not considered in matching the subjects. In our example, it is possible that a family history of misarticulation or the presence of other communicative problems may be important variables, but because of no prior research on them, they are simply not considered in matching the subjects.

Matching subjects in clinical research poses serious practical problems. It is difficult to find pairs of clients who are similar on one or more relevant variables. Many clients will have to be rejected because another client who shares the same characteristics selected for matching is not available. The clinical researcher often cannot afford this luxury. Equivalent distribution of variables in the two groups may be more feasible, but it still requires a large pool of subjects.

Theoretically, randomization assures equivalence on all of the relevant variables, known and unknown. Therefore, randomization is preferred to matching. In presenting the true experimental designs, I shall assume that randomization is the method of achieving sampling equivalence between groups, but the reader can easily substitute randomization (R) with matching (M) in the diagrams under each design.

I shall describe several true experimental designs. Some of the true experimental designs involve a single treatment (independent) variable, whereas others involve multiple treatment variables. The pretest–posttest control group design, the posttest-only control group design, and the Solomon four-group design involve a single treatment variable. On the other hand, multigroup pretest-posttest design, multigroup posttest-only design, and the several types of factorial designs make it possible to evaluate the effects of multiple independent variables.

The Pretest–Posttest Control Group Design

The pretest–posttest control group design is prototypical of the true experimental group designs. It is also the simplest. This design elegantly illustrates the logic and the strategy of the group designs. It requires two groups: an experimental group which receives treatment, and a control group, which does not.

The design is based on the logic that in order to assess the effects of an independent variable, the only difference between the groups shall be that variable. In other words, the investigator must start with two groups that are very similar if not identical. If the groups are different on some known or unknown variables other than the treatment, then the effect of that treatment variable cannot be experimentally isolated. In essence, achieving the equivalence of the experimental and control groups is the most critical task in forming the groups for this design. This task may be accomplished with randomization or matching.

The pretest–posttest control group design is illustrated in Figure 7–4. The diagram shows that the subjects were randomly selected (R) from a population and were randomly assigned to the two groups. The experimental group (E) is exposed to the treatment variable (X), whereas the control group (C) is not. The dependent variable is measured (O) twice in each group, once before and once after the experimental group has received the treatment. This basic arrangement permits a relatively unambiguous evaluation of the effects of most independent variables.

The typical pretest–posttest control group design has only one treatment variable and a true control group. However, in a variation of this design, both the groups can receive treatment, each a different one. The research question in such cases is whether one treatment is more effective than the other. A clinician, for example, may be interested in finding out whether changing stutterers' attitudes is more effective than reinforcing their fluency. In this case, we have X_1 (attitudinal therapy) and an X_2 (fluency reinforcement). Design extensions of this kind, which help analyze the effects of several treatments, are described in a later section on designs to evaluate multiple treatments.

In the analysis of the results of the basic version of the design, it is important to avoid some common mistakes. In one of the mistaken analyses, the pretest and posttest scores of the experimental group may be compared with one t test and the scores of the two tests of the control group may be compared with a different t test. These two comparisons are based on the assumption that if the experimental group's posttest mean is significantly higher than the pretest mean and the control group's pre- and posttest means are comparable, then the effect of the independent variable has been demonstrated. Actually, this analysis does not involve a direct comparison of the performance of the two groups. Sometimes investigators compare the

E R O_1 X O_2
C R O_1 O_2

Figure 7-4. The pretest–posttest control group design.

two pretest scores with a *t* test and the two posttest scores with another *t* test. This is also an inappropriate analysis of the results because it does not adequately reflect changes in the dependent variable across the conditions of an experiment.

The correct method of analysis involves either a gain score procedure or an analysis of covariance. In the former, each subject's pretest scores are subtracted from the posttest scores to obtain the gain scores. The individual gain scores are then averaged to obtain two mean scores, one for each of the two groups. The two means are then compared with either the parametric independent samples t test or the nonparametric Mann-Whitney U test. A median test may also be used to compare the two means. An analysis of covariance is a more complex and more efficient method of analysis and is preferred by many investigators.

The basic version of the design, which has a control group that does not receive treatment, is able to rule out extraneous factors relative to history and maturation. Events in the life of the subjects or maturational changes that may affect the dependent variable are assumed to be common to the two groups. Therefore, significant changes in the dependent variable, if shown by the experimental group, cannot be attributed to history or maturation.

Regression to the mean can occur, but to the extent that the groups were equal to begin with, this phenomenon will be held constant across the two groups. For example, if stuttering rate returns to the mean level in the experimental group some time after the pretest, the same thing can be expected to happen in the control group also. Similarly ruled out is the factor of subject selection as long as the samples were drawn, or at least assigned, randomly. However, if subjects are matched, then all of the sources of subject selection biases cannot be ruled out (Campbell & Stanley, 1966).

Testing as a factor of internal validity is also controlled in the design because both the groups were pretested, and therefore changes due to measurement of the dependent variable must be common across the two groups. When the same instruments are used in obtaining all measures of the variables in both the groups, the effects of the instrumentation are also not of concern.

Differential subject attrition can be a problem in the pretest–posttest control group design. The experimenter, however, would know whether attrition could have affected the results. Any drop out of subjects from the experimental group is suggestive of this potential problem. It is difficult to determine the nature or extent of the effect of attrition when it is known to have occurred, however. Unfortunately, the effects of subject attrition are "commonly swept under the rug" (Campbell & Stanley, 1966, p. 15). The loss of subjects during the course of the experiment may be reported but not handled in the data analysis. This mistake is easy to commit in a group design in which despite some subject loss, the investigator seems to have some data to be analyzed.

The external validity of this, or in fact any design, is a different matter. Most textbooks tend to advise that as long as a random sample has been drawn from the population, the results should have generality. The problem with this reasoning is that it takes into consideration only inferential generality. There is no empirical basis to assume that other kinds of generality, which are equally if not more important, are assured by even the best random sample. For instance, generality across responses, settings, and experimenters is not known unless the experiment is repeated with different responses, under different settings, and by different investigators. The position advocated here, and expanded in Chapter 9, is that generality is a function of replication, and therefore a single study using the best of the experimental designs does not assure it.

Posttest-Only Control Group Design

In the posttest-only control group design, neither the experimental nor the control group subjects are given a pretest. After randomly selecting and assigning subjects into the two groups, the treatment variable is applied to the experimental group. After the completion of the experimental treatment, the two groups are given a posttest. The design is illustrated in Figure 7–5.

A pretest is considered indispensable by many investigators. Therefore, this design is not used very frequently. However, Campbell and Stanley (1966) suggest that pretests are not at all necessary when the subjects are selected randomly. Therefore, they strongly recommend this design and consider it superior to the pretest–posttest control group design. It certainly avoids the pretest–posttest sensitization to treatment because there is no pretest. The design can also control for other sources that affect internal validity, except for differential subject attrition.

The justification for this design rests heavily on the random procedure. The argument is that when the subjects are selected and assigned randomly, the groups are equal to begin with. The pretest is only a confirmation of this fact. However, if pretests are expected to create problems, or for some reason are not possible to administer, then they can be avoided without loss of scientific rigor, since the groups are comparable anyway. A statistically significant difference in the posttest scores of the two groups must be due

$$
\begin{array}{cccc}
\textbf{E} & \textbf{R} & \textbf{X} & \textbf{O} \\
\textbf{C} & \textbf{R} & & \textbf{O}
\end{array}
$$

Figure 7-5. The posttest-only control group design.

to the experimental variable only. An analysis of such a difference usually involves a *t* test.

If the probability theory and random procedures were as practical as they are elegant, there would be no problem with this design. However, in most clinical sciences that need to evaluate the effects of treatments in persons with various diseases and disorders, randomization is the least practical of the procedures of subject selection. In other designs, the pretest will at least let the investigator know that the groups are not equal. When there is no pretest, the experimenter has no way of checking sampling equivalence of the two groups. The design places too heavy a burden on the theory of random samples and too great a confidence in its practicality. Unfortunately, the probability theory promises much at the level of theory but delivers less at the level of clinical research.

The Solomon Four-Group Design

A four-group design was originally proposed in 1949 by Solomon and quickly became one of the most prestigious of the group designs used in social and psychological research. Solomon first formally recognized the interaction of pretest sensitization and treatment as a potential threat to external validity. However, this problem must have been implicitly acknowledged by previous investigators because the design without a pretest was already available. Solomon proposed a design that provided not only an opportunity for the interaction to take place but also a method to measure its magnitude.

The four-group design is considered the most appropriate strategy for investigation when the pretest sensitization is expected to interact with the independent variable, and illustrated in Figure 7–6. It is clear from the diagram that the design is actually a combination of two previously described designs: the pretest–posttest control group and the posttest-only control group. The design has two experimental and two control groups. One of the experimental groups receives both the pretest and the posttest. The second experimental group is not pretested; it receives only the posttest. One of the two control

E	R	O_1	X	O_2
C	R	O_1		O_2
E	R		X	O
C	R			O

Figure 7-6. The Solomon four-group design.

groups receives both the tests, whereas the second control group is only posttested.

The design controls for all the factors that affect internal validity. In addition, it also demonstrates the presence and the extent of pretest sensitization as a threat to external validity. A difference between the means of the pretested groups and an absence of such a difference between the means of unpretested groups reveals the effects of sensitization. Also, from a descriptive standpoint, if the pretest sensitizes the subjects, the treatment effects are larger in the first experimental group than in the second. Because the first experimental group receives both tests whereas the second receives only the posttest, the performance of the second group is free of pretest sensitization. The two control groups also indicate any effects of the pretest on the dependent variable (a factor of internal validity). If the pretest has a direct effect on the dependent variable, the control group receiving both tests behaves differently than the one receiving only the posttest.

It has been recognized that analysis of the results of the Solomon design is difficult. A single statistical technique that can simultaneously analyze all the observations of the design is not available. Therefore, the pretest scores are ignored and a two-way analysis of variance is performed. This analysis is arranged in terms of the scores of subjects who have been pretested/unpretested × treated/untreated.

The design, though considered ideal in many respects, is of limited value. Its limitations are both practical and paradigmatic. It presents the immense practical problem of finding a population from which four groups of subjects can be drawn randomly. Because it is a combination of two designs, it is about twice as hard to implement as any of the basic group designs. Therefore, there are hardly any clinical treatment studies in which the four-group design was used. The design is simply not used often even in nonclinical social research where it is more applicable.

It can also be argued, in an admittedly controversial manner, that the design offers a methodological solution for the problem of paradigm. Obviously, the design is needed only when the pretest sensitization is a consideration. It is a consideration mostly in research that addresses reactive measures such as attitudes and opinions. In other words, the design is needed when the dependent variables are weak and at best offer indirect measures of whatever is measured. For example, we can measure the attitude of a group of speech–language pathologists toward stutterers in public schools, as several researchers have done. One would assume that this type of research is done to determine whether the clinicians are not likely to treat stutterers because of their negative attitudes or that when they do treat stutterers the outcome may not be favorable, again because of negative attitudes. Or, the researcher may wish to change the clinicians' negative attitudes with an informational package (the treatment variable). In this second instance, the researcher would need the four-group design. Incidentally, much of the research on attitudes in communicative disorders is done only to uncover negative attitudes. Hardly anything is done about them. A conceptually different approach to the issue is to find out how many stutterers are not receiving treatment in a given setting and then proceed to find out why.

The finding that some clinicians have a negative attitude toward stuttering is hardly illuminating. It is probably better to look into the clinicians' training and expertise in the treatment of stuttering, deficiencies in which may have originated a side effect described by some as negative attitudes. In essence, a conceptual solution to the problem of reactive measures is to try to avoid such dependent variables in favor of those that are less reactive, more stable, and perhaps more meaningful. Obviously, those who think that attitudes and opinions are important variables would disagree with this suggestion.

DESIGNS TO EVALUATE MULTIPLE TREATMENTS

So far we have discussed group designs in which the effects of a single treatment variable are evaluated. However, in many cases, the effects of more than one independent variable may be of interest. In clinical sciences, it is often necessary to determine whether one treatment is more effective than the other. Group designs offer some excellent options to do this. I shall describe two designs that are an extension of the designs presented earlier: multigroup pretest–posttest design and multigroup posttest-only design. Besides, I shall describe a separate class of designs, known as factorial designs, which also help evaluate multiple treatment effects on a particular dependent variable.

Multigroup Pretest–Posttest Design

In the evaluation of two or more treatment techniques, one can extend the basic pretest–posttest control group design to include the needed number of additional groups. Theoretically, several treatment procedures can be studied in multiple groups within a single design. From a practical standpoint, extensions are limited by the ease with which the groups can be formed and the data analyzed meaningfully. The extension of the basic design by a single additional treatment can introduce a considerable amount of complexity.

The multigroup pretest–posttest design with three treatment groups is illustrated in Figure 7–7. The design can evaluate the relative effects of the treatment techniques. It may be noted that the control group is placed within parentheses to suggest that it is an optional arrangement. Often, the clinicians are concerned with the *relative* effects of multiple treatment techniques, not the absolute effect of any one of them. In such cases, a control group is not necessary. However, when a control group is added, the investigator can make statements regarding the absolute effects of the treatment techniques, and the control group enhances the internal validity of the design.

180 CLINICAL RESEARCH IN COMMUNICATIVE DISORDERS ■

180   CLINICAL RESEARCH IN COMMUNICATIVE DISORDERS ■

$$
\begin{array}{lllll}
E & R & O_1 & X_1 & O_2 \\
E & R & O_1 & X_2 & O_2 \\
E & R & O_1 & X_3 & O_2 \\
(C & R & O_1 & & O_2)
\end{array}
$$

Figure 7-7. The multigroup pretest–posttest design.

The design affords a chance to determine the most and the least effective of the three techniques. Research involving this kind of design is highly desirable in areas where multiple treatment techniques are recommended by different clinicians to treat the same disorder. Such therapeutic diversity exists in the treatment of most disorders of communication.

The results of the design can be analyzed with a variety of statistical techniques, including analysis of covariance, analysis of variance based on gain scores for each subject (see pretest-posttest control group design), or a Lindquist Type I repeated measures analysis of variance. Most of these techniques of analysis simply indicate whether there is a significant difference in the performances of the groups. Therefore, when a significant difference between the groups is evident, additional analysis involving pairwise group comparisons is necessary.

Multigroup Posttest-Only Design

This is an extension of the posttest-only control group design presented earlier. In this design, two or more treatments are evaluated for their relative effectiveness in the absence of pretests. A diagram of the design with three treatments is presented in Figure 7–8. As in the original design, the subjects are selected and assigned to the groups randomly, resulting in equivalent groups that need to be pretested. Each group is exposed to a different treatment. The diagram shows an optional control group.

$$
\begin{array}{llll}
R & E & X_1 & O \\
R & E & X_2 & O \\
R & E & X_3 & O \\
(R & C & & O)
\end{array}
$$

Figure 7-8. The multigroup posttest-only design.

The results of the multigroup posttest-only design can be analyzed with a one-way analysis of variance or with nonparametric statistics such as the Kruskal-Wallis and chi-square tests.

The design shares the same strengths and weaknesses as the posttest-only control group design. It is needed when the pretest sensitization is expected to interact with the treatment variable. Unless the investigator is sure that the groups were equal to begin with, there is no assurance of internal validity. The design is as good as the random procedure in practice.

FACTORIAL DESIGNS

Factorial designs are also true experimental designs. They are an excellent example of research strategies based mostly on the method of analysis of variance. Analysis of variance is a collection of related techniques the complex forms of which can be used in the simultaneous analysis of two or more variables and their interactions. In the terminology of factorial designs, a factor is the same as an independent variable.

Factorial designs have two or more independent variables. The independent variables may be either active, assigned, or a combination of the two. It may be recalled that active independent variables are manipulated by the experimenter, whereas assigned variables may affect the results but cannot be manipulated. Assigned variables are typically subject characteristics such as age, sex, socioeconomic status, and the severity of various disorders (see Chapter 3 for details). A factorial design that includes only assigned variables is not an experimental study, but belongs to the ex post facto category. Therefore, we shall not be concerned with that type of design here. An experimental factorial design will have at lest one active independent variable. Many factorial designs have a combination of active and assigned variables.

An independent variable used in a factorial design has a minimum of two different levels. For this reason, certain factorial designs are referred to as *treatment-by-levels designs*. The levels of an active (manipulated) independent variable may be the presence or the absence of it (treatment versus no treatment). Two techniques of treatment can also be considered levels. Furthermore, a technique whose intensity is varied can create different levels.

Several examples of levels in a factorial design can be given. An investigator may wish to evaluate the manual and oral methods of teaching hearing impaired individuals. In this case, the treatment variable has two levels, which are actually two separate treatments. A third level can be created by having a control group that is not exposed to either of the two teaching methods. Another clinician may wish to test regular (twice a week) versus intensive (five times a week) scheduling of clients while using a single treatment procedure. The two schedules create two levels.

An assigned variable also typically has two or more levels. For example, hearing impaired individuals selected for a certain treatment evaluation may be grouped according to the degree of hearing loss: mild, moderate, and severe. These three categories are the three levels of the assigned variable. Most other assigned variables such as age, sex, socioeconomic class, and intelligence have two or more levels.

Within the group design strategy, factorial designs are the primary techniques of assessing the interaction of two or more variables. An interaction exists when two or more independent variables combine to produce an effect that is different from (usually greater than) the separate or independent effect of those variables. It is believed that most phenomena we study are multiply determined in an interactive fashion. in other words, most events have several causes, which in various combinations, produce the effects we normally see. The designs that manipulate single variables at a time actually simplify the phenomenon for the sake of clearer analysis. Designs that permit the manipulation of multiple variables are more powerful. They also better approximate reality.

The factorial design is also based on the random procedure. The subjects must be selected and assigned to the groups on a random basis. Once the subjects are selected randomly, however, only the active variables permit random assignment. In our example, the clinician may be able to assign subjects to the treatment and control conditions, but not either to mild, moderate, or severe categories of hearing loss. Each subject's hearing loss, not the power of randomization, determines whether he or she is assigned to one or the other category of severity.

There are several factorial designs; some are simpler than the others. The complexity of a factorial design is directly related to the number of independent variables (assigned and active) and the number of levels of each of those variables.

Randomized Blocks Design

A randomized blocks design has at least one active variable and one assigned variable. It can have more than two variables, but one of the variables must be assigned. If each variable has two levels, then we have the basic randomized design, which is often represented as the 2 × 2 (two-by-two) design. In our example, the oral and the manual methods of teaching the hearing impaired are the two levels of the active independent variable. The levels of hearing loss, if limited only to two levels (mild and moderate), are the two levels of the assigned variable that cannot be manipulated.

A 2 × 2 randomized blocks design would have four cells or conditions; a 2 × 3 design would have six. A 2 × 3 randomized blocks design is illustrated in Figure 7–9. The design has two independent variables, one a manipulated treatment variable (teaching methods) with two levels, and the other an

		Levels of Hearing Loss		
		Mild	**Moderate**	**Severe**
Treatment	**Manual**			
	Oral			

Figure 7-9. A 2 × 3 randomized blocks design.

assigned variable with three levels (hearing loss). Once the necessary number of hearing impaired individuals with mild, moderate, and severe hearing loss (defined in some operational manner) has been identified, subjects are randomly drawn from each of the levels of hearing loss and assigned to the treatment conditions. When pretests are used, testing creates another factor in the design, with two levels: pre- and posttest.

It is important to note that from each of the levels of the assigned variable, the subjects are drawn randomly and assigned to the treatments. Each level of the assigned variable is considered a "block" from which a random sample is drawn. The design can include subjects who do not receive treatment. The subjects of the control group should also represent the levels of the assigned variable.

Factorial designs can help determine the independent effects of the main treatment factors. The "main effects" in an analysis of variance of the results of a factorial design are the effects of the separate treatment variables. In our example, the oral and the manual methods of teaching can be expected to produce two main effects in the study.

The other important effect the analysis can reveal is the interaction of treatment with subject characteristics. It is possible that the oral method of instruction is most effective with subjects who have only a mild hearing loss and that the manual method is more effective with severely affected subjects. Individuals with a moderate level of hearing loss may benefit equally from the two procedures. This kind of relation is what is implied in an interaction. Obviously, discovery of such relations is important from a clinical standpoint. When such interactions exist, simpler questions that address the effects of single variables in isolation do not reflect the complexity of the phenomenon under investigation. For example, whether the oral or the manual method of teaching is more effective may not be determined unless the level of hearing loss is taken into consideration.

When the number of variables and their levels are increased, the complexity of the design increases. The need for subjects is directly proportional to the number of variables and levels in a factorial study. In the design illustrated in Figure 7–9, there are six cells, and assuming that at least 10 subjects to a cell are needed, the investigator will have to find 60 subjects to complete the study. A control group, when used, create a need for additional subjects.

Completely Randomized Factorial Design

In the previous design, one of the two factors is active (treatment) and the other assigned (levels of hearing loss). However, it is possible to design a factorial study in which all the factors are active. Such a design is known as the completely randomized factorial design. No assigned variable is included in this type of design. Hence, there is no "blocking" in a completely randomized factorial design.

It is evident that complete randomization of subjects is possible only when all the factors are active. An experimenter cannot assign subjects randomly to the experimental conditions on the basis of their sex or intelligence. Subjects can be assigned randomly only to treatment conditions that are under the experimenter's control. Therefore, completely randomized factorial designs do not address issues relative to potential interactions between treatment variables and subject characteristics.

A completely randomized factorial design is illustrated in Figure 7–10. It shows a 2 × 2 design in which two independent variables, both active, are studied. The research question of the example is whether the airflow or the syllable prolongation component of stuttering therapy is more effective in the treatment of stuttering and whether the effects depend upon the presence or absence of contingent feedback on the subjects' performance during therapy sessions. Both the forms of treatment and feedback are active; the experimenter controls all of them. The subjects are randomly assigned to the conditions of the study. In other words, who receives airflow or prolongation therapy, and who receives either of these with or without contingent feedback, are all decided on a random basis.

	Contingent Feedback	
	Present	**Absent**
Airflow		
Prolongation		

Figure 7-10. A completely randomized factorial design.

The 2 × 2 design just described would probably need at least 40 stutterers, ten to each condition. A control group, when used, would need an additional ten subjects. The design can be extended to include other independent variables.

Factorial designs are among the most powerful of the group designs. They can help answer complex and clinically significant questions. It is a common clinical observation that most treatment procedures do not seem to work equally effectively with all types of subjects. Clinicians suspect that to a certain extent the effects of treatment procedures depend upon several subject characteristics, which often reflect other variables. Some of those variables may be related to the client's learning history, the precise nature of the disorder, the past therapies that have been unsuccessful, and so on. Even such characteristics as sex and socioeconomic class may be a mixture of variables, some of which are external factors in the life of the individual. It is important to know how different variables, including those the clinician calls "treatment," come together to produce the final, desirable, effect in different clients. Factorial designs can help answer such important clinical questions.

The problems with factorial designs are mostly practical. Randomization, which is required at some or all levels, creates problems that have been discussed before. Although a factorial design can theoretically handle several variables, the complexity and the need for subjects increase in proportion to the number of variables. Finding stutterers or aphasic subjects who are willing to participate in an experimental study in enough numbers to permit random assignment to the various cells of a factorial design is difficult. Clinical conditions that are relatively rare present the same problem with a much greater magnitude. The analysis of results also becomes more and more difficult with increases in the number of variables or their levels. As a result, firm and clear conclusions regarding the interaction between several variables and levels are difficult to offer.

Summary and Summative Evaluation of True Experimental Designs

True experimental designs have a minimum of two groups. The groups are formed on the basis of either randomization or matching. Randomization is preferred because it assures sampling equivalence of the groups on known and unknown variables. In most cases, one group receives the treatment and the other does not. However, it is possible to expose both the groups to one of two treatments when the purpose is to evaluate the relative effects of those two treatments. Even then, an optional control group that does not receive treatment may be included.

The pretest–posttest control group design is the most prototypical of the true experimental designs. The posttest-only control group design and the Solomon four-group design are the other two true experimental designs that help establish the effects of a single treatment variable. The multigroup pretest–posttest design and the multigroup posttest-only design may be used to evaluate the effects of two or more independent variables. The factorial designs can be used to determine the independent and interactive effects of multiple treatment variables. Factorial designs may have some independent variables that cannot be manipulated, or they may have all manipulable independent variables.

Most true experimental designs have a pretest and a posttest. However, when the subjects are randomly selected and assigned to the groups of a study, the pretest may not be necessary, as in a multigroup posttest-only design.

True experimental designs, especially factorial designs are the most powerful of the group design strategies. They are extremely useful in isolating cause–effect relations. Also, factorial designs help evaluate interactions between two or more independent variables. True experimental designs have internal validity. Through direct and systematic replications, they may also achieve external validity.

From a clinical standpoint, a major limitation of true experimental designs is that it is not always possible to randomly draw subjects from particular clinical populations. Sampling equivalence, therefore, is difficult to achieve in clinical research that uses true experimental group designs. Besides, the group design studies may not allow an extension of results to individual clients. I shall address these and other issues more fully in a later section on group designs in clinical research.

QUASI-EXPERIMENTAL DESIGNS

Quasi-experimental designs are those experimental arrangements in which the experimenter is not able to exert full control over all the relevant variables and operations. Originally, they were suggested as a means of conducting experiments in natural settings rather than in the well-controlled laboratories (Campbell & Stanley, 1966). However, in actual practice, quasi-experimental designs are used whenever practical considerations prevent the use of better (more controlled) designs of research.

Quasi-experimental designs are weaker than true experimental designs because certain control procedures are not used. When studies are conducted in natural settings, it is not always possible to use some of the control procedures and yet the opportunity for limited experimentation may exist. For example, when an experiment on improving teaching methods is initiated in an elementary school, it may not be possible to draw a random sample of pupils. Similarly, when a new program of diet or physical exercise for the elderly is initiated in a nursing home, the investigator may not have a chance to select or assign subjects randomly. Experimental evaluation of programs in various institutions necessarily uses existing subjects and living arrangements. Therefore, some of the quasi-experimental designs do not have groups that are especially formed for the purposes of research. In such cases, the investigators often use already existing natural groups, which are called *intact* groups of subjects.

What are known as field studies are the same as, or very similar to, studies that use quasi-experimental designs. Field experiments are those done in natural conditions or in less artificial conditions than the laboratory studies. They also tend to use natural or intact groups. For this reason, they lack randomization and, as a consequence, lose control over some of the factors that affect internal validity.

Two specific quasi-experimental designs I shall describe are the non equivalent control group design and the separate sample pretest–posttest design. In addition, I shall also describe a separate class of quasi-experimental designs, known as time-series designs.

Nonequivalent Control Group Designs

The nonequivalent control group design is similar to the pretest–posttest control group design. It has two groups: one experimental and one control. Both are pretested. The experimental group receives the treatment. The posttests of the two groups follow. The nonequivalent control group design differs from the pretest–posttest control group design in only one respect: there is no random selection or assignment in the nonequivalent control group design. The design is presented in Figure 7–11. In the diagram, note the absence of R for randomization. A line of dashes separates the two groups to suggest that there is no assurance of equivalence based on the random sampling procedure.

The design can have more than two groups. Also, both the groups in a two-group nonequivalent design can receive treatment when the purpose is to evaluate the relative effects of two treatments.

The design is often necessary in such settings as schools, general and mental hospitals, nursing and extended care homes, and institutions for the retarded. Groups of patients or residents in different wards, branches, and housing units may serve as the different groups of the study. For example, all persons on the first floor of a residential facility may serve as the

$$\begin{array}{cccc} E & O_1 & X & O_2 \\ \hline C & O & & O_2 \end{array}$$

Figure 7-11. The nonequivalent control group design.

experimental group while those on the second floor may serve as the control group. This results in *intact* experimental and control groups. Which group will receive treatment and which will serve as the control is determined randomly.

Some nonequivalent control group designs may have subjects who volunteer for the study. In this case, the sample is self-selected. The investigator then has what is known as a self-selected experimental group. A control group may be created from those who do not volunteer for the study.

Intact experimental and control groups are better than the self-selected experimental groups. Possibly, those who volunteer for a study are quite different from those who do not. When the investigator forms a control group, he or she may have no knowledge about the differences between those who wish to participate and those who do not. As a result, the experimenter is likely to have two groups that are so different as to make them unacceptable even within a quasi-experimental design.

It is important to realize that the design does not recommend dispensing with the notion of preexperimental equivalence of groups. It permits an experiment under conditions of no assurance of equivalence *based on randomization*. The investigator is still expected to take every feasible step to make the groups as similar as possible. For example, an investigator may be interested in the evaluation of a treatment program designed to increase verbal behaviors in institutionalized autistic children. It is possible that the residents of one ward are more verbal than the residents of another ward. In this case, the investigator should not select the ward with more verbal autistic children for the experimental group and the ward with less verbal children for the control group. The investigator cannot use these two intact groups.

The same statistical techniques used in the analysis of the results of pretest–posttest control group design are applicable to the nonequivalent control group design. However, the use of analysis of covariance, which is based on a strong assumption of preexperimental sampling equivalence of groups, is questionable.

The most critical problem with the nonequivalent control group design is the selection biases that threaten internal validity. Other threats include statistical regression and differential subject attrition. The subjects (either selected or volunteered) may have had unusually high pretest scores to begin with, which might regress to the mean during the course of an experiment. This may lead to an erroneous conclusion that the independent variable was responsible for the change. For example, in a study designed to evaluate a new exercise program for the senior citizens, the residents who are not making progress under the treatment program may withdraw from the study, leaving only those subjects who do show improvement.

The design was originally recommended for experiments in natural settings where a better design is not suitable. However, in practice, many investigators in social and psychological research have used the design in laboratory-oriented research, partly because the requirement of randomization poses significant practical problems for all kinds of research, not just for field experiments. Nevertheless, when one of the true experimental designs can be used, the nonequivalent control group design is a poor choice.

Separate Sample Pretest–Posttest Design

Sometimes investigators wish to study certain behaviors or practices of very large natural groups such as workers in a factory, children in large schools, people living in various parts of a city, or speech–language clinicians in a large school district. In such cases, it is often not possible to select individual subjects on a random basis for the purpose of forming experimental and control groups. However, the investigators can usually use the random procedure in determining which subgroups will be observed before and after treatment. The separate sample pretest–posttest design is applicable in situations such as these.

The design is represented in Figure 7–12. Note that unlike the nonequivalent control group design, this design uses the random procedure. The two groups, therefore, are assumed to have sampling equivalence. Only one sample is pretested, and then this sample is presented with a treatment variable *not relevant* to the study: the X in parenthesis. It is the second group, not receiving the pretest, which is the true experimental group in the design. The treatment variable is applied to this group, and a posttest follows.

The design can be illustrated with a hypothetical example. Suppose a coordinator of speech–language services in a large school district wishes to find out the most frequently used articulation therapy technique before a new technique is presented to the clinicians in a workshop. The coordinator also wishes to find out if the clinicians would be more likely to change their techniques after the presentation. However, he or she needs to avoid the problem of pretest sensitization to treatment, a problem of external validity. Therefore, the investigator randomly selects two subgroups of clinicians in the district and randomly assigns the groups to the experimental and control conditions. One of the groups is pretested about the techniques of articulation therapy they use. Then they receive a presentation on the new articulation therapy whose effects are ignored. The other group, in the absence

C R O (X)
E R X O

Figure 7-12. The separate sample pretest–posttest design.

of the pretest, receives the same information. The posttest evaluates the effects of the presentation in terms of any change in the clinicians' inclination to use the new technique.

The results of a separate-sample pretest–posttest design can be analyzed with the parametric independent sample *t* test or nonparametric Mann-Whitney U or median test.

The separate-sample pretest–posttest design is one of the weaker group designs as it does not control for the effects of history, maturation, and differential subject attrition. Once again, like all of the quasi-experimental designs, it is used when a more appropriate design is not feasible.

TIME-SERIES DESIGNS

The designs described so far, including the true experimental designs, involve at the most only two measures of the dependent variable: one taken before the introduction of the independent variable and one after the introduction. The typical pre- and posttreatment measures of the dependent variable may be sufficient to demonstrate the effect of the independent variable from a statistical standpoint. However, those measures do not give a total picture of the initial stability of the phenomenon and the subsequent systematic changes caused by the changes in the experimental conditions. An alternative strategy that tracks the dependent variable more often than the pretest–posttest designs consists of time-series designs. These designs are also classified under quasi-experimental designs.

In the time-series designs, the dependent variable is observed on several occasions both before and after the introduction of the independent variable. The time-series designs are a group of flexible designs that can be used with single subjects or groups of subjects and with one or more independent variables. They can be used with independent variables that have relatively temporary or permanent effects. They are especially suited for studying changes in social behaviors that are a result of new social or legal policies.

There are many time-series designs and it is not possible to review them all here. Interested readers should consult other sources (Cook & Campbell, 1979; Glass, Wilson, & Gottman, 1974). A few of the typical time-series designs are presented here.

Single-Group Time-Series Designs

In the basic single-group time-series design, one group of subjects is observed several times before and after the introduction of an independent variable. The design has several variations. In the simplest form of the design, there is a single *temporary* treatment before and after which the dependent variable is measured several times.

The design is illustrated in Figure 7–13. The diagram shows that the treatment was applied once to a single group of subjects. The dependent variable was measured four times before and four times after the introduction of the treatment. This design is also called a *simple interrupted time-series design* (Cook & Campbell, 1979). The multiple measures before the treatment provide a better picture of the variability, if any, in the dependent variable before the application of treatment. Repeated observations after the treatment can help establish the durability of the treated behaviors over time.

A temporary treatment of the kind suggested in the design is used frequently in clinical sciences. A group of aphasic patients may be observed repeatedly by obtaining several conversational language samples before introducing a treatment program. The treatment may be continued for several days before it is terminated. Then the language samples may be resumed for the next several days or weeks in an effort to monitor the maintenance of the treatment effect.

The basic time-series design shown in Figure 7-13 has several variations. The first involves the continuation of treatment during *some* of the posttreatment measures of the dependent variable. This design is illustrated in Figure 7–14, which shows that the first four measures were taken before treatment and only the last two were truly the posttreatment measures. Measures 5 and 6 were made while the subjects were still receiving the treatment, suggested by the line under X and the respective O measures. In our earlier example of research on the treatment of aphasia, the treatment may be continued until two measures of the dependent variable have been recorded before it is withdrawn.

In a second variation of the single-group time-series design, treatment is continued while the dependent variable is measured. This design is illustrated in Figure 7–15. The measurement of the dependent variable is continuous

---

O_1 O_2 O_3 O_4 X O_5 O_6 O_7 O_8

Figure 7-13. A time-series single-group design with temporary single treatment.

O_1 O_2 O_3 O_4 $\underline{X}$ $\underline{O_5}$ $\underline{O_6}$ O_7 O_8

Figure 7-14. A single-group time-series design with continuous treatment and withdrawal.

$$O_1 \quad O_2 \quad O_3 \quad O_4 \quad \underline{X} \quad O_5 \quad O_6 \quad O_7 \quad O_8$$

Figure 7-15. A single-group time-series design with single continuous treatment.

in the design suggested by the underlining of X and all of the subsequent measures of the dependent variables.

The design is better able to track the effects of the treatment, since it measures the dependent variable during the course of the treatment. In an institution for the retarded, for example, a group language treatment program may be instituted after several measures of the clients' language have been taken. The periodic language sampling is then continued throughout the course of the treatment. In contrast, the traditional pre- and posttests are inadequate for the purposes of documenting the course of therapeutic changes that take place over an extended period of time.

The design is often used in social research. In many cases, the repeated measures of a dependent variable before treatment may have already been recorded simply as a matter of routine organizational policy. For example, a state department of motor vehicles may keep the records of bodily injuries sustained by people in traffic accidents. An investigator may gain access to such information recorded over a period of time. Incidentally, information of this kind is often called archival data. Such archival data can be used as the repeated pretreatment measures. Then the state legislature may pass a mandatory seat-belt law that requires all drivers and passengers to wear seat belts. The frequency of accidents involving bodily injury will continue to be recorded, providing the necessary repeated posttests. The treatment (the new law) continues to be applied while the dependent variable is measured. A significant reduction in the frequency of bodily injury reports in the absence of a significant change in the accident rates may be interpreted as a favorable effect of the seat-belt law.

In the example just given, it must be noted that the repeated measurements of the dependent variable do not necessarily involve the same group of subjects. The persons who had accidents before the seat-belt law went into effect may not be the same as those who had them after the law went into effect. In other words, people who get into accidents do not constitute a single static group, although some individuals may have a longer membership in that group. In all probability, it is a group whose membership keeps changing. Therefore, in such situations, the measurements of the dependent variable are taken on *replicated groups.* A replicated groups measure contrasts with a *repeated group* measure. In this latter case, subjects in the same group are measured repeatedly. This would be the case in a majority of time-series designs.

A third variation of the single-group time-series design consists of repeated measures and two or more treatments. The design is illustrated in Figure 7–16.

$O_1 \quad O_2 \quad O_3 \quad X_1 \quad O_4 \quad O_5 \quad O_6 \quad X_2 \quad O_7 \quad O_8 \quad O_9$

Figure 7-16. A single-group time–series design with multiple temporary treatments.

The diagram shows that after obtaining three measures of the dependent variable, the first treatment (X_1) was introduced. After the treatment was terminated, three more measures were obtained. Then, a second treatment was introduced (X_2), followed by three more observations of the dependent variables. The design can be extended to include additional treatments.

This design may be used in the evaluation of the temporary effects of two or more treatments on the same behavior. A program to teach language to a group of autistic children may contain two different treatment procedures. A language "stimulation" program that does not focus on specific elements of language (X_1) may be evaluated against a program in which selected grammatical features are taught (X_2). The treatments are interrupted by a series of measurements of the dependent variable. In implementing a study such as this, it is necessary to have measures of dependent variables that are independent of each other. Besides, the selected target behaviors must be equally easy or hard to learn.

The single-group time-series design with multiple treatments can be implemented with continuous treatment. After the initial set of observations, the first treatment is initiated and the measurement of the effects is continued until the treatment is terminated. The second treatment is then introduced and the measurement continued until the conclusion of the experiment.

All the single-group time-series designs described so far may be used with single subjects as well. In fact, multiple observations before, during, and after treatment are one of the most important characteristics of single-subject designs. There are, however, some important differences between the single-subject and the time-series designs. In single-subject designs, the pretreatment observations are continued until the dependent variable shows an operational degree of stability. There is no such requirement in the time-series designs. Therefore, the pretreatment measurements are made a certain number of predetermined times. Furthermore, single-subject designs typically do not use archival data. More importantly, single-subject designs differ in terms of how control is achieved. For instance, after a treatment is withdrawn, it is rarely reintroduced in a time-series design, but such reintroductions of treatment are typical of many single-subject designs (see Chapter 8 for details).

The analysis of the time-series designs involves complex statistical procedures, most of them designed especially for the kind of data generated by the strategy. The techniques are unique and involved. A set of techniques often employed uses an *integrated moving average model*. It is a statistical analysis which takes into account the change in the level of the repeated measures and change in the slope. Whether or not there was a slope may also be considered in the analysis.

A serious limitation of single-group time-series designs is the lack of control over extraneous variables, especially those included in the history. The changes recorded at the time the independent variable was introduced into a time series may have been due to some other variables in the life of the subjects. The design is not able to rule out directly the influence of extraneous variables. However, when the repeated measures are reasonably stable before the introduction of the treatment, and an abrupt and dramatic change is recorded soon after the introduction, the data may strongly suggest a relation that can be confirmed with additional research using designs that permit greater control.

The investigator has less confidence in the results of a single-group time-series design if the changes are small and gradual or highly variable, or when a clear trend in the data was evident in the predicted direction from the very beginning of the study. With regard to this last point, if the pretreatment measures of language in a language treatment research project showing an increasing trend from the beginnings of observation, the introduction of the treatment program, even when associated with a greater change than the usual, creates problems for interpretation. In such cases, one suspects an interaction of some sort whose nature and extent are not clear in the design.

Multiple-Group Time-Series Designs

The single-group time-series designs can be extended to include two or more groups. However, the groups in a time-series are not randomly drawn from a population, and therefore they do not have sampling equivalence. Usually, intact groups are used in these designs.

There are several variations of the multiple-group time-series design and it is not possible to describe them all here. A basic multi-group time-series design has two nonequivalent groups, one of which is exposed to the treatment variable. Both the groups are repeatedly measured for the dependent variable before and after the experimental manipulation in one of the groups. This design is illustrated in Figure 7–17. It shows four measures before and four measures after the introduction of the independent variable in the experimental

E	O_1	O_2	O_3	O_4	X	O_5	O_6	O_7	O_8
C	O_1	O_2	O_3	O_4		O_5	O_6	O_7	O_8

Figure 7-17. A nonequivalent two-group time-series design.

group. The dependent variable in the control group is also measured to the same extent.

The design is similar to the nonequivalent control group design (see Figure 7–11) except that the dependent variable is measured repeatedly. The suggestions offered earlier on how to form the two nonequivalent groups are relevant here also.

Compared with the single-group design, the two-group design, even without sampling equivalence, is better because the investigator has a chance to compare treatment with a no-treatment control group. If the repeated measures of the dependent variable do not show significant change, while such a change was evident soon after the independent variable was introduced into the experimental group, the possibility of a cause–effect relation is increased.

All the designs illustrated in Figures 17–13 through 7–16 can be modified into two-group or multi-group time-series designs by adding one or more groups. An added group can receive treatment when the purpose is to evaluate the relative effects of two treatments. When people in institutions or cities serve as experimental groups, people in other comparable institutions or cities may serve as the control groups.

An interesting multi-group time-series design involves two staggered treatments. The design, illustrated in Figure 7–18, shows two groups that each receive a different treatment but in a staggered sequence. Possibly, treating both the groups simultaneously may be impractical for reasons of money or personnel. In such cases, one group is treated first and the second group next. In clinical research, one group of clients may be treated first and those on the waiting list next. When measures are repeated before and after the treatment (or during it), a staggered multigroup time-series design is in effect.

Summary and Summative Evaluation of Quasi-Experimental Designs

Quasi-experimental designs are eminently practical because they do not insist upon the random selection and assignment of subjects to groups of a study. For the same reason, they are considered weaker than true experimental designs. There is usually no assurance of sampling equivalence within most of the quasi-experimental design.

$$O_1 \ O_2 \ O_3 \ O_4 \ O_5 \ O_6$$

$$O_1 \ O_2 \ O_3 \ O_4 \ O_5 \ O_6$$

Figure 7-18. A two group time-series design with two staggered treatments.

Quasi-experimental designs are appropriate for naturalistic studies conducted in nonlaboratory situations. The nonequivalent control group design and the separate sample pretest–posttest design are two of the basic quasiexperimental designs. The nonequivalent control group design is similar to the pretest–posttest control group design. However, there is no assurance of sampling equivalence in this quasiexperimental design. In the separate sample pretest–posttest design, the random procedure is used to assign subjects to the two groups of a study, but they may or may not be drawn randomly from a population. An interesting feature of this design is the presentation of an irrelevant independent variable to the control group.

Of the quasi-experimental designs, the time-series designs are probably more useful. In time-series designs, dependent variables are measured repeatedly both before and after the introduction of treatment. There are both controlled and uncontrolled varieties of the time-series design.

Time-series designs, despite their lack of sampling equivalence, are useful in showing systematic changes in the dependent variable over a period of time. The multiple measures taken before and after the treatment can demonstrate the reliability of the measures better than the single measures that are typical of the other group designs. Time-series designs are more flexible than other group designs. In terms of this flexibility and multiple measures of the dependent variables, time-series designs are similar to single-subject designs.

COUNTERBALANCED WITHIN-SUBJECTS DESIGNS

The common method of establishing cause–effect relations within the group design strategy involves two or more groups, but each group is exposed to at least one different condition of the design. In other words, the same subjects do not experience all conditions of the experiment. While measurement of the dependent variable is common to the groups, experimental manipulation is not. One group receives treatment while the other does not. Or, two groups each experience a different form of treatment. As a result, the basic strategy of analysis involves a comparison of different subjects performing under different conditions. For this reason, the group designs discussed so far are also appropriately called the between-groups strategy.

There are, however, designs within the group-strategy that do not compare the performance of different groups exposed to different conditions of an experiment. In these designs, subjects of all the groups are exposed to all the conditions of the experiment. Such designs are called within-subjects designs or counterbalanced designs. Other names for these designs include rotation experiments, crossover designs, and switchover designs. Of these, the term *crossover design* also refers to a particular type of counterbalanced within-subjects design.

In recent years, the term *within-subjects design* has been occasionally used to refer to single-subject designs. This usage is avoided here. For a long time, the term *within-subjects design* has been a part of the group-design terminology, and some of the group within-subject designs have been known since the early 1920s (Edwards, 1960; McCall, 1923). In order to avoid reference to single-subject designs, the term *counterbalanced within-subjects design* is used in this book.

There are some similarities between counterbalanced within-subjects designs and single-subject designs. In either strategy, there is no control group that does not receive treatment. Also, in both the strategies, each subject is said to serve as his or her own control. When a controlled condition is a part of an experiment, all subjects are assigned to it. Each subject experiences all the experimental conditions in both the strategies. Nevertheless, there are important philosophical and methodological differences between the two approaches. Counterbalanced within-subjects designs are a part of the group-design approach. The strategy typically uses two or more groups of subjects. It uses the random procedure in subject selection and the assignment process. The results of counterbalanced within-subjects designs are analyzed through inferential statistics. Most single-subject designs do not share these characteristics.

One-Group Single-Treatment Counterbalanced Design

The simplest form of a counterbalanced design can be seen when an investigator has only one group of subjects while evaluating the effects of a single treatment variable. The design is sometimes described as *ABBA* counterbalanced design, which should not be confused with the single-subject *ABAB* design.

The one-group single-treatment counterbalanced design has two conditions that are exposed to all of the subjects in the group: a no-treatment and a treatment condition. (In the *ABBA* terminology, the two conditions are designated *A* and *B*.) In exposing the subjects to the two conditions of the study, the investigator can follow one of three sequences: (1) all subjects first go through the control condition and then the experimental, (2) all subjects first go through the experimental and then the control condition, or (3) the subjects are divided into two subgroups, one of the subgroups goes through the first sequence, and the other goes through the second. (The two subgroups do not make it a two-group design. There is only one treatment, and the formation of two subgroups is a means of counterbalancing the experimental and control conditions.) The third sequence is the simplest form of counterbalancing, and therefore, one-group single-treatment counterbalanced designs often use it.

Suppose an investigator wishes to study the temporary effects of masking noise on stuttering with a single group of stutterers. After having selected the subjects, preferably on a random basis, the investigator forms two groups with equal number of subjects randomly. When the number of subjects is small, and typically they are in a counterbalanced design, the random procedure accomplishes very little. In any case, the two groups are then exposed to the noise and no-noise conditions in the counterbalanced order. One possible sequence of the design is represented in Figure 7–19. Of course, the sequence shown can be switched across the groups.

Whether the first group should go through the noise and no-noise sequence or vice versa may also be determined randomly. A toss of a coin may determine the initial sequence. If it is determined that the first group will experience the treatment condition (noise) first and the control condition (no-noise) next, the second group will automatically follow the opposite sequence. Thus, each half of the subjects will have been exposed to one of the two possible sequences.

The results of each of the conditions are pooled and averaged from the two groups. That is, the mean number of stutterings exhibited by all the subjects in the control condition is compared with the mean number of stutterings in the treatment condition. (This is yet another reason why the design is considered to have only one group.) If there is a significant difference between the two means as evaluated by a statistical test of significance, the possibility of an effect of the treatment variable is raised.

It must be clear that counterbalancing is done to make sure that a given order in which the conditions of a study are exposed to the subjects does not become a factor in itself. It is possible that when all the stutterers experience the noise condition first and then the control condition, their stuttering in the second condition may be higher or lower simply because of the previous condition. Counterbalancing, by having half the subjects experience one condition first and the other half experience the other condition first, seeks to balance the effects of order across the groups. In this sense, counterbalancing can be seen as a method of equating the order and sequence effects in the groups.

Counterbalancing can also be done on an individual basis. Using the random procedure, the sequence with which each subject experiences the two experimental conditions may be determined. For example, the first subject may go through the control–treatment sequence and the second subject may go through the treatment–control sequence. Care must be taken to ensure that there are equal numbers of subjects in both the sequences. This is referred

---

Sequence of Conditions

Subgroup 1   **Treatment → No-treatment**
Subgroup 2   **No-treatment → Treatment**

Figure 7-19. A one-group single-treatment counterbalanced design.

to as the *intrasubject counterbalancing.* The more typical counterbalancing of subgroups, shown in Figure 7–19, is called *intragroup counterbalancing.*

The one-group single-treatment counterbalanced design does not control for extraneous variables of history, maturation, testing, differential subject attrition, and so on. Though it includes a control condition, it does not fully control all or even most of the factors that affect internal validity. The control over the extraneous factors is increased if the same subjects, after having experienced no-treatment and treatment conditions, again experience a no-treatment condition. In this case, it becomes possible to show that changes in the dependent variables follow both the introduction and the removal of an independent variable. Such designs are typical within the single-subject strategy.

Crossover Design

Another counterbalanced within-subjects design is known as the crossover design. This design is an arrangement in which two treatment variables are evaluated with the help of two groups both of which are exposed to the two treatment variables in a crossover fashion. That is, halfway through an experiment, the subjects switch over to another treatment. The design is represented in Figure 7–20. The diagram shows that the groups are formed on a random basis and both the groups receive the two treatments selected for evaluation. Therefore, there is no control group that does not receive treatment.

A hypothetical example can clarify the design arrangement. Suppose a clinician wishes to evaluate the effects of two treatment approaches to the remediation of articulation disorders in school-age children. The clinician selects a random sample of children with multiple articulation problems and divides the sample into two randomly formed groups. The children who have specific speech sound errors may be selected, which would necessitate an access to a large number of children with those specific speech-sound errors. The subjects are pretested (O_1), for example, by standardized tests and conversational speech samples, to determine the specific speech sounds misarticulated by the children. Next, the order in which the groups will receive treatment is determined randomly. Each group then receives the two articulation treatments in a different order. The design requires an assessment

$$\text{R} \quad \text{E} \quad O_1 \quad X_1 \quad O_2 \quad X_2 \quad O_3$$
$$\text{R} \quad \text{E} \quad O_1 \quad X_2 \quad O_2 \quad X_1 \quad O_3$$

Figure 7-20. A crossover design with two treatments and two groups.

in the middle of the study when the subjects are crossed over to the other treatment. A final assessment at the end of the study is also required of both the groups.

Complex Counterbalanced Designs

When only one or two treatment variables are evaluated, the counterbalanced designs are relatively simple. Without much difficulty, the investigator can make sure that each treatment appears in the first and the second position in the sequence. However, experiments involving three or more treatments require complex counterbalanced arrangements. The basic requirement of counterbalancing is that each treatment appear at least once in each of all possible positions. To achieve this, the investigator must initially identify all possible sequences of the selected number of treatments.

A counterbalanced design involving only three treatments is already fairly complex. The three treatments *A*, *B*, and *C* combine into six sequences: *ABC*, *ACB*, *BAC*, *BCA*, *CAB*, and *CBA*. In this arrangement, each treatment appears twice in each of the initial, medial, and final positions. If the investigator were to use intrasubject counterbalancing, each subject would be randomly assigned to one of the six sequences. However, one must make sure that each order has a comparable number of subjects. This often results in ad hoc modifications in the random procedure. In intragroup counterbalancing, six comparable groups are initially formed, and each group is randomly assigned to one of the sequences.

A counterbalanced design with four treatments would have 24 sequences $(1 \times 2 \times 3 \times 4 = 24)$. However, when the number of treatments is increased by just one to a total of five, the number of sequences increases to a formidable 120 $(1 \times 2 \times 3 \times 4 \times 5 = 120)$. Obviously, arithmetic increases in the number of treatments result in factorial increases in the number of sequences that need to be counterbalanced. As a result, the need for subjects, the number of groups, or both increases dramatically. This can be a serious problem in clinical research where the required number of comparable clients with specific disorders may not be found. Because of these reasons, completely counterbalanced designs are generally limited to fewer than four treatment variables. Even then, the designs are used infrequently in clinical treatment research.

The practical difficulties involved in achieving complete counterbalancing of multiple treatment variables have led to a compromised procedure of incomplete counterbalancing. Some of the designs that use incomplete counterbalancing are also known as *Latin square designs*. In a Latin square design, each treatment in each position appears once and only once in each group. Therefore, conditions do not precede or follow each other in all sequences or in equal numbers. Therefore, not all combinations of multiple treatment variables are implemented in a Latin square design.

A Latin square arrangement is represented in Table 7–1. The numbers of groups, treatments, and positions (sequences) are all equal when a Latin square design is represented in the form of a table. Such a table has the same number of rows, columns, and cells in relation to any one group. The same four treatments (*ABCD* in the table shown) permit other combinations. A given set of treatments can be represented by different Latin squares. It must be emphasized that the arrangements of treatment sequences in a Latin square are limited. As noted before, complete counterbalancing of the four treatments shown in Table 7–1 would have required not 4 but 24 groups.

Limitations of Counterbalanced Within-Subjects Designs

When several treatments are administered to the same individual or the same group of subjects, several potential problems may make it difficult to interpret the results. One should take these limitations into consideration in designing and interpreting the studies of counterbalanced within-subjects designs. Some of these problems can be seen in a few single-subject designs as well.

Order Effects

When some or all of the effects of two or more treatments can be explained on the basis of the specific order in which they were administered, we have *order effects*. Obviously, designs with multiple treatments that are administered to the same subjects necessarily have an order. Therefore, order as a factor cannot be ruled out on a priori grounds.

The problem of the order effect can be understood clearly when two treatments are administered in a single, fixed order to all subjects. Suppose that an investigator wished to evaluate the relative (and interactive) effects of a new and an established articulation therapy. If the investigator were first to apply the traditional articulation therapy to all the clients and then to follow it with the new therapy, the results, especially of the new therapy, would be

Table 7-1.

One of the possible Latin square arrangements of four treatments in a counterbalanced design

	Order of Treatment			
Groups	1	2	3	4
I	A	B	C	D
II	B	A	D	C
III	C	D	A	B
IV	D	C	B	A

mostly uninterpretable. The effects observed during the administration of the new therapy may be due to the order in which it was administered. The investigator would not know whether the same results would be obtained if the treatments were to be administered in a different order.

The order effect is sometimes described as a practice effect. The second treatment may be more effective simply because of the increased familiarity with the experimental tasks, arrangements, and repeated practice of some of the response skills measured in the sessions. In other words, the treatment itself may not have contributed much to the changes observed in the dependent variable under treatment.

Theoretically, order effects are neutralized in a completely counterbalanced design, which provides for all possible orders in which the selected set of multiple treatments can be administered. However, when the orders included in a study do not exhaust all possible positions for all treatments, then the order effects cannot be ruled out. Generally, the greater the number of treatments, the harder it is to present each of them in every possible order, and the higher the chances of order effects.

Carryover Effects

The second problem associated with the administration of multiple treatments to the same subjects or group of subjects is known as multiple-treatment interference or carryover effects. They are also referred to as sequential confounding or sequential effects. While the order effect is due simply to the position in which a given treatment appears, the carryover effect is due to the influence of the previous treatment on the succeeding treatment. The prior treatment may have a positive or a negative effect on the succeeding treatment.

When the carryover effect is positive, the second treatment will appear stronger than it really is, and when the carryover effect is negative, the second treatment may appear weaker than it is. When administered alone, they may produce effects that are different from those observed in a sequential arrangement. The carryover effects may be cumulative over repeated phases, or they may be limited to adjacent phases. Cumulative carryover effects show increasingly larger magnitude across experimental conditions.

Whether the carryover effects have occurred or not can be assessed in a completely counterbalanced design in which each treatment precedes and follows every other treatment more than once. The presence of a positive carryover effect is suggested when the effect of a treatment is typically larger when it follows a given treatment and smaller when it precedes the same given treatment. This relationship between two treatments is illustrated in Figure 7–21. A negative carryover effect is suggested when the effect of a treatment is typically smaller when it follows a given treatment and larger when it precedes the same treatment. This relationship is illustrated in Figure 7–22.

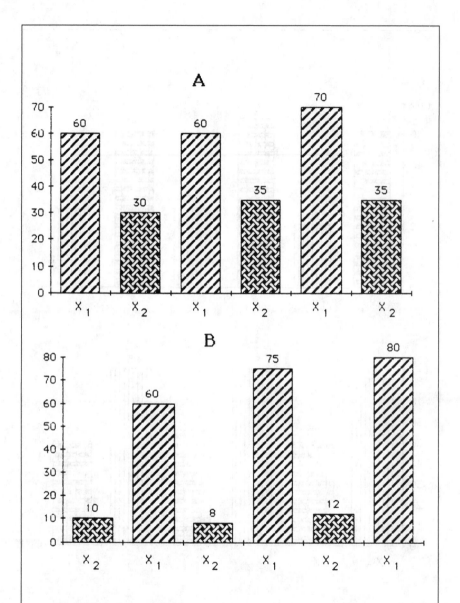

Figure 7-21. Positive carryover from treatment 1 (X_1) to treatment 2 (X_2). Note that treatment 2 had a larger effect when it followed treatment 1 (**A**) than when it preceded treatment 1 (**B**).

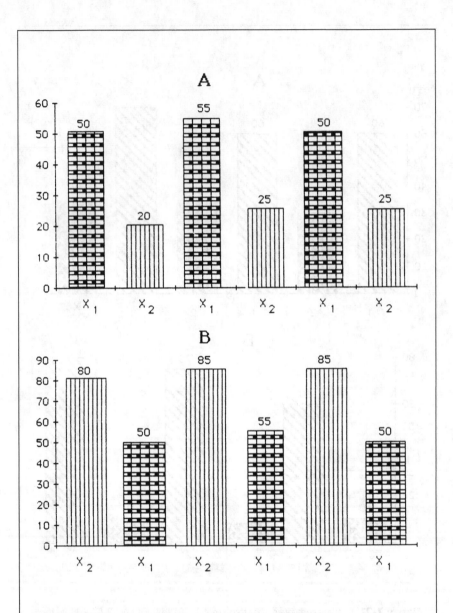

Figure 7-22. Negative carryover from treatment 1 (X_1) to treatment 2 (X_2). Note that treatment 2 had a smaller effect when it followed treatment 1 (**A**) than when it preceded treatment 1 (**B**).

Ceiling and Floor Effects

Another set of problems associated with counterbalanced multiple-treatment designs is known as the ceiling and floor effects. The ceiling effect refers to the maximum extent of change produced by a prior treatment, as a result of which the next treatment has no room to show its effect. In a study done to evaluate the effects of two treatments on stuttering, the first method may reduce stuttering to a very low level, perhaps less than 1 percent. When the second treatment is applied, only a minimal reduction in stuttering may be evident. This small change associated with the second treatment be due to the ceiling effect created by the first treatment.

As long as the first treatment has any effect at all, the second treatment in a sequence starts with a different "floor" created by the first. The floor, or the base level of performance, may be high or low, depending upon the effect of the previous treatment. This can also limit the extent of change that a variable can produce. This phenomenon is often referred to as the floor effect, which is actually a counterpart of the ceiling effect.

The ceiling and floor effects are dramatic when one treatment is stronger than the other. However, the effect can be seen when both are equally strong. In this case, the first treatment creates a ceiling effect on the second treatment, and the effect is mutual. Automatically, a new floor is created for the next treatment.

Most of the problems associated with counterbalanced designs discussed so far do not exist when all the treatments being evaluated are equally ineffective. Also, the problems are not serious when the treatments have only a temporary effect. That is, when the effects of a treatment disappear as soon as the treatment is stopped, the carryover, ceiling, or floor effects are not serious considerations. Therefore, the designs are more applicable to behaviors that take a relatively long time to change permanently but can show temporary but clear-cut changes in the short term.

Summary and Summative Evaluation of Counterbalanced Within-Subjects Designs

Counterbalanced within-subjects designs are those that expose all subjects of a group to all the conditions of a study. There are no groups that do not receive treatment within a counterbalanced within-subjects design. However, they are still a variety of group design and, as such, should not be confused with single-subject designs.

The one-group single-treatment design and the crossover design are the simpler of the counterbalanced within-subjects designs. In the one-group single-treatment counterbalanced design, the subjects are divided into two groups, and each group follows an opposite sequence of treatment and no-treatment conditions. In the crossover design, two randomly formed groups of subjects initially receive two different treatments and then cross over to the other treatment.

Complex counterbalanced within-subjects designs are not very practical in clinical research because of the difficulty involved in counterbalancing all the sequences in which different treatments are presented. Ideally, when multiple treatments are evaluated, all combinations and sequences are used so that the order effects are neutralized. This then creates a need for many subjects, who are divided into subgroups. However, complex counterbalanced designs do permit evaluations of multiple treatment variables. Problems involved in presenting all conditions of a study to all of the subjects include the order effect, the carryover effect, and the ceiling and floor effects.

CORRELATIONAL ANALYSIS DESIGN

The final type of group research design to be considered is variously called correlational analysis design, correlational design, or correlational studies. Most of the designs considered so far permit some form of manipulation of an independent variable. In a correlational analysis, there is no possibility of experimental manipulation of an independent variable. Therefore, the correlational analysis designs are not experimental designs. Many of the studies using correlational analysis are of the ex post facto variety described in Chapter 4. Therefore, our discussion of these designs will be brief.

A correlation is a statistical procedure that suggests that two events are somehow related. The relation may be positive or negative. Possibly, no relation may be revealed when a suspected relation is tested. A correlation is positive when the measured values of two variables are equally high or low; the variables seem to change in the same direction. When one increases, the other also increases, and vice versa. The negative correlation is evident when one variable is high, the other is low and vice versa. A negative correlation suggests that when one event increases, the other decreases. Two events are not related (neutral) when their measured values do not correspond in any particular way.

Such measured values of two variables may be subjected to certain statistical analysis to derive a correlation coefficient which ranges between a perfect negative correlation of −1.00 to a perfect positive correlation of +1.00. Actual correlational coefficients rarely reach these perfect values. Even if the events are perfectly correlated, the measurements are not perfect, and therefore the correlation will not reach either −1.00 or +1.00.

When an independent variable is not manipulable, one may look for natural events that seem to be related in some specific manner. Two selected variables may be measured once or repeatedly to determine if the measures reflect systematic changes in one or the other direction. A correlation coefficient is calculated for the measured values. Significant positive or negative correlations are interpreted to suggest a relation between the variables.

A correlation does not prove a cause–effect relation. Even if two events are causally related, the correlation itself does not specify which is the cause and which is the effect. Once a significant correlation is found, causes and effects are usually sorted out on the basis of prevailing theories and empirical knowledge. For example, when it is shown that academic performance and intelligence are highly (and positively) correlated, one concludes that the intelligence is the cause of better academic performance on the basis of available knowledge about these two variables. Such conclusions are not firm statements regarding functional relations between variables that are correlated. In many cases, causal relation inferred from correlation may be totally erroneous: two variables may be correlated because they are both an effect of a third variable not observed by the investigator at all.

Once significant correlations between certain events have been found, one may design experimental studies in which one of the variables is manipulated to see what effects follow. Unless this kind of experimental research is performed and the extraneous variables ruled out, it is not possible to draw firm conclusions regarding the meaning of correlations.

It is obvious that correlation is a statistical method of data analysis, not an experimental design in which variables are manipulated, controlled, and measured. As a statistical procedure, it is seen most frequently in the ex post facto type of research.

GROUP DESIGNS IN CLINICAL RESEARCH

The group design strategy described in this chapter has evolved over many years of research in several disciplines. The most significant impetus to this design strategy has come from the development of mathematical, psychological, and agricultural statistics. Research needs in agricultural, psychological, social, and biological sciences have shaped many of the methods, terms, and strategies used in the group approach. The statistical theory of probability, random selection and assignment of subjects, inferential statistical analyses of differences in the mean performance measures of groups, evaluation of the effects of independent variables against a background of "chance variability," and extension of the conclusions to the population from which the sample was drawn are all distinguishing characteristics of the group design strategy.

The group design strategy, like any other strategy, has its strengths and weaknesses. It works better with certain kinds of research problems investigated in certain settings. It does not work as well with certain other kinds of problems faced in other settings. From a theoretical standpoint, the group design approach offers an attractive and efficient strategy for investigating research questions. Various designs make it possible to isolate a cause–effect relation between events. The object of all scientific inquiry is to develop evidence of generality, though special cases are also of scientific interest. Nevertheless, most events cannot be studied in the population as a whole, and therefore we need sampling techniques. Statistics has shown that a randomly selected representative sample can help extend the conclusions of the sample to the population.

Significant problems arise when the same strategy that has worked well in large-scale social, agricultural, and certain kinds of psychological research is applied to clinical problems of treatment evaluation. To be sure, the clinician is also interested in drawing conclusions that apply to the clinical populations, not just to one or two clients that he or she may conduct research on. However, the nature of the everyday clinical business at hand and the feasible strategies of clinical research make the widespread application of statistical approach impractical.

The biggest problem a clinician faces is to achieve sampling equivalence of groups through random procedures to investigate questions of treatment effectiveness. Clinical populations are generally not accessible for random sampling. Populations with language, articulation, fluency, and voice problems are not readily available for random sampling in which every patient or client has an equal chance of being selected for the study. Assuming that this problem is somehow solved, the clinician faces the next hurdle in the implementation of the group strategy. It is difficult to evaluate clinical treatments in large groups. Much clinical work is specific to the individual. In nonclinical research the independent variables can be presented in groups. A film on attitudes or "sensitivity," a set of slides that are supposed to change subjects' rated moods, a training program designed to enhance sales clerks' skills, and so on can be easily presented in groups. However, in a treatment method with various steps in which individual clients' behaviors have to be changed to a substantial degree, group presentation of the independent variable is inefficient at best and useless at worst. Whenever it is tried, the worst case is realized more often than the best case.

Within the group strategy, the changes produced by the independent variables can be small but the study can be considered a success. Since there are statistical techniques to identify changes that are not clear when visually inspected, small changes in clients' behaviors under treatment can be considered successful. Such small changes may certainly have theoretical significance and clinical potential, but they are not of immediate clinical significance. However, in clinical sciences, the changes in stuttering or language disorders induced by experimental or routine therapies must be large enough to make a difference in the lives of the clients. A statistical difference at the .001 level may or may not correspond to the magnitude of change required by real-life conditions. Therefore, the clinician painstakingly shapes and changes individual behaviors to a point where even a lay person can recognize those changes. Once this is done, the use of statistical techniques that are especially designed to detect small changes seems unnecessary as well as unimaginative. When one can talk about individuals in a meaningful manner, the statistical average is as irrelevant as it is mythical.

The relevance of inferential generality to clinical work is typically overestimated. When a clinician reads a report on a new treatment technique in a professional journal, he or she is not especially worried about the population of clients to which the conclusions may be applied. Such a concern about the behavior of the population is real to a politician seeking a majority vote, but the clinician faces a different kind of problem. The clinician's immediate concern is whether the treatment is applicable to a few individual clients he or she may be working with. This means that the clinician's immediate concern is logical, not inferential, generality. Group designs do not offer much help in this regard.

When the group strategy is used in clinical sciences, the research tends to be nonexperimental. Ex post facto, normative, standard-group comparison studies dominate the group approach to research. Experimental research in which cause–effect relations are analyzed with randomly drawn and assigned experimental and control groups are few and far between. When the group experimental method is employed, the random sampling procedure is often not used. Therefore, the results have neither inferential nor logical generality. The difficulties involved in forming large enough clinical groups representative of the populations necessary to conduct experimental treatment evaluations have resulted in sparse experimental data.

We shall not attempt a more complete evaluation of the group research strategy here, as that will be done in Chapter 10. Because the advantages and disadvantages of a given approach are better understood in a comparative context, we shall evaluate both group and single-subject design strategies after we have considered the latter in the next chapter.

CHAPTER SUMMARY

Group designs were originally developed in agricultural and social research. They are based on the theory of probability. The group design approach requires the formation of two or more groups for the purposes of experimentation. The groups may be formed on the basis of either random selection of subjects from a defined population or by matching subjects of similar characteristics. The basic method of group designs is to initially have two or more comparable groups that represent the population from which they were drawn (especially when the random procedure is used). At the least, one of the groups receives a treatment variable and another group does not. Table 7-2 offers a summary of major group designs and the kinds of questions they can address.

Typically, the performance of the two groups is measured before and after the presentation of an independent variable to the experimental group. The

Table 7-2.

Summary of major group designs and their applications

Designs	Research Questions	Strengths/Limitations
One-shot case study (pp. 6-7)	Does the history suggest a cause?	Clinically useful; results are only suggestive.
One-group pretest–posttest design (pp. 7-9)	Is there an apparent change due to treatment?	Clinically useful; lacks control; cannot isolate cause–effect relations.
Static-group comparisons (pp. 9-10)	Does a treated group differ from an untreated group?	Uses existing treated and untreated groups; lacks pretests.
Pretest–posttest control group design (pp. 16-20)	Is a treatment effective? Is there a cause–effect relation?	True experimental design; well-controlled; can isolate cause–effect relation; often clinically impractical.
Posttest-only control group design (pp. 20-22)	Is a treatment effective? Is there a cause–effect relation?	Well-controlled when randomization is used; clinically impractical.
Solomon four-group design (pp. 22-25)	Is there an interaction between pretest and treatment, and if so to what extent?	Useful in studies on reactive variables, but impractical in clinical research.
Multigroup pretest–posttest design (pp. 26-27)	Is one treatment more effective than the other? What are the relative effects of treatments?	Well-controlled; useful to the extent practical; clinically important.
Multigroup posttest–only design (pp. 27-28)	Is one treatment more effective than the other? What are the relative effects of treatments?	Well-controlled; useful to the extent practical; lacks pretests.
Factorial designs: randomized blocks or completely randomized factorial (pp. 28-36)	What are the effects of two or more treatments? Is there an interaction between treatments or between treatments and client characteristics?	Excellent designs to study interaction; the most effective strategy to study interaction between subject characteristics and treatment. Difficult to find enough subjects in clinical research.

Designs	Research Questions	Strengths/Limitations
Single-group time series design (pp. 44-50)	Is there a change following treatment? Do multiple treatments seem to produce changes?	Multiple measures help demonstrate changes in dependent variables. Relative effects of treatment can be evaluated, but the designs are not controlled.
Multiple-group time-series designs (pp. 50-52)	Is a treatment effective? What are the relative effects of two or more treatments?	Multiple groups assure some control; multiple measures help demonstrate reliability. But, no sampling equivalence.
One-group single-treatment counterbalanced design (pp. 54-57)	Do treatment and no-treatment conditions differ significantly?	Has a control condition instead of a group. Clinically useful design.
Crossover design (pp. 57-58)	Do the same subjects react differently to two different treatments?	Useful when two treatments must be exposed to the same subjects. Control is relatively weak.
Correlational analysis (pp. 65-67)	Do the selected variables covary?	Can show covariation, not causation.

performance of the groups is expressed in terms of the statistical mean, which is used in evaluating the effects of the independent variable. Such an evaluation usually consists of various statistical analyses of data to determine if the differences in the mean posttest scores of the groups are due to the experimental variable.

True experimental designs make it possible to evaluate the effects of various independent variables. There are many designs within the group strategy, but the basic pretest–posttest control group design is the prototype of this strategy. However, when complete randomization of subject selection is assured, the posttest may be avoided. This results in the posttest-only control group design. An extended design with four groups, known as the Solomon four-group design, may be used when the pretest sensitization is expected to interact with the treatment variable.

Group designs that permit the evaluation of multiple treatments include the multigroup pretest–posttest design, the multigroup posttest-only design, and the factorial designs. In the former two designs, different groups of subjects experience different treatment variables. Factorial designs help assess not only the effects of multiple treatments but also any interactions between those treatments. Besides, they can help determine an interaction between treatment variables and subject characteristics (assigned variables).

Quasi-experimental designs are those that do not have full control on extraneous variables. Nevertheless, they are useful in identifying potential causal relations, which may be further verified through one of the true experimental designs. Of the many quasi-experimental designs, time-series designs are especially useful in clinical research. In the time-series designs, the dependent variable is measured on several occasions both before and after treatment. Therefore, the dependent variable measures may be more reliable than the single pretest and posttest measures. Time-series designs are also highly flexible. The dependent variables may be measured as often as necessary. Measures may be repeated during the treatment as well. Besides, one or more groups may be used in evaluating the effects of single or multiple treatments.

Counterbalanced within-subjects designs are a variation of group designs. In these designs, all the subjects of a study are exposed to all the experimental conditions. Each subject experiences a control condition and an experimental condition. If multiple treatments are evaluated, different combinations of treatment are presented in a counterbalanced manner. Counterbalanced designs are capable of evaluating multiple treatments although such designs tend to be complex and impractical. The limitations of counterbalanced designs include the order effect, the carryover effect, and the ceiling and floor effects. Most of these problems arise when the counterbalancing is not complete and treatments produce strong, relatively permanent effects.

Finally, the group design strategy offers correlational analysis designs based on statistical methods of correlation. These are not experimental designs because correlational studies do not involve manipulation of independent variables. The studies seek to find out if two events are related, and if so whether the relation is positive or negative. Possibly, one may find that the two events are not related in a systematic manner. Correlational designs do not permit statements on causation, but a relation found within these designs may be verified by one of the experimental designs.

Group designs are powerful tools when the requirements of the sampling equivalence based on the random procedure can be fulfilled. In clinical research, this is often not possible. Well-done group design studies are able to demonstrate internal validity, but external validity requires replication. Group designs permit inferential generality, but this type of generality may not be very useful in predicting the performance of individual clients in clinical situations. ■

S T U D Y **G U I D E**

1. Distinguish between statistics and research designs. Specify why statistics should not be equated with research designs.

2. Whose work specifies an entirely statistical approach to research?

3. What is sampling equivalence? How is it achieved in the group strategy?

4. How frequently are the dependent variables measured in most of the group designs?

5. Can a "control" group ever receive treatment?

6. What do X's, Y's O's, and R's stand for in a diagram showing experimental designs?

7. What are preexperimental designs?

8. What is the greatest weakness of a one-shot case study?

9. What statistical tests may be used in the analysis of results of a one-group pretest–posttest design?

10. Describe how a one-group pretest–posttest control group design would not be able to demonstrate internal validity of its results.

11. Give a hypothetical example of the static-group design. Use a clinical problem for illustration.

12. What are the limitations of preexperimental designs?

13. What is the main mechanism through which true experimental designs rule out the influence of extraneous variables?

14. Describe two methods of drawing a random sample from a population.

15. Why is randomization considered the best method of achieving sampling equivalence?

16. Distinguish between random selection and random assignment of subjects. What different functions do they serve?

17. Describe two methods of matching subjects. What are the limitations of matching?

18. Draw a diagram of the pretest–posttest control group design.

19. A clinician wishes to evaluate the effects of a language treatment procedure with the help of the pretest–posttest control group design. The subjects are school-age children. Design this study and justify its procedure.

(continued next page)

Study Guide *(continued)*

20. Specify one incorrect and one correct method of analyzing the results of the pretest–posttest control group design.

21. Describe the factors of internal invalidity the pretest–posttest control group design does and does not control for.

22. Are pretests absolutely necessary in a true experimental design? Why or why not?

23. What specific problem is the Solomon four-group design thought to avoid?

24. What are the limitations of the Solomon four-group design? What is your alternative to using that design?

25. Suppose you wish to evaluate the effects of three treatment techniques used in the management of stuttering. What would be your experimental design? Draw a diagram of the design.

26. What are factorial designs? What purposes do they serve?

27. Describe a randomized blocks design. Give an example, complete with all the variables involved.

28. How many conditions or cells does a 2×3 factorial design have?

29. Define a "block" and a "level" in a factorial design.

30. Describe a completely randomized factorial design. Identify all the levels, variables, and cells. How many subjects do you need? How do you plan to get them?

31. What are quasi-experimental designs? When do you use them?

32. In what respect does the nonequivalent control group design differ from the pretest–posttest control group design?

33. What is meant by intact experimental and control groups? Give examples.

34. Illustrate the use of a separate sample pretest–posttest design with an example of your own.

35. What is the most important characteristic of time-series designs?

36. A clinician evaluated a certain treatment procedure used in the management of language disorders. The clinician measured the language performance of the clients four times before starting treatment. The treatment was then applied for three months. Finally, the clinician took four more measures of language behaviors in the absence of treatment. What kind of design did the clinician use? What kinds of conclusions were possible?

37. Draw a diagram of a single-group time-series design with continuous treatment and withdrawal.

38. In a time-series design, can treatment be continued while the dependent variable is measured? If so, what is the name of the design?

39. Demonstrate how you can evaluate the effects of two or more treatments in a time-series design. Illustrate your answer.

40. Show how a control group can be built into a time-series design.

41. What are counterbalanced within-subjects designs?

42. As described in the text, are within-subjects designs the same as single-subject designs? Justify your answer.

43. Illustrate a one-group single-treatment counterbalanced design. Identify your variables, experimental conditions, and the sequences.

44. What is a crossover design? Do you evaluate a single treatment or multiple treatments in this design?

45. What is a Latin square design? What are its limitations?

46. Define "order effects." How do you handle them in a counterbalanced within-subjects design?

47. Distinguish between positive and negative carryover effects. Give examples.

48. Distinguish between ceiling and floor effects. Under what conditions are they significant in a study?

49. What are the limitations of correlational analysis designs?

50. Evaluate the usefulness of group designs in clinical treatment research.

■ CHAPTER 8

Single-Subject Designs

■ Basic terminology and characteristics of single-subject designs, 217

■ Control mechanisms in single-subject designs, 221

■ Preexperimental single-subject design, 241

■ The ABA designs, 242

■ The BAB design, 246

■ The ABAB designs, 247

■ The multiple baseline designs, 250

■ Multiple treatment comparisons, 259

■ The ABACA/ACABA design, 259

■ The alternating treatments design, 261

■ Ineffective treatments in multiple treatment evaluations, 265

■ The interactional design, 266

■ The changing criterion design, 270

■ Designs to assess response maintenance, 271

■ Other single-subject designs, 273

■ Single-subject designs in clinical research, 275

■ Chapter summary, 276

■ Study guide, 279

I n the previous chapter, I described a research strategy in which the data represent the performance differences between groups of subjects. In this chapter, I shall describe a different strategy of research in which the data represent the performance of single subjects. The designs are therefore known as single-subject designs.

The single-subject design strategy is now well established, though the group strategy is still the most widely known and traditionally taught approach to research. Several outstanding books on this strategy are now available (Barlow, Hayes, & Nelson, 1984; Barlow & Hersen, 1984; Johnston & Pennypacker, 1980; Kazdin, 1982; McReynolds & Kearns, 1983; Sidman, 1960). The book by McReynolds and Kearns is the first one to be devoted entirely to the single-subject research strategy in communicative disorders. A series of three papers published in the *Journal of Speech and Hearing Disorders* offers an excellent overview of the single-subject methodology as well as single-subject clinical research in communicative disorders (Connell & Thompson, 1986; Kearns, 1986; McReynolds & Thompson, 1986). Clinicians should consult these sources, starting with the Sidman classic.

BASIC TERMINOLOGY AND CHARACTERISTICS OF SINGLE-SUBJECT APPROACH

Before we consider some of the technical aspects of single-subject designs, it is necessary to understand the basic characteristics of, and terminology used in, the single-subject approach. The single-subject designs are also described as single-case designs, intrasubject replication designs, and designs of behavioral analysis. As noted in Chapter 7, occasionally they are also referred to as within-subjects designs, a name not used here because of the existence of a variety of group designs to which it has been historically applied.

The single-subject approach, though fully developed by behavioral scientists, was used by early psychologists who studied psychophysics; physiologists and neurologists who studied individual differences in anatomy, physiology, and neurology; and psychiatrists who studied behavior disorders and their unique manifestations in individual clients. In fact, Broca's classic work in 1861 on the motor speech center in the brain was a single-subject study. However, most of the currently used single-subject designs were developed in the process of experimental and applied behavioral analysis.

The basic strategy of extended observation of a single organism and experimental manipulation came from animal laboratory research involving operant conditioning. Several of the currently popular designs were subsequently developed in the course of applied behavioral research. Most of the specific designs to be described were therefore necessitated by practical clinical considerations. The kinds of dependent and independent variables manipulated in these designs have been influenced to a great extent by behavioral philosophy. Nevertheless, the designs themselves are strategies of research, which can be used to answer questions that may or may not have come from behavioral philosophy.

One of the mistaken notions about single-subject or single-case designs is that only one subject can be used in a study. Though some reported studies may have had single subjects, the designs themselves are not restricted in this manner. Typically, multiple subjects, perhaps three to six, are used in most single-subject designs. In any case, the number of subjects used in single-subject designs is much smaller than in a group design.

The main concern of the single-subject approach is the behavior of an individual. Therefore, variations in an individual's behavior, or among a few individuals, are not treated as "errors" as they are in group designs. Such variations themselves may be subjects of experimental analysis. In any case, an effort to control or eliminate an individual person's behavioral variability under controlled conditions so that the effect of an independent variable becomes evident is one of the important characteristics of single-subject designs.

Because of its interest in behaviors of individuals, the single-subject strategy does not involve group comparisons. Instead of comparing the mean performance of subjects receiving treatment with the mean performance of subjects not receiving treatment, the single-subject strategy compares the same individual's performance under treatment and no-treatment conditions. Therefore, when several subjects are used in a study, the results are not averaged across individuals. Each subject's results are described separately.

The single-subject strategy places a heavy emphasis on the experimental methodology and philosophy of natural sciences. Theoretically, this should be true of group designs as well, but in practice, the enormous impact of statistics on that approach often detracts from the task of producing strong experimental effects in individual cases.

Single-subject designs must be distinguished from case studies in which one or a few individuals are researched. The typical case study is an ex post facto analysis of factors that may have been responsible for an effect, but it lacks experimental control. Case studies rely heavily on the method of correlation, not experimentation. On the other hand, single-subject designs are experimental and therefore attempt to establish cause–effect relations between events.

Single-subject designs require repeated measurement of the dependent variables. There are no pre- and posttests, as in the group design approach. Both the terminology and the practice of pre- and posttests are determined mostly by educational research and methods. The dependent variables are not tested but measured continuously: before, during, and after treatment. Such continuous measures give a better picture of the course of changes in the dependent variables than the two-point measures of pre- and posttests.

The repeated measures made before the introduction of treatment are typically known as baselines or steady-states, and some measures made after treatment are known as probes.

In the single-subject strategy, the subject selection process is not dependent upon the random theory and procedure. With a few restrictions, available individual subjects are considered appropriate for experimental analysis. Since no effort is made to have a representative sample of a population, the conclusions of the study are not extended to the population on the basis of a single study or a few studies. The approach is based on the assumption that generality, including inferential generality, is a matter of replication. Since even the most representative sample is not likely to have all kinds of generalities, it is not critical to strive for the mostly unmet but always recommended goal of a randomly selected representative sample.

The results of single-subject designs are generally not analyzed with the help of statistical techniques. There are at least two reasons for this. The first is that the experimental effects produced in single-subject designs are large enough to support conclusions without statistical analyses. Most statistical techniques are designed to detect small changes in dependent variables against a background of poorly controlled natural variability. In other words, single-subject designs depend upon empirical significance in differences in conditions, not statistical differences. When conditions of an experiment differ markedly, visual inspection of data will reveal the effects of experimental manipulations. Therefore, in reading and evaluating single-subject studies, visual inspection plays a major role.

Figure 8-1 shows the difference between the group and the single-subject data of a hypothetical study. If a certain treatment of stuttering is evaluated within a two-group study and also a single subject study, the kinds of results that are depicted in Figure 8-1 are likely . The data in the single-subject design, (A), make the effects of treatment visually obvious. On the other hand, whether the difference in the mean frequency of stutterings of the two groups, (B) is due to the treatment or chance fluctuations is better determined by statistical analysis.

The second reason for not using statistical procedures in the analysis of single-subject designs is that a majority of techniques are based on the random theory and require both random sampling and groups of subjects. Such techniques may not be appropriate for evaluating data of individual subjects. However, for those who prefer them, there are several special statistical techniques that can be applied in the analysis of single-subject studies (Barlow & Hersen, 1984; Kazdin, 1982).

Mostly because of the characteristics just described, the single-subject strategy is highly suitable for clinical research. The need to work with a small number of clients, the problem of not being able to form large groups of clinical subjects, the ethical implications of having to deny treatment to a control group that needs it, and the clinical requirement of having to produce

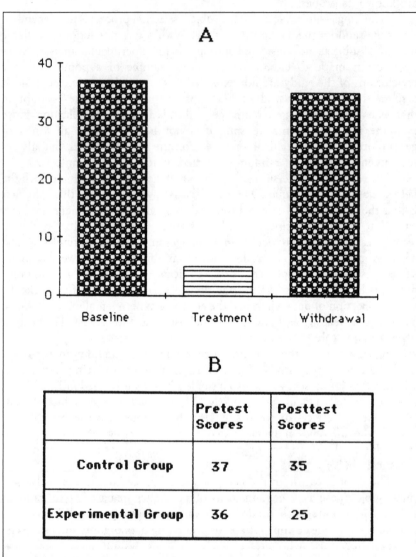

Figure 8-1. Differential visual effects of single-subject (A) and group design studies (B) of a hypothetical treatment effect on stuttering.

large effects in individuals who receive treatment underscore the value of single-subject strategy for clinical professions.

CONTROL MECHANISMS IN SINGLE-SUBJECT DESIGNS

In most group designs, the control group that does not receive treatment provides the basic control mechanism to rule out the influence of other variables. Because the single-subject designs generally do not use control groups, they rule out extraneous variables in other ways.

There are several conceptual and procedural control mechanisms within the single-subject strategy. Together, they provide a comprehensive tactic of isolating the effects of independent variables on dependent variables. The control mechanisms variously employed in the single-subject strategy include replication, withdrawal, reversal, reinstatement, criterion-referenced change, rapid alternations, baselines, and simultaneous multibaselines.

Replication

One of the important characteristics that distinguish the single-subject strategy from the group strategy is the replication of treatment effects within individual subjects. The group designs typically introduce the treatment once, and when it is discontinued, there is no reintroduction of treatment. Therefore, within the group design strategy, there is no recapturing of a state after the dependent variable has been changed. The experimental group that shows change, remains changed, and the control group that does not, remains unchanged. Therefore, there is no replication of conditions in the group strategy.

In the single-subject strategy, the treatment condition, the control condition, or both are changed from one state to the other. Equally important is the fact that one or more of the earlier states are recaptured. In other words, the effects of the independent variable are shown once by introducing it and thereby changing the dependent variable; and again by removing it thereby changing the dependent variable a second time. A preexperimental state or an approximation of it is recaptured. The simplest of the single-subject designs, the *ABA* design which involves a baseline (*A*), treatment (*B*), and withdrawal of treatment (*A*), replicates the original steady-state.

In the *ABAB* design, a baseline is first established (*A*), a treatment is then introduced (*B*), which is subsequently withdrawn (*A*), and finally reintroduced (*B*). This design replicates the pretreatment steady-state or baseline once (the two *A* conditions). In addition, the design replicates the treatment effects as well (the two *B* conditions).

When the relative effects of two or more treatments are evaluated, the single-subject designs repeatedly present and withdraw treatment variables. A series of replications may thus be achieved to observe different patterns of responses under the two treatment procedures. When the interactive effects of two treatments are evaluated, one treatment is withdrawn and reintroduced against the background of a constant treatment variable. In this manner, target response rates under treatment and no-treatment are established repeatedly.

The intrasubject replication, by itself, is not the strongest of the control procedures. However, when an effect is repeatedly demonstrated and repeatedly neutralized, the experimental operations gain credibility. When replication is combined with other control procedures, it can be a significant factor in ruling out extraneous variables.

Intrasubject replication must be distinguished from intersubject or intergroup replication. Most single-subject designs involve both intrasubject and intersubject replication of treatment effects. When multiple subjects are used in a single-subject study involving a design such as the *ABAB*, the same treatment effects are demonstrated repeatedly both within and across subjects. Intergroup replications are achieved when different groups of subjects react similarly under the same treatment condition.

Withdrawal of Treatment

After a period of application, the treatment variable is withdrawn in some of the single-subject designs. Such a withdrawal can also demonstrate control of the independent variable over the dependent variable. In the withdrawal strategy, the experimenter simply stops the application of treatment and continues to measure the dependent variable.

In a clinical research study, for example, the clinician may wish to find out whether production of morphological features can be reinforced by verbal praise. After the baseline production levels of selected morphologic features have been established, verbal praise may be made contingent on the production of those features in phrases or sentences. When an increase in the production of these behaviors becomes evident, the clinician may withdraw verbal praise. The selected stimuli are presented continuously in an effort to evoke relevant verbal responses to see if the production of the morphemes decreases. If they do, the clinician is able to conclude that the treatment variable was responsible for the initial increase and the subsequent decrease in the morpheme productions. Figure 8-2 shows the visual effects of the withdrawal procedure in which a target behavior increases under treatment and decreases under withdrawal.

Withdrawal of treatment in single-subject designs is not the same as the termination of the treatment followed by the posttest in a group design. The withdrawal of treatment is a sensitive operation in that it is supposed to demonstrate both the effects of the independent variable as long as it is present and the absence of the same effect as long as it is withheld. In the group strategy, the treatment is not terminated to show that the effects disappear. Also, the researcher in the group strategy does not need to have the treatment

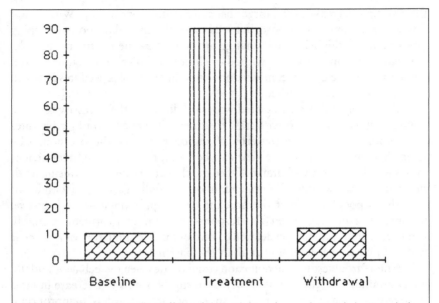

Figure 8-2. The controlling effects of the withdrawal procedure. A behavior which is stable under baseline, increases under treatment, and decreases under withdrawal.

effect neutralized; he or she has the control group to show that when there was no treatment, there was no effect.

Withdrawal of treatment and the resulting decrease in the response rate help rule out the effects of history and maturation. If events in the life of the subjects are responsible for the changes observed during treatment, then the withdrawal of treatment should have no effect on the response rate. If the behavior increases when the treatment is applied, and decreases when it is withdrawn, then the probability that events in the life of the subjects are responsible for the changes is reduced greatly. Similarly, if biological or other internal changes taking place in the subjects are responsible for the increase in the behavior during the treatment condition, then such an increase should at least be maintained, if not continued, when the treatment is discontinued.

As a control strategy, withdrawal has its disadvantages. It can be clinically undesirable because the treatment effects are neutralized even if only temporarily. This poses no serious problem in basic laboratory research in which various independent variables are introduced and withdrawn to created and neutralized effects of variables. For example, in animal research, some response such as barpressing can be increased by reinforcing it and decreased by withholding the reinforcer. This way, the experimenter can bring the barpressing response under experimental control and rule out the influence of other variables. In clinical situations, however, withdrawal of treatment and the resulting decrease in the target behavior is not appropriate. Withdrawal serves an experimental purpose, but it damages the clinical purpose of keeping and enhancing the behavioral change introduced by the treatment variable. Therefore, it is not a control method of choice in clinical research. However, withdrawal can be used in combination with other control procedures in which the treatment is reestablished.

The other problem associated with withdrawal is the necessity to make a judgment as to when to withdraw treatment. There are no objective rules on this issue, but certain patterns of responses dictate the decision. The researcher must see a change that can be so judged when the treatment is introduced before it is withdrawn. Once the change reaches a convincing level, the treatment should not be continued. In other words, it should be withdrawn as early as possible so that the baseline or an approximation of it can be recaptured. However, when the response rate under treatment is highly variable, withdrawal may be delayed to find out if a continuation of treatment will stabilize it at a level higher than the baseline.

A more troublesome phenomenon could occur when the behavior initially increases under treatment but slowly or abruptly begins to decrease in later treatment sessions. While this is happening, withdrawal is inappropriate because it will only show a continuation of the trend already established during the treatment phase. The investigator once again may wish to continue treatment for a while to determine if the declining rate of response can be checked or even reversed. A point may still come, however, when the treatment is withdrawn in spite of a declining rate of response that persists. Although the results cannot be interpreted clearly in this case, the suggestion is that the treatment perhaps has had only a temporary effect or actually no effect at all. The issue must be addressed in additional research.

Finally, if the response rate does not approximate the baseline rate when the treatment is withdrawn, the results cannot be interpreted. The possibility that some extraneous variable is responsible for the change observed during the treatment condition cannot be ruled out.

Reversal of Treatment

Reversal of treatment is an alternative to withdrawal. Sometimes, the terms *withdrawal* and *reversal* are used interchangeably. However, this practice is avoided here because of the procedural differences between them (Barlow & Hersen, 1984; Leitenberg, 1973). In withdrawal, the treatment is simply discontinued. In reversal, on the other hand, the treatment variable is applied to an alternative, incompatible behavior. That is, the treatment is not withdrawn altogether; it is withdrawn from the particular behavior for which it was applied only to apply it on some other behavior.

Another way of looking at the distinction between withdrawal and reversal may be helpful. While withdrawal is a short- or long-term termination of treatment, reversal involves an intrasubject but interbehavior replication of treatment. Initially, the investigator hopes to show that the application of the treatment variable to behavior A resulted in an increase in that behavior. The treatment of behavior A is then discontinued. Next, the investigator demonstrates that an application of the same treatment to behavior B (reversal), increased behavior B while decreasing behavior A. This documents experimental control on both the behaviors, resulting in interbehavior/intrasubject replication. In essence, withdrawal is a singular procedure, but reversal includes withdrawal because before the treatment is applied to an incompatible behavior, it is withdrawn from the original behavior.

A hypothetical example can be given here. Suppose a clinician treats a stuttering client by reinforcing durations of fluency in conversational speech. A stable baseline of fluency and stuttering is established before the initiation of treatment. Reinforcement of fluent durations in speech results in a marked increase in fluency. At this time, the clinician cannot conclude that the reinforcement is responsible for the change, since the factors such as history and maturation have not been ruled out. At this point, the clinician stops reinforcing fluency and starts to reinforce stuttering. As a result of the reversal of the treatment contingency, fluency decreases and stuttering increases. This then demonstrates that the reinforcing contingency is indeed responsible for the changes in fluency as well as stuttering.

As a control procedure, reversal has some of the same problems as withdrawal. Initially, the investigator must decide when to withdraw treatment from the first behavior according to the suggestions offered earlier. Then the investigator must select a behavior that is incompatible with the first behavior. Unless the behavior to be reinforced next is incompatible with the original behavior, a partial replication of the treatment effect may be all that can be achieved. The original behavior may or may not show a swift and concomitant change when the treatment is applied to a compatible behavior.

For example, in the treatment of a client with a language disorder, the clinician may first apply the treatment to the production of regular plural allomorph /s/ in words. After having seen a substantial increase in the production of this allomorph, the clinician may decide to reverse the treatment. Now, the clinician must make sure that the behavior to be treated next is incompatible with the plural allomorph. The best strategy is to reinforce the production of the same words used in training the plural allomorph but in their singular form while showing the plural stimulus items. When the plural responses to plural stimulus items decrease, the singular responses to the same stimulus items increase. Should the clinician reinforce the present progressive *ing* or some other behavior that is not incompatible with the plural allomorph, the production of the latter may not show a concomitant change under the reversal condition.

Reversal presents special problems in clinical research. Therefore, other control procedures are preferred. The procedure requires that the clinician increase the frequency of an undesirable behavior after having increased its counterpart—a desirable behavior. Whenever it is used, the treatment for the original, desirable, target behavior is reinstated in the next phase. This then shows that the undesirable behavior decreases and its counterpart increases a second time. Thus, the treatment achieves its clinical goal.

When it takes several sessions to increase an incompatible, undesirable behavior, the experimental strategy is inefficient and perhaps totally unacceptable from the clinical standpoint. The parents or other members of the client family may react negatively to the clinician who first teaches a correct response and then spends a considerable amount of time and energy teaching the incorrect response. In institutional research, staff members who are asked to reverse the treatment may be reluctant to do so (Barlow & Hersen, 1984). For example, aides in an institution for the retarded who are now asked to reinforce gestures instead of word responses may not be willing to follow through this reversal procedure.

In a more conservative use of the reversal strategy, the clinician can make sure that both the reversal and reinstatement of treatment are achieved in a single session. If the clinician is not sure of this, the reversal strategy may be avoided. In our example of language treatment research, if the clinician is not confident of increasing the production of the singular morpheme in relation to plural stimulus items (reversal) and then an increase in the correct production of the plural allomorph in relation to plural items (reinstatement)—all in a single session—reversal may be avoided.

In many cases, it is possible to reverse and reinstate treatment in a single, perhaps a little extended session. Also, the wrong responses need not be increased to the 100 percent level and stabilized there. Though there are not quantitative guidelines on this, an increase from a low 10 to 15 percent error rate to a moderately high 40 to 50 percent may be considered adequate for the purposes of control. The clinician can then reinstate treatment for the correct response. The correct response rate under reinstatement cab also be achieved quickly. When reversal and reinstatement are thus achieved in a single session, the client is not sent home with an increased or increasing rate of wrong response.

Reinstatement

Reinstatement of treatment is yet another strategy of control within single-subject designs. Technically, reinstatement is possible or necessary only when the treatment has been either withdrawn or reversed. Thus, it is a contingent control condition that has a cumulative control effect within a design. It is contingent upon withdrawal or reversal that will already have demonstrated some control over the dependent variable. The reinstatement of treatment then adds additional control.

Reinstatement can be considered an optional control strategy in basic research. In nonclinical settings, a behavior shaped or taught can be eliminated by withdrawal. Along with this, another behavior may be increased with reversal. However, in clinical research, reinstatement of effective treatment is almost mandatory when the control procedures of withdrawal or reinstatement are used.

The concepts and procedures of withdrawal, reversal, and reinstatment, though separate, are closely interrelated. They also converge on the concept of replication. A single withdrawal replicates the baseline condition by showing an initial increase from, and then a decrease to, the baseline response rate. A single reversal replicates the treatment effect twice, first by showing that the initial target behavior increases and then by showing that the incompatible behavior increases under reversed contingencies.

When a treatment is withdrawn and then reinstated once, the effects of treatment are demonstrated thrice: first when the treatment is initially applied, second when the treatment is withdrawn, and third when the treatment is reinstated. In the first and the third case, an increase in the frequency of the target behavior is demonstrated. In the second case, decrease in the frequency is demonstrated. Together, the three demonstrations strengthen the possibility that the extraneous variables were controlled. Figure 8-3 shows the effects of a single withdrawal and reinstatement of a treatment.

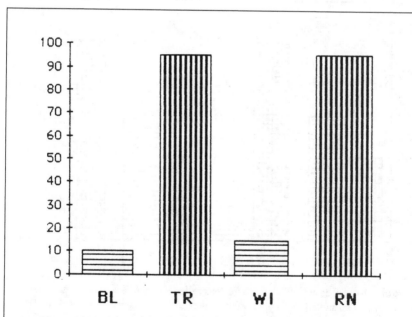

Figure 8-3. The controlling effects of a single withdrawal and reinstatement of treatment. A stable and low rate of the target behavior observed during the baseline (BL) increases during treatment (TR), which then decreases during withdrawal (WI), which again increases during reinstatement of treatment (RN).

When a treatment is reversed and then reinstated once, the treatment effects are demonstrated six times. The first demonstration occurs when the treatment is first applied to the target behavior which shows an increase; the second occurs when the treatment is withdrawn and the target behavior decreases; the third occurs when the treatment is reinstated for the target behavior which shows an increase again; the fourth occurs when the incompatible behavior decreases when the target behavior is treated; the fifth involves an increase in the incompatible behavior when the treatment is applied to it; and the sixth is evident when the incompatible behavior decreases under reinstatement of treatment for the target behavior. Figure 8-4 shows these demonstrations with the hypothetical example of fluency (target, 1) and stuttering (incompatible behavior, 2).

A combination of reversal or withdrawal with the reinstatement procedure can provide a convincing demonstration of the treatment effect by making it difficult to explain the results on the basis of extraneous variables. When systematic changes are associated with the experimental manipulations of withdrawal or reversal on one hand and reinstatement on the other, the probability that the changes are due to those manipulations increases.

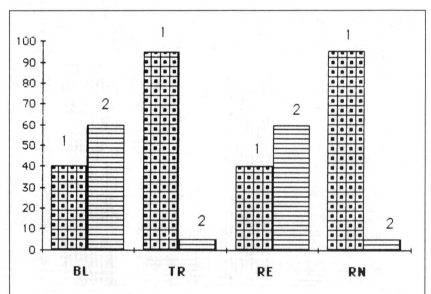

Figure 8-4. Six demonstrations of a treatment effect with a reversal and reinstatement. Fluency (1) and stuttering (2) are baserated (BL) and then fluency is treated (TR). The treatment is reversed (RE) and finally reinstated for fluency (RN). Note the corresponding changes in the two incompatible behaviors.

Criterion-Referenced Change

In one of the single-subject designs, some level of control of extraneous variables is achieved by showing that the dependent variable changes in relation to a criterion, and the criterion is changed several times in subsequent stages of the experiment. This kind of control is called the criterion-referenced change here.

The criterion-referenced change has not been used frequently in demonstrating the experimental control of independent variables (Barlow & Hersen, 1984). The basic idea is that if changes in a dependent variable approximate a preset criterion, and if whenever the criterion is changed, the dependent variable also changes in accordance with the new criterion in force, then the experimental control is demonstrated. In this case, the changes in the dependent variable follow a more predictable pattern that corresponds to the changing criteria.

A hypothetical example can illustrate the criterion-referenced change. An investigator may wish to find out if the amount of home work done by a child is a function of the reinforcement contingency. In order to rule out the influence of factors other than the reinforcement contingency, the investigator may devise a series of changing criteria that the dependent variables may track. For example, initially the child may be asked to complete five academic tasks in a given time. This is the initial criterion to which the dependent variable is held. The investigator will continue to measure the number of tasks completed. Reinforcement is provided for task completion. Suppose that in due course, the child stabilizes at the five completed tasks required by the criterion. After this, the investigator changes the criterion to eight tasks, and the child's behavior reaches and stabilizes at this level. In subsequent stages, the criterion is changed to 10, 14, 16, and 18 tasks. If the number of tasks completed by the child reaches and stabilizes at each new criterion in force, a certain degree of control over the dependent variable becomes evident.

If the dependent variable does not reach the criterion or stabilize at that level, then the control is not evident. Capricious changes unrelated to the criterion in force will also invalidate the data. In order to demonstrate an acceptable degree of control, the dependent variable should closely parallel the criterion in force.

The criterion-referenced change is probably the weakest of the control procedures available within the single-subject strategy. By itself, it does not provide for a no-treatment control condition, which is inherent to withdrawal and reversal. However, such control procedures can be incorporated into the criterion-referenced change. Treatment may be withdrawn at some stage to determine if the behavior returns to at least one of the previous levels. Or, by periodically switching back and forth to a higher and a lower criterion, bidirectional control over behavior may be demonstrated. This also provides replication at the repeated criterion levels. The control function demonstrated by criterion-referenced change is illustrated in Figure 8-5.

The criterion-referenced change is involved in a design known as the changing criterion design. This design is described in a later section of this chapter.

Rapid Alternations

Another form of control used in some of the single-subject designs is the rapid alternation of two or more conditions. The conditions may include treatment and no treatment, or two or more treatments. Of course, two or more treatments may be alternated along with no-treatment conditions as well.

Rapid alternation of conditions can be considered a control procedure because of the possibility of showing dependent variable changes that are equally rapid and consistent with the alternations of conditions. For example, when treatment and no treatment are alternated, the dependent variable may show appropriate increases and decreases. When the treatment is repeatedly introduced and withdrawn with results showing appropriate changes, the investigator increases the probability that the changes are due to the rapidly changing conditions of the experiment.

Rapid alternation of treatment and no-treatment conditions is not the same as treatment conditions interspersed with baseline conditions. In the latter strategy, one can initially baseline a behavior and introduce a treatment that will be continued for a certain length of time. After the behavior shows a convincing change, the treatment may be withdrawn until the client returns to the baseline. This second baseline may also be continued until the behavior shows a change toward the baseline. Then once again the same or even a different treatment may be introduced and maintained for an extended time. This strategy attempts to expose the subjects to treatment and baseline conditions for a duration needed to produce changes that do differentiate the conditions.

On the other hand, in rapid alternation of treatment and no-treatment, there is no attempt to continue either the treatment or the no-treatment condition until some change is judged to have occurred. Each session involves a different condition, and the treatment and no-treatment conditions may be alternated even within sessions. In rapid alternations, the investigator expects to show a data trend over a time involving several alternations.

In the rapid alternation of two or more treatments, an initial baseline may be established, although it is not always required. The purpose of such a strategy is to determine the relative effects of two or more treatments, not the absolute effect of either of them. Therefore, baseline or any other form of control procedure is not necessary, though it is desirable. The control function of rapid alternations involving two treatments (X_1 and X_2) is

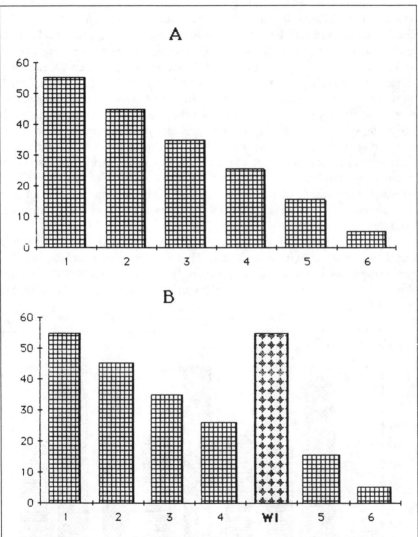

Figure 8-5. Criterion-referenced change showing control over an undesirable target behavior with an initial baseline and 5 decreasing criteria (A). The (B) portion shows the introduction of withdrawal (WI) as one of the criteria which results in a temporary increase in the response rate.

illustrated in Figure 8-6. Note that treatment *1* is more effective than treatment 2 in increasing the target behavior from its baseline level.

A clinician, for example, may wish to evaluate the relative effects of two kinds of stimulus items in teaching the vocabulary items to a mentally retarded child. The stimulus variables to be evaluated in the study may be actual objects and pictures that represent the words to be taught. During the training, objects and pictures may be rapidly alternated. However, through such alternations, training trials on a given word will have a constant type of stimulus. Each stimulus type may involve several target words. Over several rapid alternations, several words may be taught with each of the two types of stimulus materials preceding specific targets. The data may be analyzed in terms of the number of training trials (or sessions, or both) needed to achieve an operationally defined training criterion for the set of words taught with objects versus pictures as stimulus antecedents. Or, when the number of sessions is held constant, the number of words learned within the two procedures can also be analyzed. Such analyses can reveal the differential effects of the two stimulus variables.

Rapid alternation of two or more treatments, by itself, does not provide for strong controls within a design. That is why it is more suitable for evaluating relative, not absolute, effects of two or more treatment variables. When the alternations involve treatment and no-treatment conditions,

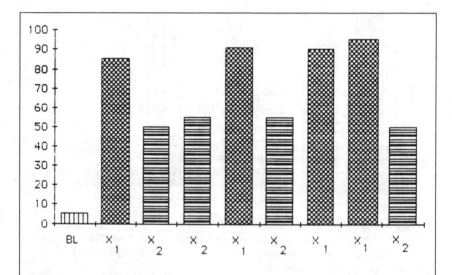

Figure 8-6. The demonstration of experimental control with rapid alternations of two treatments (X_1 and X_2). Note that in increasing the frequency of the target behavior, treatment *1* was more effective than treatment 2.

appropriate controls to rule out extraneous variables exist. Lacking such a control condition, the multitreatment alternations can only identify which one had a greater effect on the dependent variable. However, control conditions such as a withdrawal of all treatments can be built into the alternating sequence. In that case, question whether treatments had any effect at all when compared to no-treatment can also be answered.

Baselines

An important control strategy within single-subject designs is the baselines or baserates of responses. Baselines are rates of responses in the absence of the independent variable whose effects are the subject of experimental analysis. They can also be described as "natural" rates of responses and the operant level of responses. Baselines document the frequency of the dependent variable before the independent variable is introduced. The absence of treatment during baseline condition makes it the control condition within the single-subject designs. The dependent variable measures obtained in the treatment and baseline conditions can be compared to assess the treatment effects.

It must be noted, however, that a mere baseline at the beginning of the experimental manipulation does not rule out extraneous variables. If a study includes only the baseline and treatment conditions, it has the same deficient control that is seen in one-group pretest-posttest design. In the single-subject terminology, this is an *AB* design which cannot rule out the influence of history or maturation. The improvement shown by the subjects under a treatment condition within an *AB* study may be due to the events in the life of the subjects or to the intrasubject biological changes. Therefore, what is needed in addition to a baseline is either withdrawal of treatment, reversal of treatment, rapid alternation, or criterion-referenced change. Baselines serve a control purpose only in conjunction with one of these procedures. Most frequently, baselines and either withdrawal or reversal are used to demonstrate the internal validity of experimental operations.

There is an exception to the rule that baselines must be combined with other control procedures to eliminate or minimize the influence of extraneous variables. The exception constitutes simultaneous multi-baselines, which are described in a later section.

Baseline Criteria

Baselines established before the introduction of treatment must fulfil certain criteria of acceptability. An overall consideration is whether the baselines are adequate to evaluate the treatment effects in conjunction with the treatment and other control conditions. There are three criteria that must be applied in evaluating the adequacy of baselines.

The first criterion to be applied is *reliability through multiple observations*. Unlike pretests in a group design, which normally involve a single observation of the dependent variable, baselines are held to an initial criterion of multiple observations. A single measurement of the dependent variable is inadequate because of its unknown reliability. By definition, reliability is consistency across measures, and therefore, multiple measures are needed to make sure that the frequency with which the dependent variable naturally occurs has been documented. It has been suggested that at least three separate observations are needed before the adequacy of a baseline can be evaluated (Barlow & Hersen, 1984). In fact, three observations may suggest that either additional measures are needed or the behavior has stabilized so that the treatment can be introduced.

The second criterion to be applied is that of *stability of the measures*. A highly variable baseline does not permit a valid comparison with the response rate under the treatment condition. If the rate of response is constantly fluctuating from observation to observation, then the treatment effects may be buried in this variability. However, variability itself can have some patterns, and it is important to note them.

If the response rate is variable in a predictive fashion, it then has a pattern, which is better than the kind of variability with no pattern whatsoever. For example, the behavior may show a consistent increase in one session and decrease in the other session, and the overall data may show this duplicating pattern. Or, the measures may show no pattern in the first few observations, and then a pattern either of stability or of alternating increases and decreases may emerge. Yet another possibility is that the variability may be too high in the beginning, but gradually its extent may be reduced though no pattern emerges. Baselines with no pattern and unpredictable variability are not acceptable.

A stable response rate is the one *without a trend* and without unpredictable variability. A trend is evident when the rate of responses either increases or decreases over time. A stable response without a trend is considered the ideal baseline. When the pretreatment baseline is stable, it is relatively easy to detect the effects of the independent variable.

A stable baseline is difficult to obtain in many cases, and fortunately it is not the only acceptable baseline. Baselines with certain trends are acceptable, as long as the trends themselves help establish a strong effect of the independent variable. Therefore, baselines with a clear trend in the direction that is opposite to the changes to be created by the experimental manipulations are acceptable. For example, in a study designed to evaluate the effects of timeout on stuttering, the clinician observes the rate of dysfluencies in conversational speech over several sessions. The measures of dysfluencies may show an increasing trend over the baseline sessions. This is sometimes referred to as a "deteriorating" baseline (Barlow & Hersen, 1984), as the problem to be reduced is getting worse. Such a baseline is acceptable because the treatment is expected to produce an opposite trend in the data. If timeout is effective, it will not only check the deterioration in stuttering but will also reverse the trend. Indeed, a treatment that reverses a deteriorating baseline can be considered a strong one.

A trend that is clearly not acceptable is one in which the behavior to be increased shows consistent improvement over the baseline sessions. For example, when a clinician measures fluency in a baseline session, it may be found that there is a clear trend toward improvement. In such cases, treatment cannot be instituted simply because the positive effects of the treatment, if any, will be confounded with the baseline trend of improvement in fluency. With such a trend, one will have to assume that fluency would have improved in the absence of treatment.

The best course of action to take when baselines are unstable without a pattern is to continue measurement until an acceptable pattern or trend emerges. Basic research has repeatedly shown that when the conditions are well-controlled and observations are repeated, variability eventually dissipates. It is easier to take this course of action in basic research than in clinical research, however. In clinical settings, baselines cannot be extended indefinitely. The clients who serve as subjects are also seeking treatment for their problem, and since one of the strengths of the single-subject designs is an integration of treatment and clinical service, the treatment must be introduced as soon as possible. At the same time, a highly variable baseline will not permit conclusions regarding the effects of treatment being evaluated. Therefore, one has to make a judgment regarding both the acceptability of the baselines and the duration for which they can be extended. The clinical researcher will have to weigh the advantages and disadvantages of continuing the baseline measures or introducing the treatment variable.

Another way of handling the variability, which has proved successful in basic research, is to make variability itself the subject of experimental analysis. For instance, when a stutterer's dysfluency rates do not stabilize in spite of repeated observations, the clinician may begin to wonder why and think of strategies to find out. It is possible that the conditions of observation are not constant. The time of making observations, the method of evoking speech, or the topics discussed may have been variable. If the conditions have been constant, then perhaps factors in the life of the individual are affecting the dysfluency rates. Are there patterns of events that are related to the changes in the dysfluency rates? Such an inquiry is also relatively easily conducted in basic research, where the entire life and genetic history of an experimental animal is under the control of the investigator. However, a serious attempt to find out the sources of variability may be fruitful, though difficult, in applied settings. Possibly, it may be found that a female stutterer's variability in stuttering is related to premenstrual and menstrual conditions. Another stutterer's variability may be due to the frequency with which he or she has meetings with the boss before coming to the baseline sessions. Still another stutterer's variability may be due to fluctuating marital problems at home.

Although tracking the variability of behaviors is worthwhile because it can lead to new information, it does involve taking a step back from the immediate clinical task at hand. The treatment will have to be postponed until the question of baseline variability is resolved. Obviously, this is not always desirable in clinical situations.

The third criterion to be applied in evaluating the baseline adequacy can be called a *potential for contrast*. This criterion is often described as the level of a baseline response rate (McReynolds & Kearns, 1983). A very high or very low baseline can be either acceptable or not acceptable, depending upon the direction in which the dependent variable is expected to be changed by the treatment variable. For example, a high rate of stuttering is acceptable, since the treatment is supposed to lower it. However, a high rate of fluency (with a negligible rate of stuttering) may not be acceptable because there is not much room to show the effects of treatment.

The best baseline provides a good contrast to the treatment condition. The behavior that is very low in the baseline condition may be shown to be very high in the treatment condition. When the reversal procedure is used in the later part of an experiment, the rates of manipulated behaviors may contrast with each other. One of the incompatible behaviors manipulated by the experimenter will be high and the other will be low.

In some cases, the potential for contrast may make it possible to accept a highly variable response rate after all. Once again, a hypothetical example from stuttering may help. Assume that the stuttering is highly variable with no clear pattern. But the clinician may find out that although there is a wide range to the variability, the lowest level of stuttering, replicated a minimum of three times, is still considerably high. Let us say that over repeated observations, the least amount of dysfluency ever recorded is 15 percent, with a variability range of 15 to 37 percent. In this case, the clinician may decide to introduce treatment in spite of the variability, on the assumption that the treatment will bring stuttering to less than 1 percent. When a treatment is successful in virtually eliminating the disorder along with its variability, then the resulting contrast will have justified the introduction of treatment at a time when it would normally be considered undesirable.

Introduction of treatment on the basis of a potential for contrast in the face of high variability can be risky, of course, but taking risks is a part of all research activity. It is appropriate to introduce treatment when the variability gives the clinician a clear and solid floor so high that the treatment can be expected to lower it to a level that would provide a good contrast. In this case, one guideline that a clinician may use is the expected amount of change in the dependent variable. If a large effect that comes close to eliminating the behavior is expected (and supported from past research or experience), the clinician may be able to introduce treatment in spite of a range of variability. However, if only a small degree of change is expected of the treatment, the clinician should continue baseline observations or seek an analysis of the reasons for variability. If either of these options is precluded, for whatever reason, the study may be abandoned and the client may be treated.

The basic strategy of analysis used in the single-subject designs requires contrasting levels of response rates in the adjacent conditions of most experiments. A contrastive shift in the rate of response must be evident in the treatment condition compared with the baseline condition. When the treatment is withdrawn, the declining (and decreased) response rate should provide a contrast with the increasing (and increased) response rate found in the treatment condition. Or, when the reversal follows treatment, the behaviors that changed in the opposite directions should contrast.

Although contrast helps demonstrate experimental control, a lack of contrast between certain conditions is also part of the analysis in single-subject designs. The baseline and the withdrawal conditions are expected to show a lack of contrast. In reversal designs, the behavior from which the treatment is withdrawn is expected to show the same lack of contrast, although its counterpart would provide increased contrast.

The various baseline patterns that illustrate stability, pattern, and the presence and the absence of contrast are illustrated in Figure 8-7.

Ideal baselines are rarely achieved in clinical fields unless one is willing to extend the observations to extents that are often impractical or unethical. Therefore, in the final interpretation of the data, a variety of factors, not just the stability of the baseline, must be taken into consideration. Such factors as the degree of variability, the existence of helpful patterns in variability, the presence of a high and stable floor, the expected magnitude of treatment effects, the degree of contrast in conditions that should be contrasted, and a similarity of patterns in conditions that need to be comparable help evaluate the internal validity (control) of given experiments.

Simultaneous Multibaselines

The final form of control used in the single-subject strategy involves simultaneous multibaselines. Normally, a single, stable baseline of a single target behavior is established before the treatment is started. This is the kind of baseline that was discussed in the previous section. In simultaneous multibaselines, several behaviors are observed before the introduction of treatment, and baselines are established on all of them. The baselines are repeated throughout the course of the experiment.

As noted earlier, the single pretreatment baselines do not demonstrate control by themselves; they must be combined with one of the other control strategies. On the other hand, the simultaneous multibaselines can

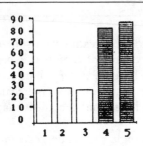

A. Stable baseline, dramatic increase in the response rate under treatment, and a good contrast.

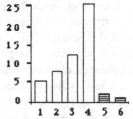

B. High but stable baseline, a notable decrease in the response rate under treatment, and a good contrast.

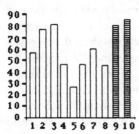

C. A variable baseline with an unclear treatment effect due to poor contrast.

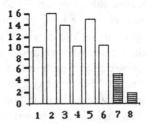

D. A deteriorating baseline (increasing frequency of an undesirable behavior) with a reversed trend under treatment with good contrast.

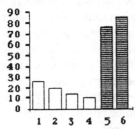

E. A decreasing baseline (decreasing frequency of a desirable behavior) with a reversed trend under treatment with good contrast.

F. A variable but acceptable baseline because of a high floor (10 percent) that provides good contrast with the treatment effect.

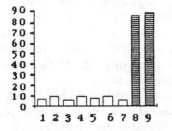

G. A variable desirable behavior, providing a low floor for a high contrast when the behavior increases dramatically under treatment.

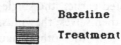

☐ Baseline
▤ Treatment

Figure 8-7. Seven patterns of baselines showing variability, stability, low and high floors, and presence and absence of contrast.

demonstrate experimental control by themselves. For example, an investigator may obtain baselines of four grammatical features in an effort to establish the effectiveness of a language treatment program. Suppose that each of the behaviors is at zero percent baseline. The clinician then treats one of the grammatical features and increase its production to 90 percent accuracy. Then, the other three morphemes are baserated again to show that their frequency did not change since they were not treated. The second morpheme is trained next, and the remaining two morphemes are baserated to document their unchanged status in the absence of treatment. In this manner, every time a behavior is brought under control, the baselines of unchanged behaviors help document the effects of treatment. The visual effects of the control feature of the simultaneous multibaselines on four target behaviors are illustrated in Figure 8-8.

The multibaselines can be behaviors of the same or different subjects. The baselines may also be situations where a particular behavior of a given individual is measured. When different subjects constitute simultaneous multibaselines, subjects are treated in sequence and baselines are repeatedly established on untreated subjects. Unchanged behaviors of untreated subjects help rule out the influence of extraneous variables. When different situations are the multibaselines, the same behavior is treated in sequence in different situations, and the rate of that behavior in untreated situations helps demonstrate the effects of the treatment. These three versions of the simultaneous multibaselines correspond to the three versions of the multiple baseline designs described in a later section of this chapter.

The logic of the simultaneous multibaselines comes close to that of the group-design strategy. In group experimental designs, untreated subjects serve the control function. In simultaneous multibaseline strategy, untreated behaviors, subjects, or situations serve the same function.

The simultaneous multibaseline control procedure has been used extensively in clinical research because it does not require clinically questionable strategies of withdrawal or reversal.

Summary of Single-Subject Control Procedures

Unlike group designs, single-subject designs arrange treatment and control conditions that are exposed to all the subjects of a study. The designs use several control mechanism to rule out the influence of extraneous independent variables. These control mechanisms include replication of treatment effects within subjects, withdrawal of treatment after it shows some effect, reversal of treatment that shows changes in two incompatible behaviors, changes in behaviors that approximate changing performance criteria, rapid alternations of treatments that show corresponding changes in behavior, various patterns of baselines, and multibaselines that are treated sequentially.

As noted earlier, control procedures in the single-subject strategy are multiple and replicative. More than one control procedure is typically involved

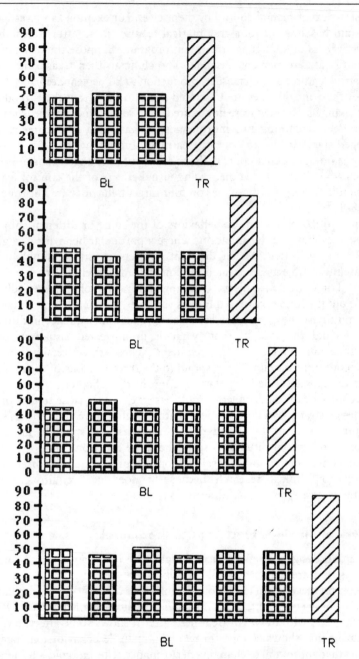

Figure 8-8. Simultaneous multi-baselines (BL) and treatment (TR). Baselines are longer for behaviors that are treated later in the sequence and each behavior increases only when treated.

in many designs. They are all applied to the same individuals in most of the designs. When combinations of control procedures support the treatment effects in replicated series, the investigator can claim internal validity for his or her experimental findings.

SINGLE-SUBJECT DESIGNS

Preexperimental Single-Subject Design

Preexperimental designs, as described in Chapter 7, do not have adequate control for the factors that affect the internal validity of an experiment. There is a single-subject design that parallels the group preexperimental one-shot case study. In the terminology of single-subject designs, this is known as the *AB* design.

The *AB* design is not unlike traditional case studies. A case study is a rather detailed study of a single patient or client who undergoes a form of treatment. Such case studies are common in many clinical fields, including medicine, clinical psychology, psychiatry, and speech–language pathology.

In the *AB* design, a baseline of the target behavior is first established. The treatment is then applied and the dependent variable is measured continuously. When the treatment objective is achieved, a report is made on the recorded changes in the client behaviors. The design is illustrated in Figure 8-9.

It is obvious that the *AB* design lacks experimental control of extraneous variables. Therefore, it is not classified as an experimental design. It is similar

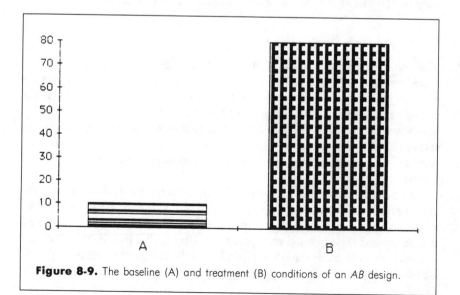

Figure 8-9. The baseline (A) and treatment (B) conditions of an *AB* design.

to the traditional case study. The observed changes in the dependent variable may or may not be due to the influence of treatment. There is no assurance that in the absence of treatment, the behaviors would not have improved. Therefore, history and maturation, among other factors, may explain the results of case studies and *AB* studies.

AB studies do not require control procedures that consume extra time and energy. Although they do not permit statements on cause–effect relations, *AB* studies are thought to suggest ideas for more controlled research while providing for a certain degree of confidence in the treatment procedure. If an *AB* study fails to show improvement, that is considered a significant finding, because a treatment that does not produce an effect under uncontrolled conditions may not produce an effect under controlled conditions either.

Many researchers believe that the matter of control is not an either-or phenomenon and that different designs have varying degrees of control. The *AB* designs can also vary in terms of the degree of confidence one can place in the results. Some of them can be more trustworthy than others. Multiple observations before, after, and during treatment with stable measures and good contrast can enhance the validity of *AB* studies.

The *ABA* Design

The basic experimental paradigm of the single-subject strategy is known as the *ABA* design. The *ABA* design was developed in the context of basic laboratory research. It is most appropriately used in demonstrating the control of variables that are not expected to produce lasting treatment effects. Nevertheless, this design reveals the basic logic and the strategy of single-subject designs. It has two versions: withdrawal and reversal.

The *ABA* Withdrawal Design

The *ABA* withdrawal design, illustrated in Figure 8-10, is the original experimental design within the single-subject design strategy. In the laboratory research involving animal behavior, subjects are typically run for an extended period of time to establish the operant level (baseline) of selected behaviors. It is not uncommon to run subjects for several weeks to achieve behavioral stability. Following a stable response rate, various kinds of stimulus and response-consequent contingencies are applied to assess the effects on behavior patterns.

Depending on the research question, the experimental contingencies are also applied over extended time. A marked shift in the response rate creating a contrast between the baseline and the treatment conditions is the goal of this prolonged experimental manipulation. After such a shift is observed, the independent variable is withdrawn, and the subjects are allowed to respond. Normally, the response rate gradually decreases until it approximates the

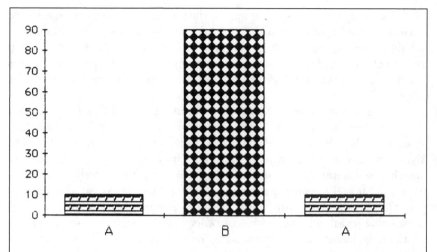

Figure 8-10. The *ABA* design in which the positive effects of a treatment is cancelled by withdrawal.

original baseline level. When the independent variable investigated is a reinforcer, the withdrawal condition is also known as the extinction condition.

In Figure 8-10, note that the first two conditions of the design show a comparable response rate. The response rate is higher under the treatment condition, which contrasts with the baseline and extinction conditions.

The *ABA* withdrawal design is a reasonably well-controlled design. When a stable response rate, documented by baseline measures, changes dramatically when the treatment is introduced but returns to the baseline level when the treatment is withdrawn, a convincing demonstration of the treatment effect will have occurred. The basic logic of the design is that when a variable is present, it produces an effect, but when the variable is absent, the effect disappears. When this happens, other factors cannot account for the presence and absence of the effect.

Much of the basic information we have regarding the principles of learning and conditioning, including reinforcement, punishment, and the effects of various reinforcement schedules, has been generated by this *ABA* withdrawal strategy. It continues to be one of the most important experimental strategies of research in behavioral analysis.

It is clear that the final phase of the *ABA* withdrawal design does not involve treatment. When it is used in clinical settings, the improvement shown by the client in the treatment condition is neutralized in the final *A* condition. Therefore, it is not a clinical treatment design. However, the design has a place in clinical research. Its use in clinical research can be justified on certain discriminated grounds.

The design is certainly not appropriate when a clinician expects to use a treatment procedure until the clinical goals of complete habilitation or rehabilitation are accomplished. However, the *ABA* design is appropriate when the effects of a new technique of treatment must be evaluated and there is no evidence yet that it will be the long-term treatment for the disorder under investigation.

There is a more important reason for using the *ABA* design. Whether a variable has any effect at all on a given behavior is an important research question. The effects may be temporary, in which case they may not lead to the development of a treatment effect. They may be relatively permanent, in which case the possibility of developing a new treatment technique exists. When the initial research question is whether a particular variable has any effect at all, the ABA withdrawal design is appropriate. For instance, it is reasonable to ask whether verbal or other kinds of stimuli have any effects at all on dysfluencies, misarticulations, vocal pitch breaks, or other kinds of speech–language problems.

If the answer produced by an *ABA* withdrawal design is positive, more clinically appropriate designs can be employed to develop treatment techniques. For example, much of the operant research on stuttering involving such aversive stimuli as shock, noise, and verbal stimuli was done with the *ABA* design. Hindsight would now justify the use of the *ABA* withdrawal strategy, since stimuli such as shock and aversive noise have not led to routine clinical treatment procedures.

The *ABA* Reversal Design

The reversal operation described in an earlier section can be used in the *ABA* format. It is illustrated in Figure 8-11. In terms of the baseline and treatment, the design is the same as the *ABA* withdrawal design. However, during the second *A* condition, the experimental contingencies may be reversed. Instead of simply withdrawing the treatment from the target behavior (*1*), another, incompatible behavior (*2*) may be treated. As a result, it can be shown that the first behavior returns to the baseline and the second behavior shows new and systematic changes. This would help rule out extraneous variables.

For example, if the design is used in evaluating a treatment procedure for articulation disorders, the clinician first increases the correct production of selected phonemes and then reverses the contingencies to increase the original incorrect productions of the same phonemes. In the treatment of language disorders, subjects' production of selected grammatical features may be first increased, and then the same treatment may be used to increase the production of phrases or sentences without those grammatical features. For instance, if a child initially omits the auxiliary *is*, resulting in such responses as *boy running* and *girl writing*, the reversal involves a reinforcement of these responses.

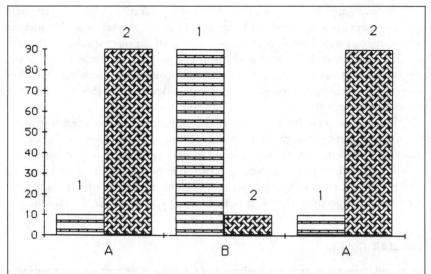

Figure 8-11. The *ABA* reversal design. Note the corresponding effects of treatment (B) and reversal (the second A) on a target (1) and its incompatible (2) behavior.

From a clinical standpoint, it may appear that *ABA* reversal is more problematic than *ABA* withdrawal. An initial thought may be that in a withdrawal design the client is no better or no worse than his or her initial standing, since at the end of the experiment his or her response rate will approximate the pretreatment baseline. The same client in a reversal design may appear to be worse off at the end of the experiment because the clinician reinforced the wrong response in order to increase it. These initial reactions may not be valid, however. Especially as the two designs are used in communicative disorders, clients in either case are in the same position: they are roughly at their baseline at the end of the experiment.

When a reversal is used, there is no need to increase the error response to a level that is higher than that observed at the baseline. When the baseline is at zero, and the treatment increases the target behavior to 90 percent or higher, then the reversal need not be continued until the target behavior reaches zero. A reduction from 90 percent to 30 or 40 percent may be convincing. As such, reversal and withdrawal are both mechanisms to either recover the baselines or force the target behaviors in that direction.

In withdrawal, the baseline is recovered rather slowly because the main mechanism is extinction of the treated behavior. It is known that extinction is a slow process. In reversal, the baseline may be recovered faster because it is a more active process. It increases an incompatible behavior, which indirectly decreases the treated target behavior. In this sense, reversal may be a more efficient control procedure.

As was suggested in the context of the withdrawal design, when there is no expectation of producing lasting effects, reversal may be just as appropriate as withdrawal. Questions of effects of various stimulus conditions on communicative behaviors and disorders may be researched within the reversal strategy because they have important theoretical implications. Whether eventually a treatment procedure will be developed out of this research may be an extraneous or a later consideration.

It must be noted that when either the withdrawal or the reversal strategy is used, the client participates in an experiment with no change in his or her problem situation. Taking appropriate human subject protection steps (see Chapter 12), the investigator can recruit clients for this kind of research. However, at the end of the experiment, it must be possible to offer those clients a treatment procedure that will remedy their specific clinical problem.

The *BAB* Design

In the *BAB* design, which is a variation of the basic *ABA* format, the treatment is introduced in the very first phase of an experiment. In this case, there is no initial baseline. The three conditions of the design, as shown in Figure 8-12 are the treatment (*B*), baseline (*A*), and treatment (*B*). From a technical standpoint, it may be more appropriate to use the terms *withdrawal* or *reversal* for the second condition because it is unlike the original baseline, which precedes treatment.

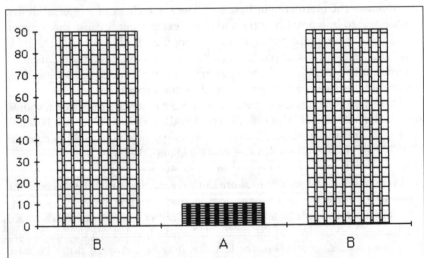

Figure 8-12. The *BAB* design with the initial and final treatment conditions that increase a target behavior.

One of the strengths of this design is that the experiment ends with treatment, and therefore the design is more suitable than the *ABA* design for clinical evaluation of treatment techniques. Another strength is that the design involves intrasubject replication of treatment effects because the treatment is applied twice. However, the problem with this design is that there is no pretreatment baseline against which to compare the treatment effects. The treatment effects can be evaluated only in relation to the response rates under reversal or withdrawal of treatment. Nevertheless, the reversal or withdrawal in the second phase and the reintroduction of treatment in the third phase should provide a reasonable justification to evaluate the efficacy of the treatment variable. The feature of treatment replication should enhance the internal validity of the experimental findings.

The *ABAB* Design

To evaluate clinical treatment procedures, the *ABAB* design and its variations are considered better alternatives to the basic *ABA* design. It is similar to the *BAB* design in that the treatment is the final condition of the experiment and that it is replicated. In this respect, it is better than the *ABA* design. It is also better than the *BAB* design in having a pretreatment baseline against which to compare the treatment effects.

The *ABAB* design starts with the establishment of an acceptable baseline of the dependent variable (the first *A* condition). The treatment is then introduced in the first *B* condition and continued until the experimenter observes an unmistakable change in the dependent variable, or concludes that a change is unlikely to take place. If found effective, the treatment is either withdrawn or reversed in the second *A* condition. The effects of this withdrawal or reversal are measured for an appropriate period of time. Finally, the treatment is reintroduced to replicate and continue the treatment effects in the second *B* condition. The withdrawal version of the *ABAB* design is shown in Figure 8-13.

Assuming that the treatment is effective in changing the behavior when it is first introduced, a change in the opposite direction during the withdrawal or reversal (the second *A* condition) must be evident. When the treatment is reintroduced a second time, the response rate must change again in the opposite direction. If the treatment is expected to increase the rate of response, then the rate of response in the two treatment conditions should be higher than that in the two no-treatment conditions. If the treatment is expected to decrease a behavior, the rate of response should be lower in the two treatment conditions than in the two no-treatment conditions.

Let us suppose that a clinician wishes to assess the effects of verbal reinforcers on the production of selected grammatical features by a language disordered child who is producing those targets at a low rate. The clinician initially baserates the production of the selected morpheme by presenting it

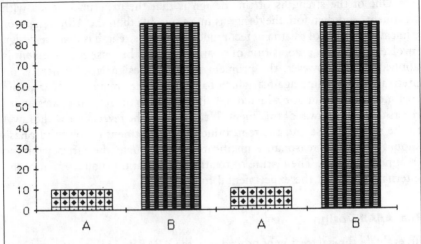

Figure 8-13. The baseline (A), treatment (B), withdrawal (A), and reinstatement of treatment (A) conditions of an *ABAB* withdrawal design.

in the context of several sentences to be evoked by pictorial stimuli and an appropriate question. This is the first *A* condition, which may show that the morphemes are produced with 15 percent accuracy. Then the clinician shows selected pictures to evoke particular responses and reinforces the correct production of the target morpheme in sentences. This is the first treatment condition, B. During this condition, it may be observed that the production of the morpheme has increased to 86 percent. At this point, the clinician withdraws the verbal praise and continues to evoke the target responses on a series of trials. This is the second *A* condition, during which the response rate decreases to 21 percent. Finally, the clinician reintroduces the verbal praise for correct production of the morpheme, which may increase to 95 percent or better. This is the second *B* condition, in which the treatment is continued until the client has generalized and maintained the production of the morpheme in conversational speech evoked in naturalistic settings.

Introduction of additional treatment features such as generalization and maintenance during the latter part of the second *B* condition does not affect the conclusions that can be drawn from the study. The data needed to evaluate the effects of verbal praise on the production of the selected morpheme have been produced by the time such additional procedures are introduced. However, no firm conclusions regarding the effects of the additional procedures are permissible since those procedures have not been evaluated experimentally. For example, one cannot assume that because the child maintains the production of the morpheme after a maintenance program is implemented, the program is indeed effective. We shall discuss the issue of evaluating maintenance programs in a later section.

In the *ABAB* reversal version, the experiment just described involves reinforcement of productions that does not include the target morpheme but should. In other words, the contingency is placed on an incompatible behavior. In this case, the responses that do not include the morpheme would show an increase. In the final treatment condition, the reinforcer would be made contingent again on the correct production of the target morphemes.

A variation of the *ABAB* design is known as the *ABCB* design. In this design, the target behavior is baserated and a treatment applied, as in the *ABAB* design. However, the next condition involves neither withdrawal nor reversal. Therefore, this third condition is known as *C* instead of *A*. In this *C* condition, the reinforcer may be delivered on a noncontingent basis. In other words, the reinforcer does not follow correct production of the target behavior, but it may happen to follow any of the nontarget behaviors that happen to be produced. This may also result in a decrease in the target behavior, essentially showing the controlling function of the reinforcer. The amount of reinforcer delivered noncontingently is the same as that in the previous treatment condition.

The *ABAB* design permits the reinstatement and continuation of treatment until the clients are ready to be discharged. However, the design does require the use of either withdrawal or reversal of treatment in order to show that no other variable is responsible for the changes in the behavior. In this respect, it shares all problems associated with withdrawal and reversal. When the treatment is withdrawn, the rate of the target behavior may not show a decline. Reversal may take an unduly long period of time, raising questions of ethical justification concerning "teaching the wrong response."

Reversal or withdrawal may be totally undesirable when the behavior reduced during the treatment is either self-injurious or abusive of other persons. In such instances, reversal or withdrawal of successful treatment leads to injury to the self or to other persons. In many cases and especially in communicative disorders, however, withdrawal and reversal are achieved in a relatively short time so that the treatment is reinstated quickly and without any negative effects on the client or other persons. When treatment is withdrawn, faulty articulation, dysfluencies, inappropriate vocal qualities, and inappropriate language responses show a relatively quick return to the near-baseline level, and reinstatement of treatment can result in equally quick recovery of the appropriate target responses. The *ABAB* design has been used extensively in modifying a variety of problem behaviors in clinical and educational settings.

In spite of its limitations, some clinical research questions require the *ABAB* strategy. When one wishes to evaluate the effects of treating one behavior on another behavior that is not treated, the *ABAB* is an excellent choice. This kind of research is able to identify behaviors that belong to distinct groups, called response classes. The clinician often faces the problem of not being able to identify target behaviors that are apparently different but are empirically the same. Conversely, the clinician may also face the problem of having a single category of responses that are actually a collection of different behaviors. The issue is important because a resolution of it often clarifies the number of clinical target behaviors in given treatment situations.

Take, for example, the question of subject noun phrase and object noun phrase. Are they separate clinical targets or are they one and the same? Are verbal auxiliary and copula one and the same or are they different clinical targets? In other words, what is the effect of training subject noun phrase on object noun phrase (and vice versa), and training verbal auxiliary on copula (and vice versa)? Questions such as these are appropriately answered by the *ABAB* design, in which one of the pairs in question is trained, the treatment is then withdrawn or reversed, and then it is reinstated while the production of both the responses is measured. For example, the object noun can be trained, reversed, and reinstated to see if the subject noun phrase is also produced, reversed, and reinstated without a direct application of the treatment variable. Such an outcome would suggest that the two are not separate clinical targets in spite of the structural distinctions between them. A study of this kind has suggested that subject and object noun phrases belong to the same response class (McReynolds and Engmann, 1974). Similarly, there is some evidence to suggest that the verbal auxiliary and copula belong to the same response class (Hegde, 1980b).

In the study of communication and its disorders, there are many structural categories such as semantic and pragmatic notions whose status as empirically valid responses is not clear. The *ABAB* design provides an excellent means of determining whether such structural categories are independent responses that can be clinically taught.

The Multiple Baseline Designs

The multiple baseline designs are among the most desirable of the single-subject designs because they avoid the problems of withdrawal and reversal. The structure of the multiple baseline designs includes a series of baseline and treatment conditions across different behaviors, persons, settings, and some combinations of these. The design is essentially a multiple *AB* series. It is still able to control for the extraneous variables by arranging a series of simultaneous multibaselines in such a way that the dependent variables change *only* when they come under the influence of the treatment variable.

The multiple baseline design has three standard versions: multiple baseline design across behaviors, across subjects, and across settings. We shall consider these standard versions as well as some variations.

Multiple Baseline Across Behaviors

Since its formal recognition in 1968 by Baer, Wolf, and Risley, the multiple baseline across behaviors has been used extensively in clinical research involving treatment evaluation. This design requires that the investigator have several dependent variables for experimental manipulation in a single subject or client. In most clinical situations, this is easily accomplished, since clients usually need treatment for several target behaviors. For example, clients with articulation disorders typically need treatment for multiple phonemes, and clients with language disorders for multiple grammatical, semantic, pragmatic, or response class targets. Also, in most clinical situations, the clinician is not able to treat all target behaviors simultaneously. Single behaviors or just a few behaviors may be targeted for treatment at any one time. When the training is accomplished on certain behaviors, other behaviors are targeted for further training. This typical clinical situation is well suited for multiple baseline evaluation of treatment.

In the evaluation of a given treatment procedure with multiple baseline across behaviors, the clinician selects a client who needs treatment on several behaviors. To begin with, all of the target behaviors are baserated. When a stable response rate is established for at least one of the target behaviors, the treatment is applied to that behavior. The treatment is withheld from other behaviors that are still at baseline. The first behavior is trained to a specified criterion, say 90 percent accuracy on probe trials that do not involve treatment (no reinforcement, for example). Then the remaining behaviors are once again baserated to make sure that the behaviors not trained did not change relative to the original baseline. The second behavior is then trained to the selected criterion. The other target behaviors remain in baseline, which is repeated before the third behavior is trained. After obtaining another baseline of untrained behaviors, the fourth behavior is trained. In this manner, every time a behavior is trained, the untrained behaviors are baserated to demonstrate a lack of change in them in the absence of treatment.

The typical results of a multiple baseline design involving four target behaviors are illustrated in Figure 8-14.

There are two important considerations in the use of the multiple baseline design across behaviors. The first consideration is the number of target behaviors that are sequentially treated and the second is the independence of those behaviors. Both the considerations have a potential for creating problems for interpreting data generated by the design.

It is generally thought that to demonstrate the controlling effects of the experimental manipulation, a minimum of three to four behaviors must be included in the design (Barlow & Hersen, 1984). Three to four behaviors give an adequate chance to show that the behaviors change only when treated and not when in baseline. In this case, the experimenter can establish a clear trend in the data that demonstrate the effect of an independent variable.

The second question, the independence of the behaviors selected for experimental manipulation, is more difficult for a priori judgments. The problem is that when two behaviors in a multiple baseline design are not independent of each other, then the treatment applied to one behavior may affect the other, which is supposedly still in the baseline. Changes in untreated

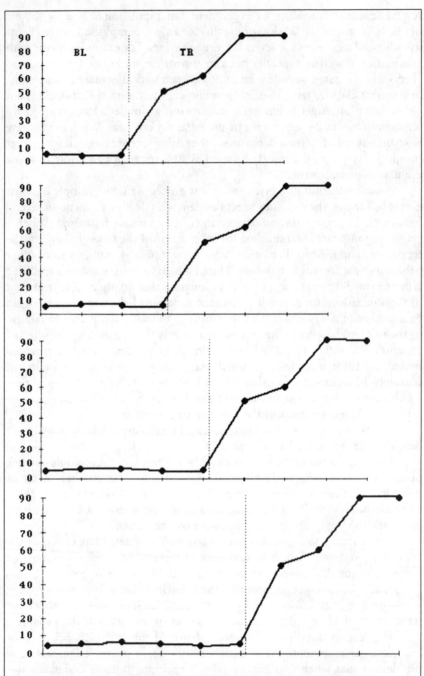

Figure 8-14. The multiple baseline design involving four target behaviors. Each behavior increases only when brought under the influence of the treatment.

behaviors may be due to either uncontrolled independent variables or a dependence between the treated and changed, though untreated, behaviors.

The independence of behaviors selected for a multiple baseline design is often judged on the basis of theory, clinical experience, or empirical evidence. In given cases, these bases may or may not be valid. In this respect, untested theoretical grounds are the most risky, and the experience less so. The best empirical basis is provided by past evidence. In the field of speech–language pathology, the independence of behaviors is one of the most troublesome issues for clinical researchers because speech and language behaviors are often distinguished on the basis of response topography only. Behaviors are independent when they have different independent variables. However, distinctions among behaviors that are insensitive to the independent variables may prove misleading under conditions of experimental manipulations.

The misleading nature of behavioral distinctions based on untested theoretical grounds is evident in research on language treatment. The grammatical, semantic, and pragmatic theories of language have identified an endless variety of response categories that are based solely on the basis of *form* of responses. Distinctions between various grammatical categories, semantic notions, and pragmatic rules are based on structural theories with very little evidence regarding their empirical validity.

My associates and I had an opportunity to find out the hard way that some of the grammatical categories may be unreal. An experiment on language training was designed to discover certain forms of contextual generalization (Hegde, Noll, & Pecora, 1978). A multiple baseline design across behaviors was selected to demonstrate the effectiveness of the treatment variable. The selected multiple target behaviors included contractible auxiliary (e.g, *he's* riding), contractible copula (*she's* happy), uncontractible auxiliary (*he was* painting), and possessive morpheme /s/ (*lady's* hat). Initially, the four behaviors were baserated in a mentally retarded language handicapped child, 3 years and 9 months old. The correct production of the behaviors on the initial baseline was 0 percent. The contractible auxiliary was trained first, and a second set of baselines were then obtained on the remaining three target behaviors. During this baseline, the correct production of the second target morpheme, contractible copula, was produced with 100 percent accuracy. This raised the possibility that either contractible auxiliary and copula were not independent of each other or some extraneous variable was responsible for changes in the first target behavior.

Fortunately, two other baselines did not show any change when measured a second time (uncontractible auxiliary and the possessive morpheme). This supported the possibility that the contractible copula changed not because of an extraneous treatment but because it is not independent of contractible auxiliary. However, we could not be sure, since within a multiple baseline design, change in an untreated behavior *must* be considered to represent weakened experimental control. We decided to see if we would get similar results by first treating contractible copula and then testing contractible auxiliary in a multiple baseline design applied to another client. This client was a 4-year-old boy who did not produce contractible copula, contractible auxiliary, uncontractible auxiliary, uncontractible copula, and the possessive /s/ morpheme. In this case, there were five baselines.

After establishing the initial baselines on all five morphemes, we first trained the contractible copula and found that the production of the contractible auxiliary also increased to 100 percent on the second baseline. However, the three remaining untrained behaviors showed no change, and they continued to show no change until each of them was brought under the influence of the treatment contingency. This once again suggested that the contractible auxiliary and copula probably belong to the same response class and hence are not independent behaviors. However, switching the sequence of the two morphemes across two subjects was not considered a crucial test of the independence of the auxiliary and copula, since a multiple baseline design could not provide such a test. An altered sequence was applied to another subject in the hope that some additional suggestive evidence might emerge. And it did. Eventually, an appropriate test of the independence of the two behaviors was made within the *ABAB* reversal design (Hegde, 1980b).

When the design includes four or more baselines (target behaviors), a potential interdependence between two of them may not be very damaging. The other baselines that do not show changes until treatment is applied to them will continue to serve the control function within the design.

It is obvious that a lack of independence between behaviors, though troublesome, can provide interesting hints on responses that belong to the same class. When such hints are taken up for experimental analysis, a more specific information on clinical target behaviors is likely to emerge. In this sense, interdependence of behaviors shown by a multiple baseline design, when confirmed, can be considered worthwhile accidents in research.

Multiple Baseline Across Subjects

When a given target behavior is baserated across individuals rather than across different behaviors of the same individual, we have the multiple baseline across subjects. Thus, a speech–language clinician may baserate a single grammatical morpheme such as the plural /s/ across four individuals. Then the language treatment to be evaluated may be given to the first individual while the other individuals remain in baseline. When the first subject's production of the plural morpheme reaches the training criterion, the baselines are repeated on the remaining subjects. Assuming that the untreated subjects are still not able to produce the morpheme, the clinician applies treatment to the second subject. The third and the fourth subjects remain untreated until the second one is treated. After another set of baseline measures, the third subject receives treatment, and the fourth subject is baserated for the last time and then receives treatment.

Typically, the same behavior is baserated across different individuals. This practice is considered a standard and perhaps safe strategy. However, the basic logic of the design permits baselining different behaviors across different individuals (Barlow, Hayes, & Nelson, 1984). For example, four different morphemes such as the plural /z/, present progressive *ing*, regular past tense /ed/, and possessive /s/ can be the four respective targets across four individuals. As long as the behaviors of subjects who are not yet treated do not change from the baseline, the design is able to demonstrate that the treatment is effective.

Another variation of the multiple baseline design across subjects is to apply treatment sequentially to groups of subjects. For example, three groups of children, all language disordered, may be treated sequentially. The selected target behaviors are initially baserated in all subjects in the three groups, and then the treatment is applied to the subjects in the first group. After repeating the baselines on the two remaining groups, the treatment is given to subjects in the second group. After an additional baseline, the third group receives treatment in the final stage of the experiment. If subjects in each group change only when treated, potential external variables are ruled out.

When groups of subjects are used in the multiple baseline format, it is necessary to present evidence of change in individual subjects as well. The philosophy of single-subject designs does not allow a mere reporting of statistical means based on group performances. For this reason, large groups are not practical in this format.

It is recommended that the subjects selected for a multiple baseline across subjects be similar to each other and that they be living in the same or similar environmental conditions. If one follows these recommendations, the design presents some of the same problems of a majority of group designs that require matching in the absence of randomization. Finding matched clients living in the same environment or similar environments can be difficult. Moreover, "environmental similarity" is not easy to determine. However, when the individuals can be described separately, and the treatment effects are evaluated in relation to an individual subject only, the need for matching is not as strong as in a group design. The behavior that changes in an untreated subject affects the control of the design negatively, but such changes can be observed in homogeneous as well as heterogeneous subjects. The assumption that such changes are more likely in heterogeneous subjects is logically appealing, but its empirical status is not clear.

Demonstration of an experimental effect in individuals who are different from each other in terms of the clusters of problem behaviors (symptoms) or in terms of one or more of assigned variables (subject characteristics) can actually enhance the generality of experimental data. Therefore, unmatched subjects can be used as long as the experimenter is aware of the potential risk involved. The risk of having a behavior change in a subject who is still in baseline must be weighed against the potential of producing data with enhanced generality. However, as noted earlier, the risk is logically justified, but it may be empirically weak enough to allow some creative risk-taking on the part of the experimenter.

Multiple Baseline Across Settings

When a given behavior of a single subject is measured in different settings and when the treatment is applied sequentially in those settings, we have the multiple baseline across settings. In the most typical version of this design, the same behavior of the same subject exhibited under different settings provides the multiple baselines. The treatment is applied in one of the settings. When the target behavior shows the treatment effect in this setting, the baselines are reestablished in the untreated settings. The treatment is extended to the second setting, and so on until the behavior is independently established in all of the settings.

The design can be illustrated in the treatment of an articulation disorder. A child's misarticulation of a given phoneme may be measured in different settings such as the office of the clinician, the classroom, the school cafeteria, and the playground. The treatment contingency may be positive reinforcement of correct production of the phoneme in single words. After the initial baselines have been established in those settings, the treatment may be started in the clinician's office. When the treatment is successful in this setting, the behavior is baselined in the untreated settings. The treatment is then applied in the classroom setting with the cooperation of the teacher. Baselines are repeated in the cafeteria and the playground. In this manner, the clinician applies treatment sequentially in different settings, showing that in each setting, the correct production of the phoneme increases only when treated in that setting.

The correct production of the phoneme in one or some of the untreated settings creates design problems. Such a production may be due to generalization of the treatment effect or to some uncontrolled variables. Therefore, just as in the other versions of the multiple baseline design, independence of baselines is necessary for unambiguous interpretation of data. The design depends upon the discriminated responding in different settings. It assumes a lack of generalization of treatment effects across settings until treatment is applied in those settings. This assumption may or may not hold in given situations. In some cases, behaviors established in one setting can generalize to other settings although they may or may not be maintained over time. In other cases, the production of target behaviors may be restricted to the setting in which it is supported. Speech–language clinicians typically find that at least in the initial stages, target behaviors are situation-specific. The stuttering client who is fluent in the clinic may still be very dysfluent at home, in the office, or at the supermarket. In such cases, the design can demonstrate experimental control by showing that changes in the target behavior are associated with treatment in different settings.

The application of treatment in different settings can pose practical problems. Treatment may be inefficient or even impossible in some settings, such as the cafeteria or the playground in our example. The design is probably more efficiently used in certain institutions such as those for the mentally or neurologically handicapped. In such institutions, different settings may all be under the control of the researcher to an extent necessary to carry out the experiment.

Typically, the multiple baseline across settings involves single subjects, but it can be used with a group of subjects whose behavior is measured and treated in different settings. In this variation, it must be possible to apply the treatment contingency to the group as a whole. For example, a special education specialist may be able to apply a group token system for "quiet behavior" during the class, in the library, or in the cafeteria. When a group of subjects is used, the clinician must still present data on individual subjects to show that changes reported are not based on the group averages that mask individual differences. For this reason, a large group may be impractical from the standpoint of data analysis and presentation.

The Problem of Repeated Baselines

As noted throughout our discussion, multiple baseline designs require repeated measures of target behaviors. This is one of the cumbersome aspects of the design. The last behavior, subject, or setting to be treated will have been measured repeatedly. The greater the number of series in a design, the more often the baselines need to be measured. Most behaviors studied within the designs are not reactive, but those that are can pose problems because of the repeated baseline measures. Obviously, reactive changes make it difficult to isolate the effects of treatment.

A partial solution offered to the problem of repeated measures is to treat more than one behavior in the multiple baseline across behaviors. For example, if six phonemes are targeted for treatment within a multiple baseline across behaviors, two phonemes may be simultaneously treated, resulting in only three sets of phonemes to be baserated instead of six individual phonemes. This limits the number of baseline measures. Similarly, in the multiple baseline across subjects involving eight subjects, baseline and treatment may be alternated with sets of two subjects. In the multiple baseline involving multiple settings, treatment may be given in two settings while two sets of two settings each are kept in baseline.

Another solution offered to the problem of repeated baseline measures is known as the multiple probe technique (Horner & Baer, 1978). This technique was originally described as a means of verifying the status of untreated target responses that are a part of a behavioral chain. Complex skills, such as the use of a hearing aid, for example, need to be taught in terms of specific target responses that are chained (Tucker & Berry, 1980). The child may be taught to remove the hearing aid from its box, place it behind the ear, turn the power on, adjust the volume, and so on. Each of these responses constitutes a chained element in the total behavior under training. In cases such as this, it is not necessary to spend much time measuring the subsequent behaviors of the chain when the prior responses that need to be mastered earlier have still not been learned by the client. For example, trying repeatedly to measure the response of adjusting the volume of the hearing aid when the client has not even learned how to put the aid on is a waste of time.

The probe technique, however, can be used in the treatment of independent behaviors as well. Instead of continuous measurement of the behaviors yet to be trained, they may be probed periodically to see if they are stable. A probe is a quick test of a given response, generally used to assess generalization of treatment effects. A more detailed measure of a particular behavior just before treatment is considered the baseline. If there are additional behaviors in the baseline, they can be probed without detailed measurement. For example, in the treatment of four grammatical features, the clinician may establish baselines (more detailed measurement) on all of them. Each feature may be baserated in the context of 20 sentences, each presented on a modeled and evoked trial. The first feature is then trained. Then the second feature is baserated with the 20 sentences whereas the third and the fourth features are probed with only a few sentences. The second feature is then trained. The baseline is repeated on the third feature, but the fourth feature is only probed. Finally, the fourth feature is trained after a full baseline measure on it has been obtained. Especially in the treatment of language and articulation disorders, periodic probes are all that are needed. Full baseline measures must be established initially on all behaviors and on every behavior just before it is treated.

Additional Control Within the Multiple Baseline Designs

As noted previously, the multiple baseline designs arrange a series of *AB* conditions. Control is demonstrated by either the untreated behaviors, the untreated subjects, or the "untreated" settings. Each subject, however, experiences only two conditions: the baseline and the treatment. Therefore, multiple baseline designs are considered somewhat weaker than the reversal or withdrawal designs.

A multiple baseline design can be combined with either reversal or withdrawal, however. When this is practical to do, the control aspect of the design is increased significantly. In the multiple baseline design across behaviors and subjects, treatment can be withdrawn for a brief period of time as soon as a particular treated behavior or subject shows a considerable change from the baseline. The treatment can then be reinstated. Reversal and reinstatement can also be used in the same manner. In the multiple baseline across settings, treatment can be reversed or withdrawn in each of the settings in which the treatment is applied and then reinstated in that setting before moving on to the next setting.

Although withdrawal/reversal and reinstatement can add additional control to the multiple baseline designs, they also neutralize many of the advantages of these designs. The designs are thought to be more suitable for clinical purposes precisely because they do not require reversal or withdrawal to demonstrate experimental control. When a multiple baseline design includes four or more baselines (behaviors, subjects, or settings) and each baseline changes only when treatment is applied, the experimental control so exhibited can be considered reasonably satisfactory.

Multiple Treatment Comparisons

A basic question about treatment procedures is whether they are effective when compared with no treatment. Within the single-subject strategy, the *ABA*, the *ABAB*, and the multiple baseline designs are useful in answering that basic question. However, these designs can evaluate only one treatment at a time. We have seen in Chapter 7 that within the group design strategy, options are available to evaluate multiple treatments in a single study. Factorial designs are especially useful in this regard. Within the single-subject strategy, there are some designs that permit an experimental evaluation of multiple treatments.

Generally speaking, a study compares two treatments only when independent evaluations of them have produced some evidence that each is effective to a certain degree. When nothing is known about the effects of a given treatment, a logical start is to find out if it is effective at all. In this case, the design is more likely to be an *ABA*, *ABAB*, *BAB*, or multiple baseline. In the next stage of the experiment, the two treatments that have produced favorable effects in separate studies may be evaluated within a single study. I shall describe two methods of evaluating the effects of two or more treatments within the single-subject strategy.

The *ABACA/ACABA* Design

A clinician may be interested in evaluating the effects of two treatments on a single behavior produced by one or several subjects. For example, a clinician may be interested in evaluating the effects of two methods of teaching alaryngeal speech, articulation, or language responses. The two procedures, X_1 and X_2, may be applied to the same subject or subjects interspersed by baselines (*A*). The resulting design is known as the *ABACA/ACABA* design. The two portions of the design are needed to counterbalance the two treatment variables. Each portion of the design (*ABACA* or *ACABA*) is applied to one or more subjects. For a given subject or set of subjects, either the *ABACA* or the *ACABA* design applies. The first treatment (X_1) is represented by *B* in the design and the second treatment (X_2) by *C*. The design is illustrated in Figure 8-15 with its two sequences of treatment presentations, *(1)* and *(2)*.

The two sequences (*ABACA* and *ACABA*) counterbalance the order of presentation of the two treatments. If only one of the two sequences is used in a study, the potential order effects cannot be ruled out. If the investigator

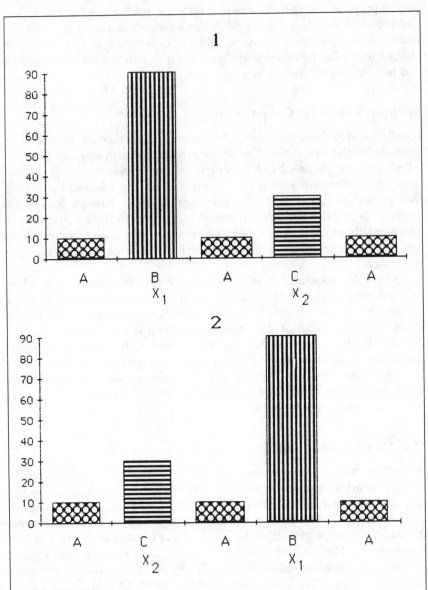

Figure 8-15. The *ABACA/ACABA* design. The first sequence (1) shows the administration of treatment 1 followed by treatment 2 with an interspersed baseline. The second sequence is opposite to the first. In either case, treatment 1 had a larger effect than treatment 2.

were to use four clients in a study designed to evaluate the effects of two treatment procedures, then the first two subjects would undergo the first sequence, and the second two subjects, the second sequence. This way, each treatment precedes and follows the other treatment. It may be noted that the counterbalanced crossover group designs are similar to this single-subject design.

In this design, baselines separate the treatments. Therefore, the design can incorporate withdrawal or reversal. Either version of the design can demonstrate whether one or both the treatments are effective. Once it becomes clear that one or both of them are effective, the clinician can reinstate a treatment to achieve the clinical goals.

The results generated by the design can be suggestive of the *relative* effects of the two treatments but do not permit firm conclusions. In other words, whether one treatment is more effective than the other is a difficult question to handle within this design. Any suggestion regarding the relative effects of treatments from this design must be evaluated within other design formats. In the single-subjects strategy, the relative effects of two or more treatments are compared only when they are administered in *adjacent* conditions. Interspersed baselines result in treatments that are separated in time, and data points that are separated in time are not considered reliable for analysis of the relative effects of two or more treatments (Barlow et al., 1984). For this reason, the alternating treatments design, to be described shortly, is considered the most appropriate strategy to analyze the relative effects of two or more treatments.

A potential problem with the *ABACA/ACABA* design is that the first treatment may be so effective as not to leave any opportunity for the second treatment to show its effects. This is the ceiling effect, described in Chapter 7. The clinician should know when this happens, however. When the wrong response rate is reduced dramatically to near-zero levels by the first treatment, the application of the second treatment may not serve any purpose. The design may also suffer from some carryover effects in spite of the interspersed baselines. In other words, some of the effects of the first treatment may be carried over to the second treatment. The second baseline may give some indication of a carryover, however.

The Alternating Treatments Design

Once it has been determined that several treatment techniques are all effective with a given disorder, the clinician faces a different question. Can it be that one treatment technique is *more* effective than the other? The question, then, does not concern the absolute effects of a given treatment, but the *relative* effects of two or more treatments. Alternating treatments design offers a strategy to answer such questions.

The design can also help answer other questions of relativity. For example, is one therapist more effective than the other? In answering this question, a *single* treatment may be administered by two different therapists whose participation in treatment sessions is alternated. Or, two treatments may be administered by both the therapists alternately. Another question that can be answered by the alternating treatments design is whether the time of treatment can make a difference. The design can help answer this question by arranging treatments at different times of the day, while making sure that each treatment is administered in all of the selected time periods equally often.

The alternating treatments design has also been called multiple schedule design, multi-element baseline design, randomization design, and simultaneous treatments design (Barlow & Hersen, 1984). Of these, simultaneous treatments design is clearly inappropriate because there is another design by the same name that does not involve alternation of treatment. The term *alternating treatments* (Barlow & Hayes, 1979) seems to describe the logic and the strategy of the design accurately. The basic arrangement of the design involving two treatments is illustrated in Figure 8-16.

The design is based on the logic that when two or more treatments are alternated rapidly in the treatment of the same subject, the relative effects of the treatments can be determined in a fairly short duration of time. The treatments may be alternated in a single day, with the number of daily treatment sessions corresponding to the number of the treatments being compared. However, as pointed out by Barlow et al. (1984), rapidity of alternations is determined by the nature of the clinical phenomenon under investigation. If the daily measurement of the phenomenon is not appropriate, and weekly measurement is most likely to reveal changes, then the weekly alternations may be acceptable.

In the treatment of stuttering, for example, a clinician may examine the relative effects of stuttering-contingent aversive noise and verbal punishment involving "No." Let us assume that both the procedures have been evaluated in separate studies showing that they are capable of reducing the frequency of stuttering to varying extents. The clinician can then evaluate the relative effects of the two procedures by applying both to the same client or clients. The two punishment procedures are alternated in the treatment sessions. In the analysis of the results, the rates of stuttering observed in the treatment sessions are separated according to the two procedures. The stuttering

Sessions							
1	2	3	4	5	6	7	8
X_1	X_2	X_2	X_1	X_2	X_1	X_1	X_2

Figure 8-16. Arrangements of experimental conditions of an alternating treatments design involving two treatments.

rate under the aversive noise sessions are compared with those under verbal stimulus.

Typical results of an alternating treatments design are represented in Figure 8-17, which shows that treatment 1 (X_1) was more effective than treatment 2 (X_2).

Order Effects and Counterbalancing. The reader may have noticed in Figure 8-16 that the treatments were not alternated systematically. If one treatment systematically follows another treatment, treatment effects may be confounded by the order effect described in Chapter 7. Therefore, the order of treatment presentation is counterbalanced. Each treatment precedes and follows every other treatment applied in the design. Each treatment can be made to precede and follow every other treatment *equally often*, although this is not always done, nor is it always necessary. As long as the treatments precede and follow more than once and the sequences are roughly comparable in number, the order effects can be minimized.

When two or more clinicians administer the same treatment, the order in which the two clinicians treat the client must be counterbalanced. When two clinicians administer two or more treatments, both the treatments and the clinicians must be counterbalanced. When two treatments are evaluated by the same clinician, it is possible that the sessions are held during a morning and an afternoon session. In this case, each treatment must be administered in roughly the same number of morning and afternoon sessions. Such

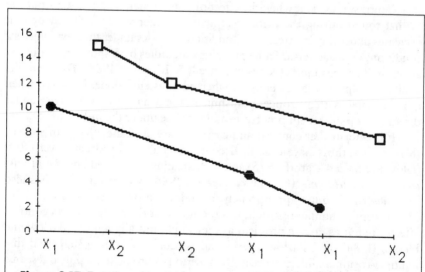

Figure 8-17. Typical graphic representation of the results of an alternating treatments design. The graph shows a larger effect for treatment 1 than for treatment 2.

counterbalancing avoids the potential for a given treatment to be more effective because it is administered by a particular clinician or at a certain time.

Counterbalancing requires multiple subjects. For example, if the clinician counterbalances the time of treatment, he or she may apply the first treatment to the first subject in the morning session and the second treatment to the same subject in the afternoon session. From then on, the order of presentations is semirandomized and counterbalanced. In a second subject, the second treatment may be given in the first morning session and the first treatment in the first afternoon session. As in the first subject, the treatment presentations from then on are counterbalanced. In this case, the two treatments and time periods are also counterbalanced across the two subjects.

Carryover and Contrast Effects. In addition to a potential order effect, the alternating treatments design can pose two additional problems: carryover and contrast effects. Both these effects create problems for an unambiguous interpretation of data. In either case, the effects of a second treatment are partly determined by the effects of the first treatment.

As described in Chapter 7, the term *carryover effects* refers to generalization of the first treatment effect to the second treatment. In this case, the observed effects of the second treatment are larger than what might be expected if the second treatment were administered alone. In terms of our earlier example of the relative effects of aversive noise and verbal "No," a stutterer's fluency in the verbal punishment condition may be higher because of the carryover effects of the aversive noise condition.

Contrast is evident when the effect of a subsequent treatment is opposite to that found during the prior treatment. In other words, a behavior that decreases under the first treatment condition increases under the next, adjacent condition, and vice versa. Some punishment studies have shown the contrast effects in human subjects (Newsom, Favell, & Rincover, 1983). For example, a mild punishment may be effective when administered alone. However, when it is alternated with a stronger punishment, the behavior may decrease under the stronger punishment procedure and increase under the milder procedure.

It is evident that contrast and carryover are opposite effects. In spite of this, some authors have described contrast as a variety of carryover effect (Ulman & Sulzer-Azaroff, 1975) and both are often subsumed under *multiple-treatment interference* (Barlow & Hersen, 1984). Carryover effect has also been described, quite appropriately, as induction or generalization.

In applied human research, it is thought that the carryover and contrast effects are not as great a problem as they might initially appear. Barlow and Hersen (1984), and Barlow, Hayes and Nelson (1984) have suggested that multiple-treatment interference is not as serious a problem in applied research as in basic research. Nevertheless, the clinician wishing to use the alternating treatments design should take at least two steps to counteract its potential problems. First, the clinician should counterbalance the treatment conditions.

This will help minimize both the order effects and the carryover effects. Second, the treatment sessions must be separated in time, and only one treatment must be administered in a given session. Originally, it was suggested that within a single session, two treatments may be alternated.

It is possible that even when there is a carryover effect from one treatment to the next, the relative effectiveness of the two treatments may still be the same as it would have been in the absence of carryover effects (Barlow & Hersen, 1984). In any case, should an investigator be concerned with the carryover effects in a particular study, he or she can proceed to analyze such effects by making them the object of further experimental inquiry. Procedures to analyze the carryover effects are described in Sidman (1960) and Barlow and Hersen (1984).

One issue raised in early discussion of the alternating treatments design was whether the clients should discriminate the two treatment procedures that are alternated in order for a differential effect to appear. It was originally suggested that some external stimulus must clearly signal the particular treatment in effect in any given session. The current thinking, however, is that the clients may be simply told what treatment is going to be applied in a given session. At the beginning of each treatment session, the clinician can tell the client that "in this session, we will be using the treatment procedure _____." No additional steps to insure discrimination are considered necessary (Barlow & Hersen, 1984; Barlow et al., 1984). In laboratory research, when similar treatment variables (reinforcement schedules that are close to each other) are alternated rapidly (often by the minute), differential effects may not emerge because of a lack of discrimination. This has not been a major problem in applied research, in which clients are usually able to discriminate treatment procedures.

The alternating treatments design does not require a formal baseline before the treatment variables are introduced. For this reason, it is thought that the alternating treatments design is especially useful in case of behaviors that are inherently variable (Ulman & Sulzer-Azaroff, 1975). The alternating treatments design is considered to be relatively insensitive to background variability in behaviors. True differences between treatments can emerge against a background of variability.

Most investigators do establish baselines of target behaviors before introducing treatment. That is still a desirable, though not required, feature of an alternating treatments design. Such baselines give an opportunity to analyze the effects of different treatments in relation to baselines as well.

INEFFECTIVE TREATMENTS IN MULTIPLE TREATMENT EVALUATIONS.

Sometimes the clinician may find out that one or more of the treatments in a multiple treatment evaluation are ineffective. In an *ABACA/ACABA* design, for example, it may be found that treatment B does not affect the behavior at all. In such cases, there is no point in returning the client to a period of baseline measurement. The B "treatment" condition, for all practical purposes, is comparable to the baseline in that there were no changes in the response rate. The next treatment can then be introduced without the second, formal baseline. In such cases, the design is redesignated as an $A=BCA$ design, which means that the first treatment was treated like a baseline because of lack of effect. If in the second sequence, treatment C is ineffective, treatment B may be introduced without a preceding baseline, resulting in a $A=CBA$ design.

Because ineffective treatments are functionally equivalent to baselines, single-subject strategies allow modifications in treatment procedures within a single study. Such modifications typically are not done within the group-design strategy. Even when the experimenter realizes that the treatment is not producing changes in the behavior, the study is completed as planned. However, within the single-subject strategy, a clinician can introduce another treatment without baselines or make modifications in the original treatment (Connell & Thompson, 1986). For example, if a 5-second timeout proves ineffective in reducing the frequency of stuttering, a 10-second timeout contingency may be applied. No baselines need to be interspersed between the treatment variations as long as the first treatment does not result in a changed baseline. If verbal praise does not act as a reinforcer for the correct production of target phonemes, a token system may be implemented. Of course, the treatment variable that produces changes in the baseline will have to be evaluated with such controls as untreated multiple baselines, withdrawal, or reversal.

The Interactional Design

Clinicians know that in most cases, what is considered a single treatment for a given disorder is actually a combination of several treatment components. For example, an articulation treatment program may consist of certain stimulus presentation, modeling, reinforcement for the correct production, and punishment for the incorrect production. In this case, the stimulus, modeling, reinforcement, and punishment constitute four components, each of which can be manipulated independently. Similar components are used in language treatment. In the treatment of stuttering, instructions, modeling, reduced rate, altered airflow, gentle phonatory onset, counseling, attitudinal changes, increased self-confidence, reinforcement of correct responses, and punishment of incorrect responses may all be treatment components. In fact, such therapeutic packages that combine different components are quite popular in speech–language pathology.

In controlled studies, one can demonstrate the overall effectiveness of a treatment package. Such a demonstration, however, is no testimony to the effectiveness of the individual components included in the package. In our example of the stuttering treatment package, one or many of the components may contribute very little or nothing at all. There may be just one or two effective components, which then create the impression that all components are effective.

When two or more treatment components within a package are effective to any degree at all, then the question of interaction, discussed in Chapter 7, emerges. Single-subject interactional designs are strategies to study such interactional effects of two or more treatment components of therapeutic packages. In addition, the design can help isolate components that are effective to any extent from those that are not at all effective. The importance of such a design strategy in the task of developing a clinical science is obvious.

The basic interactional strategy has a pair of sequences with two experimental arrangements in each sequence. At the least, one complete sequence must be completed in a given study. Suppose that a clinician wishes to study the independent and interactive effects of two treatment components in remediating stuttering: reduced speech rate (X_1) and modified airflow (X_2). The two components can be tested under four experimental arrangements created by the two sequences.

Let us further suppose that the clinician wishes to use the first sequence with two experimental arrangements. In the first experimental arrangement, the baselines of stuttering are established (A), and then the rate reduction strategy is applied in the initial treatment (B) condition. After several sessions of rate reduction, the modified airflow component is *added* to the existing rate reduction component. This combined treatment condition $(BC$ or $X_{1+2})$ is in effect for a certain number of sessions. In the next condition, the modified airflow is withdrawn, leaving only the rate reduction as the treatment component (the second B or X_1 condition). Finally, the modified airflow is added a second time to the rate reduction component (the second BC or X_{1+2} condition).

In the second experimental arrangement, which is used in a *different* set of stutterers, the modified airflow is applied in the first treatment condition. The rate reduction is added in the next condition and subtracted in the following condition. In the final condition, the rate reduction is once again added to the modified airflow component. The two experimental arrangements of this sequence of an interactional design are illustrated in Figure 8-18.

The two experimental arrangements result in an A-B-BC-B-BC design. These arrangements, each applied to two individual subjects or two different sets of subjects, can help determine the independent and interactive effects of rate reduction and airflow. The first arrangement will demonstrate the effects of rate reduction alone as well as rate reduction plus modified airflow. The second arrangement can demonstrate the effects of airflow alone as well

Conditions

1.	**Baseline**	X_1	X_{1+2}	X_1	X_{1+2}
	A	**B**	**BC**	**B**	**BC**
2.	**Baseline**	X_2	X_{2+1}	X_2	X_{2+1}
	A	**B**	**BC**	**B**	**BC**

Figure 8-18. The first sequence of an interactional design.

as airflow plus rate reduction. The independent effects of airflow cannot be determined in the first arrangement because it is not tested independently. Similarly, the independent effects of rate reduction cannot be determined in the second arrangement. It is for this reason that both the experimental arrangements must be used in a given study.

Assuming that the rate reduction results in some decrease in stuttering frequency, the addition of airflow may show a further decrease. When the airflow is subtracted, the stuttering frequency may increase, and once again decrease when the airflow is added. Similarly, addition of rate to the airflow may enhance the effect on stuttering, which would show a decline when the component is withdrawn. On the other hand, it may be evident that one of the components has a greater effect than the other. Adding one component may not make a big difference, whereas adding the other component may result in a more dramatic decrease in stuttering. In essence, the results may show that both the components are equally effective or equally ineffective, or that one is more effective than the other. The results may also show that each of the two components is weak by itself but that the two in combination can produce notable effects.

The first sequence involves the presentation of only *one* of the treatments during the initial treatment condition. However, the clinician can just as appropriately introduce the *combined* treatment during the initial treatment condition. Then, in the next treatment condition, one of the components is subtracted, then added, then once again subtracted. This results in a an *A-BC-B-BC-B* design with two experimental arrangements, as illustrated in Figure 8-19. In one of the arrangements, the first treatment component is subtracted and added, whereas in the other arrangement, the second component is subtracted and added.

In our example of an evaluation of rate reduction and airflow components, the clinician first establishes the baseline (*A*) in either of the two experimental arrangements shown in Figure 8-18. Then, while following the first arrangement, the clinician applies both the rate reduction *and* airflow components (X_{1+2}) in the first treatment condition (*BC*). In the next

Conditions

1.	**Baseline**	X_{1+2}	X_1	X_{1+2}	X_1
	A	**BC**	**B**	**BC**	**B**
2.	**Baseline**	X_{1+2}	X_2	X_{1+2}	X_2
	A	**BC**	**B**	**BC**	**B**

Figure 8-19. The second sequence of an interactional design.

condition (B), the clinician subtracts the airflow component (X_2) and leaves only the rate reduction (X_1) in force. In the following condition (BC), the airflow is added to the rate reduction component (X_{1+2}). In the final B condition, the airflow is once again subtracted. It must be noted that in all of the treatment conditions, the rate reduction is constant.

The second experimental arrangement of the same sequence involves the subtraction and addition of rate reduction instead of airflow. In this case, airflow is constant across the treatment conditions.

The second sequence can also determine the effects of the two treatments in combination and of either of them alone. In other words, whether the two components are both strong and equally so, whether both are weak and equally so, and what happens when the two are combined in either case can be determined within the design.

The two sequences differ in terms of whether in the initial stage of treatment the entire package or only one of the components is applied. If the entire package is applied, one of the components is *subtracted* and added in subsequent conditions. If only one of the components is applied initially, another component is *added* and then subtracted in subsequent conditions. As noted before, any one sequence can be considered satisfactory as long as both the experimental arrangements are used. However, both the sequences, when applied with both the arrangements, can strengthen the conclusions.

In using either of the sequences, it is important to remember that the same variable is added or subtracted. For example, if the clinician starts with the rate reduction as the first treatment condition, then the airflow is added and subtracted. One cannot add airflow in one condition and subtract rate reduction in the other. In other words, the first treatment component stays constant; the second component is added or subtracted. When the clinician starts with the airflow component, rate reduction is added and subtracted and airflow stays constant. When both the components are applied in the initial treatment condition, only one of them is subtracted and added in any one or a set of subjects. The other component is subtracted and added only in another subject or set of subjects.

Interactional designs have not been used frequently in communicative disorders. The design deserves greater application because many untested treatment packages exist in the treatment of articulation, speech, language, voice, and fluency disorders. Even when a total package is known to be effective, we need to determine the independent and interactive effects of each of the components of the package so that ineffective components can be discarded and more effective components can be combined.

The Changing Criterion Design

It must be clear to the clinician by now that a critical element of the experimental strategy is to demonstrate that the behavior varies in accordance with a specific experimental manipulation. A design that retains this feature but does not use the control features of the previously described designs is known as the changing criterion design (Hartman & Hall, 1976). In this design, the clinician tries to have a behavior repeatedly approximate a preset criterion. Whenever the clinician changes the criterion for which the behavior is held, the behavior changes and approximates that criterion. The previously discussed criterion-referenced change is the control mechanism in the changing criterion design.

The design has not been used in communicative disorders, and has had limited use even in behavioral research. Still, the best example of the design comes from the original Hartman and Hall (1976) study on controlling smoking behavior with response cost based on the number of cigarettes smoked and bonus for reduced smoking. A baseline level of smoking was established over several days, and then the multiple treatment phases were initiated. In each phase of the treatment, a new criterion was imposed. A criterion allowed the client a certain number of cigarettes a day. In successive phases, the criterion was lowered so that the client was asked to smoke less and less. The study showed that every time a new (and lower) criterion was imposed, the client's rate of smoking approximated the criterion in force. The smoking behavior changed only at times when the criterion was changed. This fact helped rule out the influence of extraneous variables.

The changing criterion design is helpful when the behavior changes slowly and over a period of time. From a logical standpoint, it must be possible to use the design in the reduction of such behaviors as dysfluencies, errors of articulation, and, as noted by McReynolds and Kearns (1983), vocal abuse. After the establishment of a baseline, the clinician requires a certain reduction in the frequency of undesirable behaviors over the next several days and uses appropriate reinforcement procedures to help the client move toward the new criterion. When the behavior approximates the criterion, a new criterion with a lower frequency of the undesirable behavior is established. Such progressive reduction in the behavior in accordance with changing criteria helps establish experimental control.

In the use of the changing criterion design, the clinician must make sure that the baseline phase is not too short when compared with any of the single treatment phase. Also, the clinician must implement multiple criterion changes to demonstrate the experimental control. If additional control procedures are considered necessary, the treatment can be totally withdrawn in one of the phases to show that the behavior returns to the original baseline. A more practical strategy is to return the client to an earlier criterion. In this case, the target behavior would reverse and approximate the earlier criterion. Following this, the new criterion may once again be imposed.

Designs to Assess Response Maintenance

An important clinical question concerns the durability of treated behaviors. Whether the target behaviors established in the clinical and educational settings are produced in other situations and over time is an important question, an answer to which will determine the eventual success of treatment. Within the clinical tradition, the follow-up procedures are designed to assess the maintenance of treated behaviors over time. Follow-up, however, can only demonstrate whether the response is maintained or not. Variables responsible for either the loss of established behaviors or those that are responsible for the maintenance cannot be determined in a follow-up assessment.

The question of maintenance is often confused with that of generalization in most of the clinical literature. Generalization is a temporary phenomenon of declining response rate when the independent variable is suspended (Hegde, 1985). Generalization is measured in relation to situations, persons, and responses that are not a part of treatment in a given study. It is typically measured through probes, which were described in Chapter 5. Generalization, however, is not the same as maintenance. A response that shows an initial generalization may not be maintained over time. For example, the client who is fluent in the home may not maintain that fluency 6 months after the treatment is terminated. Whether treatment effects are maintained over time in different settings, in interaction with different individuals, and in the kinds of responses that were not specifically trained by the clinician calls for a different approach.

An experimental analysis of response maintenance requires an identification of the independent variables that are responsible for such maintenance. Some clinicians seem to assume that the maintenance of target behaviors subsequent to the termination of treatment is still due to the treatment effects. However, there is no evidence to support this view. To assume that an absence of treatment variables is the required condition of response maintenance is to assume that effects are produced without causes. Perhaps there is an absence of the treatment variables manipulated by the investigator, but not necessarily an absence of any kind of independent variables, since no dependent variable can exist without independent variables. Therefore, response maintenance is a question of transferred control. Initially, the response is controlled by the independent variables manipulated by the clinician, and this fact can be documented by any one of the several group or single-subject designs described so far in this book.

When the treatment is discontinued, the target responses must be maintained by independent variables that are operative in the client's everyday environment. Those variables may be similar to the ones manipulated by the clinician, or they may be of entirely different kinds. In any case, those variables are a part of the client's living environment, and they are knowingly or unknowingly administered by the people surrounding the client. An experimental analysis of maintenance should look at the independent variables that are operative in the client's natural environment and administered by persons that interact with him or her.

The technology of response maintenance is in its earliest stage. Rusch and Kazdin (1981) have proposed three design strategies that they believe will help assess response maintenance. First, when a treatment procedure consists of multiple components, such as modeling, reinforcement, informative feedback, and tokens, the clinician can withdraw each of the components, one at a time and in sequence. Any time a given component is withdrawn, whether the response is maintained or not is carefully assessed. If it is, the next component is withdrawn. In this manner, all the components are withdrawn while care is taken to insure that the target behavior is not lost. This design is known as the sequential-withdrawal design.

Second, when a clinician is using a multiple baseline design to evaluate the effects of a treatment package, either the entire package or one of the components can be withdrawn from one of the subjects, or behaviors, or the settings used in the design. This is known as the partial-withdrawal design. Of course, the treatment is withdrawn only after the behaviors show change under treatment. In the multiple baseline across subjects, if the subject for whom the treatment is withdrawn continues to respond appropriately, the treatment is withdrawn from other subjects as well. If a particular response in the same subject continues at a high rate in spite of treatment withdrawal, then the treatment can be withdrawn from other behaviors of the same client when the design used is the multiple baseline across behaviors. Similarly, if the withdrawal of treatment in one setting proves to have no negative effects, then it can be withdrawn in other settings when the design is the multiple baseline across settings.

Third, a treatment component or a package can be first removed from one behavior, subject, or setting and then, if the data warrant, removed from all of the behaviors, subjects, or settings. Once again, the basic design used to demonstrate the treatment effects will be the multiple baseline design. This strategy is a combination of the first two, and therefore it is known as partial-sequential withdrawal.

The strategies suggested by Rusch and Kazdin (1981) do not necessarily address the issue of response maintenance as described here. Obviously, when a treatment is withdrawn, the response rate may or may not be sustained. If it is not sustained, the treatment is clearly still needed for the response to be made and no other variable has come to control it. If the response rate is sustained when the treatment variable is withdrawn, then either the response is under the discriminative stimulus control, which may fade in time, or independent variables other than the one manipulated by the clinician are controlling the response. The withdrawal strategies described by Rusch and Kazdin (1981) are not able to make a discriminative experimental analysis of these possibilities.

Further developments in the technology of response maintenance may be possible when research attention is focused on the mechanisms by which the response controls initially exerted by the clinician are transferred to other individuals and other settings. It may be a mistake to assume that the end of a clinician's treatment is the end of response control. This assumption implies that once created, an effect does not need a cause to sustain itself.

It would appear that no new technology is needed to begin an experimental analysis of response maintenance in nonclinical settings. What is needed is a study of contingencies managed by other individuals in natural settings and over time. Existing experimental methodologies are capable of handling these concerns.

Other Single-Subject Designs

Of the several other single-subjects designs that exist, two deserve to be mentioned: the simultaneous treatments design and the periodic treatments design. In the *simultaneous treatments design* (Browning, 1967), two or more treatments are simultaneously available to a client, but because of the nature of the design, the multiple treatments are not administered an equal number of times. The design is suitable to measure the client's preference of treatment.

In the simultaneous treatments design, multiple treatments are made available to a client who then chooses the treatment and thus controls which one is administered more often. This is the main difference between the alternating treatments design and the simultaneous treatments design. In the former, selected treatments are counterbalanced and administered equally often. In the simultaneous treatments design, the client eventually determines which treatment is administered more often.

The design has not been applied widely, even in behavioral research, where it originated. Clinicians who are interested in finding out the relative efficacy of two or more treatments while permitting a choice on the part of the client use the design in the following manner. Suppose that two clinicians wish to evaluate the usefulness of attitudinal therapy and fluency reinforcement therapy in the treatment of stuttering. Each clinician administers each treatment in a counterbalanced order. One clinician administers the attitudinal therapy first and the fluency reinforcement therapy next, whereas the other clinician follows the opposite sequence. A given clinician administers a particular treatment for a certain number of days. Both the clinicians are simultaneously available to administer treatment. The stutterer initially experiences both the treatments from both the clinicians but eventually may seek out the clinician who administered one of the two therapies, thus rejecting the other. A preference on the part of the client is thus evident. From then on, the preferred method is likely to be administered more often.

A potential problem with the design is that preference and effectiveness may not be the same. Most children, for example, love to go to "speech" when it is fun and play with no particular contingencies on any behaviors. More formal therapy procedures designed to produce systematic changes in the client behaviors may not necessarily be preferred. However, the design can be useful in evaluating the preference of two equally effective techniques that can be administered with equal ease. In such cases, one of the procedures may be more reinforcing to particular clients, resulting in faster change in target behaviors.

The *periodic treatments design* (Hayes, 1981) has not been used frequently either, but it offers an interesting opportunity to assess treatment effects in such settings as private practice and in any settings where other, more stringent control procedures are not practical. The design is based on the logic that in comparison with the times preceding treatment, a greater change in behavior would be evident following treatment. If the treatment sessions are scheduled once a week or less often, it is possible that the treatment effects are most visible soon after therapy and may show a gradual decline until the next therapy session. Once again, following the therapy session, the treatment effects would be clearly evident.

Most clinicians probably notice some deterioration in their clients' target behaviors during the session scheduled after a break in the services. Sometimes, differential changes of smaller magnitude may be noticed when the treatment sessions are scheduled twice weekly, say on a Monday-Wednesday schedule. During the very first portion of the Monday session, the behavior may be at a relatively lower frequency compared with the initial portion of the Wednesday session. However, the periodic treatments design requires that the target behaviors be measured more often than the number of treatment sessions. That is, measures of the dependent variable must be obtained on a continuous basis.

Continuous measures can be obtained by the cooperation of parents or clients. When parents audiotape the speech of the child at home on a daily basis and submit this for the clinician's evaluation, the measures are continuous. The clinician has data to track the differences in the dependent variable before and after therapy and any time in between. It may become evident that soon after therapy, the target behaviors are produced at a high level at home and that they begin to decline with the passage of time until the next therapy session. Again, after the next therapy session, the frequency of target behaviors may increase noticeably. If such changes are replicated several times, then the clinician has a basis on which to conclude that the treatment was probably responsible for the changes.

The control feature of the design is rather weak. Practicality is also a serious concern in using the periodic treatments design. Continuous measurement of client behaviors during periods of no treatment can pose problems. Also, the design is perhaps more appropriately used in evaluating treatments whose effects are documented in designs with stronger control procedures.

SINGLE-SUBJECT DESIGNS IN CLINICAL RESEARCH

The application of single-subject designs in communicative disorders has increased in the past few years. Many clinicians have found that the method is more applicable than group designs in evaluating treatment effects. It is more relevant to clinical research because it frees the clinician from seeking the unattainable random samples of clients and from the pursuit of the unrealistic goal of inferential generality.

Single-subject designs are especially suited for clinical treatment evaluation. Clinicians can use the clients they serve as subjects in experiments that seek answers to significant clinical questions. The single-subject experimental methodology can integrate clinical service and research. The clients who serve as subjects in experiments designed to evaluate treatment effects receive their clinical services as well. Therefore, such experiments help bridge the gap between research and clinical services.

If practicing clinicians were to use the single-subject designs on a large scale, the amount of in-house knowledge regarding the effectiveness of treatment procedures would be increased to a great extent. There is an urgent need to use the experimental methods of science and an equally urgent need to establish the treatment effects under controlled conditions. Although theoretically the group designs can offer the same opportunities for experimental-clinical research, it is the single-subject strategy that can actually make it happen.

Single-subject designs help generalize from research studies to individual clients. Thus, they provide for the much-needed logical generality. Detailed descriptions of individual client characteristics and treatment effects can help establish the generality of treatments across a wide variety of clients.

Single-subject design studies are more easily replicated than group design studies. A treatment known to be effective can be relatively easily replicated by clinicians while serving their clients. Designs such as the multiple baselines across subjects, behaviors, and settings provide a practical means of producing additional information on the generality of treatment effects.

A more detailed comparative evaluation of both the group and the single-subject strategies is made in Chapter 10.

CHAPTER SUMMARY

Single-subject designs are experimental designs that help establish cause–effect relations based on individual performances under different conditions of an experiment. They permit extended and intensive study of individual subjects and do not involve comparisons based on group performances. Instead of the pre- and posttests of the group designs, single-subject designs measure the dependent variables continuously. The subjects are not necessarily selected with the random procedure, and the results are not always analyzed statistically. Typically, the magnitude of effects produced within single-subject designs are large enough to be appreciated via visual inspection.

Single-subject designs use a variety of control mechanism to rule out the influence of extraneous variables, including replication, withdrawal of treatment, reversal of treatment, reinstatement, criterion-referenced change, rapid alternations, baselines, and simultaneous multibaselines.

Table 8-1 summarizes information on the major single-subject designs along with the kinds of questions they can answer.

The *AB* design is a preexperimental single-subject design, which lacks internal validity. It is similar to the traditional case studies.

The prototype of the single-subject design is the *ABA* design, which involves a baseline, treatment, and either withdrawal or reversal of treatment.

TABLE 8-1.

Summary of major single-subject designs and their applications

Designs	Research Questions	Strengths/Limitations
AB design	Is there an apparent change due to treatment?	Clinically useful; results only suggestive
ABA design	Is treatment effective? Is there a cause-effect relation?	Controlled experimental design; can isolate cause–effect relations; not a treatment design
BAB design	Is a treatment effective? Is there a cause-effect relation?	Controlled experimental design; can isolate cause–effect relations; not a treatment design
ABAB design	Is a treatment effective? Is there a cause-effect relation?	Controlled experimental design; can isolate cause–effect relations; not a treatment design

TABLE 8-1 (continued).

Designs	Research Questions	Strengths/Limitations
Multiple baseline across behaviors	Do only the treated behaviors change? Do untreated behaviors remain at baseline? Is treatment effective?	Fairly well-controlled design; clinically useful; is a treatment design; problems of repeated measurement
Multiple baseline across subjects	Do only the treated subjects change? Do untreated subjects remain at baseline? Is a treatment effective?	Fairly well-controlled design; clinically useful; is a treatment design; some need to find homogenous subjects; problems of repeated measurement
Multiple baseline across settings	Does the behavior change only in the setting in which it is treated? Does the behavior remain at baseline in untreated settings? Is a treatment effective?	Fairly well-controlled design; clinically useful; is a treatment design; problems of repeated measurement
ABACA/ACABA design	Are two or more treatments effective? Is one treatment more effective than the other?	Well-controlled design; can assess the independent and relative effects of two treatments; need to use counterbalancing
Alternating treatments design	What are the relative effects of two (or more) treatments?	Control relatively weak; clinically useful; is a treatment design; can help identify effective and ineffective treatments
Interactional design	Is there an interaction between two or more treatments? What are the relative effects of different treatment variables?	Fairly well-controlled design; clinically useful; excellent for studying interaction; can separate effective components from ineffective ones
Changing criterion design	Is a treatment effective? Do behaviors approximate changing criteria?	Control is relatively weak; useful only for certain kinds of behaviors; not well-researched yet

It can demonstrate the effects of a treatment variable clearly, but it is not a clinical design because it does not end with treatment. A variation of this design is the *BAB* design, which does end with treatment.

The *ABAB* design is an extension of the *ABA* design and is useful in clinical research. The conditions of this design are the baseline, treatment, either withdrawal or reversal, and reinstatement of treatment. An effective treatment can be continued until certain clinical objectives are met.

A set of clinically appropriate designs that do not involve either the withdrawal or reversal of treatment is known as the multiple baseline designs. These designs are based on the logic that when multiple dependent variables change only when each of them is brought under the control of an independent variable, then the extraneous variables are ruled out. The multiple baselines may be either behaviors, individuals, or physical settings.

Single-subject designs that permit evaluations of multiple treatments include the *ABACA/ACABA* design and the alternating treatments design. In both the designs, treatment conditions are counterbalanced. In the *ABACA/ACABA* design, the effects of two treatments (*B* and *C*) are compared. The treatment sequence is counterbalanced so that each treatment is preceded as well as followed by the other treatment. The treatments are separated by baselines. In the alternating treatments design, two (or more) treatments are rapidly alternated with the same subjects to evaluate the relative effects of those treatments. Most single-subject designs that expose the same subjects to multiple treatments have the potential problems of order effects and carryover effects.

The interactional design permits the assessment of interaction between two or more treatment components included in a treatment package. The design can also help isolate effective components from ineffective or less ineffective components.

In the changing criterion design, behaviors are forced to approximate changing criteria of performance. The design seeks to demonstrate that whenever the performance criteria change, the behavior also changes to fulfill the criteria in force. Such systematic criterion-referenced changes help establish control within the design.

Designs that help assess response maintenance after successful treatment include the sequential-withdrawal design, the partial-withdrawal design, and the partial-sequential withdrawal design. However, these designs do not necessarily shed light on the mechanisms of response maintenance in natural environments.

Single-subject designs are eminently practical in clinical settings. Their philosophical bases are compatible with clinical philosophies. They permit the assessment of treatment effects with individual clients who seek clinical services. The designs help blend the needs of science with those of clinical services. ■

(continued next page)

S T U D Y G U I D E

1   Distinguish between case studies and single-subject design studies.

2   In the single-subject strategy, what kinds of measures are substituted for the pre- and posttests of the group design strategy?

3   What are the six control mechanisms used within the single-subject strategy?

4   Illustrate how in a given study, more than one control mechanism may be used to demonstrate the experimental effects.

5   Distinguish intrasubject replication from intersubject replication.

6   Distinguish between reversal and withdrawal of treatment.

7   What are the limitations of withdrawal and reversal when used in clinical treatment research?

9   Design a study in which you would use the reversal procedure to demonstrate the effects of an articulation treatment program.

10 What is a "conservative use of the reversal strategy"?

11 Why is reinstatement a contingent control condition?

12 How many times is a treatment effect demonstrated when that treatment is reversed and reinstated once?

13 Why is criterion-referenced change the weaker of the control strategies?

14 Describe how rapid alternations can demonstrate the controlling effects of an independent variable.

15 Define baselines. What are the baseline criteria?

16 Describe how a good potential for contrast can make it possible to use a variable baseline in evaluating treatment effects.

17 In an *ABA* design, what conditions are not supposed to show contrast?

18 How do simultaneous multibaselines help rule out the influence of extraneous variables?

19 What are the limitations of an *AB* design?

20 Suppose you wish to evaluate the effects of delayed auditory feedback on stuttering. Describe a study with the *ABA* design. Specify the design aspects of the study.

Study Guide *(continued)*

21 In evaluating the effects of a treatment procedure, what design will permit you to start with the treatment condition?

22 Describe the *ABAB* design and point out its advantages and disadvantages from the clinical research standpoint.

23 What kinds of research questions require the use of the *ABAB* design?

24 Describe the three variations of the multiple baseline design.

25 What problems do you face when the multiple behaviors used in a multiple baseline design are not independent of each other?

26 What additional controls can you introduce to a multiple baseline design? What problems do these additional controls create?

27 Suppose you wish to evaluate two methods of teaching basic vocabulary to mentally retarded clients. What design would you use? Justify your answer.

28 Compare and contrast the *ABACA/ACABA* design with the alternating treatments design.

29 Why do you need both the *ABACA* and the *ACABA* sequences?

30 What kinds of questions are answered by the alternating treatments design?

31 Describe the carryover and contrast effects.

32 What is an $A = BCA$ design? When do you use it?

33 What is an interaction? How do you study it within the single-subject strategy?

34 Find two methods of teaching correct articulation in young children. Then, design a study to evaluate the independent and interactive effects of the two methods with a single-subject interactional design. Use both the sequences described in the text.

35 Describe the difference between the *A-B-BC-B-BC* design and the *A-BC-B-BC-B* design.

36 In an interactional design, can you change more than one variable at a time while moving from one experimental condition to the other? Why or why not?

37 Describe the changing criterion design. Illustrate the design with a hypothetical study.

38 What kinds of behaviors are especially suited for the changing criterion design?

39 Distinguish between generalization and maintenance.

40 When can you say that you have made an experimental analysis of response maintenance?

41 What is the sequential-withdrawal design? What is its purported use?

42 What is a partial-withdrawal design? How would you use it in clinical research?

43 Do the strategies suggested by Rusch and Kazdin necessarily address the issue of response maintenance? Justify your answer.

44 Suppose you wish to study whether clients prefer one treatment over the other, assuming that both are equally effective. What design would you use in answering this question?

45 What is a periodic treatments design? What are its limitations?

46 Summarize the advantages of single-subject designs in clinical research.

■ CHAPTER 9

Generality Through Replications

■ Direct replication, 283

■ Systematic replication, 287

■ Conditions necessary for systematic replication, 290

■ Failed replications, 291

■ Treatment variables and treatment packages, 294

■ Homo- and heterogeneity of subjects, 296

■ Study guide, 298

The various group and single-subject designs described in the previous chapters help establish cause–effect relations between selected independent and dependent variables. Necessarily, any experimental study is done in a given setting, by one or a few investigators, and with a few subjects. A laboratory study may isolate a cause–effect relation between two variables. A clinical study may demonstrate that a given treatment technique is effective in a few clients. Such clinical studies also demonstrate a cause–effect relation. As long as cause–effect relations are demonstrated under well-controlled conditions, internal validity (described in Chapter 6) is assured. Once a cause–effect relation emerges within a single study, the next question of concern is whether the same relation can be verified by other investigators, in other settings, and with other subjects or clients. As noted in Chapter 6, this is the question of generality of research findings.

In Chapter 6, various types of generality were described. In this chapter, we shall be concerned with the *procedures* of establishing generality of research data. The emphasis will be on the generality of data relative to clinical treatment research.

The clinical importance of the question of generality is obvious. Clinicians wish to know whether a given procedure, demonstrated to be effective in a particular study, will be equally effective when used by other clinicians, on other clients, and in other settings. The question of generality is related to both reliability and the range of conditions under which a demonstrated cause–effect relation holds good.

Replication is the method of establishing generality of research findings. A single study, no matter how well done, is not able to establish generality. This is true even of group designs that draw random samples from the population, because sampling equivalence should not be equated with generality. A study must be repeated in order to find out if the evidence holds under different circumstances. A study can be replicated in different ways, and different replication strategies are used in different stages of research. The questions and strategies of replication have received much attention from behavioral scientists, who have described two major kinds of replications: direct and systematic (Barlow & Hersen, 1984; Sidman, 1960).

In Chapter 8, it was pointed out that single-subject designs replicate the treatment effects within the same study. This is known as intrasubject replication. Such intrasubject replications are typically done with similar subjects. Such replications help increase the confidence one can place in the experimental findings, but they do not necessarily suggest significant generality. Both direct and systematic replications are necessary to establish generality.

DIRECT REPLICATION

In direct replication, the same experiment is repeated by the same researcher in the same physical setting. Direct replication involves a different set of subjects who are similar to those in the original study. Therefore, direct replication is homogeneous intersubject replication by the same investigator in the same setting.

When a clinician finds out that a given form of treatment is effective with a set of clients with a particular disorder, direct replication must be initiated. It does not matter whether the single-subject or group design strategy was used in the original study. A given report of experimental findings does not establish generality; it is the repetition of the experiment that does. Therefore, the investigator is expected to find additional subjects who are similar to the original set of subjects and repeat the experiment. If the treatment shows similar effects with this new set of clients, the first step toward achieving generality of findings will have been taken.

Direct replication of treatment effects requires that everything except the subjects be the same as in the original experiment. The treatment, the client disorder or behaviors, the experimental arrangements, the physical setting, the clinician-experimenter, all stay constant through the direct replication series. The same experimental design is used in a direct replication.

The new subjects used in a direct replication must be similar to those in the original study. In other words, the investigator needs to find clients who are homogeneous with regard to the disorder as well as the relevant assigned variables. For example, when it has been determined that a given language treatment procedure is effective with four to six aphasic patients, the speech–language clinician may find other aphasic patients who are similar to the original set of patients and repeat the experimental treatment program.

Homogeneous intersubject replication is considered the safest initial strategy because if the method does not work with a heterogeneous set of subjects, then it is difficult to determine the source of the problem. Continuing our example of treatment evaluation involving aphasic patients, it is possible that compared with those in the original study, a replication study may have aphasic patients who are different in terms of the severity of aphasia, preonset educational and intellectual levels, postonset duration before therapy is introduced, age of the patients, and other such variables. In this case, if the investigator fails to replicate the original effects of the treatment procedure, it is difficult to determine whether the failure was due to differences in one, some, or all of the variables that were different in the second set of subjects. Thus, heterogeneous intersubject replication is considered risky because failures are difficult to account for. Nevertheless, such heterogeneous intersubject replication is the essence of systematic replication. It is the success with homogeneous intersubject direct replications that justifies taking such a risk. Even then, given systematic replications do not involve subjects who are different on multiple variables. If they are, the same difficulty in interpreting the results arises.

Problem of Finding Homogeneous Subjects

It is clear that by definition, direct replication requires subjects who are similar to those used in the original investigation. This requirement can pose one of the most difficult problems for the clinician who wishes to replicate the effects of a particular treatment. In some respects, this requirement is based on a theoretical, and hence an ideal, progression of research through various stages of original and replicated series of investigations.

Ideally, the investigator has either strictly homogeneous or strictly heterogeneous subjects in the original investigation. In the single-subject strategy, the subjects are expected to be homogeneous; in the group strategy, they are expected to be heterogeneous. When the subjects in the original study are homogeneous, the subjects in direct replication are expected to be similar to those in the original study and homogeneous among themselves. When the subjects in the original study are heterogeneous, the subjects in the direct replication are expected to be similarly heterogeneous.

It is relatively easy to find homogeneous animal subjects. The animal subjects' genetic and environmental history may be controlled by the investigator to produce a homogeneous as well as heterogeneous set of subjects that can then be used in the original, direct, and systematic series of experiments. In human research, especially in human clinical research, this ideal sequence of original, direct, and systematic research is not achieved. Consequently, those sequences are not as well distinguished in human clinical research as in animal research. Therefore, we shall have to consider direct as well as systematic replications from the standpoint of practical exigencies that dictate clinical research.

In practice, neither a single-subject design study nor a group design study is likely to have the kinds of subjects they are supposed to have. The subjects in a single-subject design study, though few, may still be heterogeneous. The subjects in a group clinical study are less heterogeneous than expected because of the difficulty in obtaining a random sample. In essence, clients in clinical research are neither ideally homogeneous nor ideally heterogeneous. If the target is a heterogeneous sample, the clinician does his or her best to increase the diversity of subjects. If the target is a homogeneous sample, the investigator takes all practical steps to minimize differences in subject characteristics. In either case, the eventual sample is likely to be other than the ideal.

Another difficulty with subject selection for either an original or a replicative study is that it is one thing to strive for an ideal sample of subjects, but it is an entirely different thing to *know* what is an ideal sample. Homo- or heterogeneity of subjects is a matter of judgment based on past research and clinical experience. Investigators judge the similarities and differences between individuals on the basis of known variables, but unknown variables may make subjects either similar to, or different from, each other. Obviously, such similarities and differences do not enter into judgments of homo- and heterogeneity of subjects selected for a study. Assume, for example, that an aphasic patient's age at which schooling is started is a variable that determines the rate of improvement in therapy. Lack of information on this variable also means that it will not be considered in judging homo- and heterogeneity of subjects for a given study. The result may be that subjects who are similar on this variable may be considered different, and vice versa.

Practical difficulties in obtaining subjects for a study often lead to compromises in the application of subject selection criteria adopted by an investigator. Age ranges may be stretched to accommodate available subjects. Differences in health history may be ignored. Although initially planned to have subjects of only one sex, the eventual sample may contain both the sexes. Such compromises are made sooner or later by most investigators. Though justified on practical grounds, such compromises may create difficulties for interpreting data and for planning replications.

When the subjects in the original study were about as homogeneous as expected, and all of them reacted the same to the treatment variable, the investigator may search for similar subjects for a direct replication. There is no guarantee, however, that the subjects selected for the direct replication will be very similar to those in the original study. They are likely to be more or less homogeneous among themselves and more or less similar to the subjects in the original study. If the subjects selected for direct replication are about as similar to those in the original study as can be expected, another replication may be attempted. In some cases, the investigator may decide that it is time to initiate systematic replications, which involve subjects who differ from those in the original as well as direct replication studies.

To a certain extent, an original study that contains heterogeneous clients and produces consistent data is already a systematic replication. In other words, although ideally the initial study involves homogeneous subjects, in practice the subjects may be heterogeneous. For example, the investigator wishing to evaluate the effects of a new treatment for aphasic patients may not have been able to select patients of the same age, health history, and severity of aphasia. Though it is not prudent to have heterogeneous subjects in an initial study, the alternative course of not conducting the study may not be considered a good choice. Therefore, the investigator, trying his or her best to minimize the differences between subjects, may go ahead with the study. If the results are consistent across those somewhat different subjects, the original study itself can be considered a systematic replication. Such a study will have demonstrated that different subjects react the same to the same treatment variable.

Research philosophies generally discourage such studies in the initial step because when the results are not uniformly good or bad, an unambiguous interpretation of results is not possible. However, when practical considerations force the selection of available clients for an initial study, the next attempt often depends upon the judgment of the particular investigator. If the sample is thought to be relatively heterogeneous and the results are consistent, replications may be either direct or systematic. However, when the results are inconsistent across clients while there is reason to believe that the sample was heterogeneous in some respects, then the investigator will have learned a lesson. He or she will not try too hard to interpret the data in any global manner and instead will look at individual differences that might have accounted for divergent data. In further studies, a more serious attempt may be made to obtain homogeneous sets of subjects. In essence, there are very few rigid rules that an investigator can follow in determining the exact nature of replication.

Direct replication need not be lengthy. When the effect of an independent variable is replicated across a few subjects, systematic replication may be initiated. Within the philosophy of single-subject designs, Barlow and Hersen (1984) recommend that when a procedure has been directly replicated in four different subjects or clients, systematic replication must be started. Continued direct replication may not be productive beyond that point. What is needed at that point is information on whether the procedure has the same effects in subjects of different characteristics, in different settings, and when implemented by different investigators.

SYSTEMATIC REPLICATION

Direct replication can only demonstrate that the causal relation found in the original study may have some homogeneous subject generality. It does not, however, provide any information on the potential problems one might face when the relation is studied in new settings, by other investigators, and with clients who may be in some ways different from those in the original study as well as in the direct replications. Information of this kind can be generated only by systematic replications.

Systematic replication involves varying one or more variables at a time to see if the results of the direct replication series can still be duplicated. For the sake of clear interpretations, it is necessary to vary only one or two variables at a time. If too many factors are varied simultaneously, a failure to replicate the findings of the direct replication series is difficult to understand, although a success in such cases results in significant economy of effort.

It is possible that the initial systematic replication is made by the same investigator. Once it has been determined that a given functional relation is reliable and that it has some degree of subject generality, the investigator may wish to find out if the same relation can be found in a different setting or with subjects who are in some specific way different from those in the earlier studies. A clinician who has found that a given treatment procedure is effective with a number of clients showing a particular disorder may be curious about its effects in (1) a different setting, involving similar clients; (2) the same setting, but with clients who show a variation of the same disorder; (3) in the same setting with clients who have the same disorder but different assigned variables; (4) a different setting, also involving subjects who show a variation of the same disorder; (5) in the same setting, with clients who have an altogether different disorder; and (6) in a different setting, also with clients who show a different disorder. These possibilities are not exhaustive, but they illustrate the basic nature of systematic replication.

Systematic replication of clinical treatment effects is a time-consuming process because the diagnostic categories are not strictly homogeneous. Intersubject variability among such clinical groups as stutterers, hearing or language impaired individuals, aphasic patients, and apraxic patients is considerable. The variability regarding such background variables as age, sex, education, and socioeconomic status of clients within diagnostic categories is well known. Besides, clients within and across diagnostic categories vary in terms of the severity of the disorder, subtypes within the disorder, the degree and types of prior treatment experiences, etc. A treatment procedure that works well with young language handicapped individuals may or may not work with older clients having the same disorder. Clients with multiple misarticulations may not react as favorably to a treatment procedure as those with single-phoneme misarticulations. A procedure that is effective with mild stutterers may not be equally effective with severe stutterers. A technique found to be effective with stutterers who have marked respiratory abnormalities may be useless with those who do not show such abnormalities.

On the other hand, certain treatment techniques may be effective within and across diagnostic categories. Obvious differences between clients such as age, sex, severity, and diagnostic categories and subcategories do not necessarily mean that they will react differently to the same treatment procedure. There are many well-researched behavioral treatment procedures that are known to be effective across clients, disorders, age groups, and diagnostic subgroups (Barlow & Hersen, 1984; Hegde, 1985). As Barlow and Hersen (1984) have shown, behavioral techniques such as differential attention (reinforcing one behavior with attention while not reinforcing another behavior) is known to be effective with a variety of behavior disorders treated by many professionals and paraprofessionals under many different settings. However, an extensive series of systematic replication can point out conditions or disorders for which a given technique with a certain degree of known generality may not be appropriate. In case of differential attention, systematic replication series have noted that while its generality is quite impressive, the technique is not particularly effective in case of self-injurious behavior and children's oppositional behavior (Barlow & Hersen, 1984).

Systematic replications are needed to establish that a given treatment procedure works when implemented by other clinicians. Assuming that other clinicians are equally capable of administering the treatment procedure in question, the results must be comparable to those of the original investigator.

If it is proved that some dramatic results obtained by a clinician cannot be replicated by other clinicians, the reported effects must be attributed not to the described technique but to some extraneous factors. Those extraneous factors may include such variables as the "personality" or the special interpersonal skills of the original clinician. What is more important is the possibility that the original investigator may not have described all of the therapeutic manipulations. Certain critical elements of the procedures may not have been included in the description, and hence those who try to replicate the study may not do precisely what the original clinician did.

It is likely that other clinicians will replicate a treatment procedure in a setting different from that of the original setting. In this case, successful replicative attempts demonstrate generality not only across subjects and clinicians, but also across settings.

Successful replication across clients, clinicians, and settings is essential to a widespread practice of therapeutic techniques, although this has rarely been a condition required by many clinicians in speech–language pathology. A treatment procedure can be recommended for general application only when it is shown that a variety of clients can benefit from it. In speech–language pathology, most of the therapeutic practices are neither replicated nor experimentally tested in the first place.

When a therapeutic technique designed to remedy a particular disorder has been replicated in other settings, by other investigators, and on a number of different clients, the question that arises is whether the technique can be equally effective with different disorders. A successful language treatment technique or components of the technique may be useful in the remedying of articulation or voice disorders. For example, components such as modeling, shaping, and differential reinforcement are known to be useful components of therapy for many different kinds of verbal as well as nonverbal behavior disorders.

Unfortunately, replication of a technique across disorders may be discouraged by the fixed notions of nosology. There is an implicit assumption that different diagnostic categories necessarily require treatment techniques that are independent of each other. This assumption may not be valid in speech–language pathology, in which diagnostic categories are not strictly etiologic, but are often descriptive. As a result, topographically different behaviors such as high vocal pitch or dysfluency may be susceptible to the same treatment variables. Furthermore, there is no compelling reason to believe that different instigating causes of communicative disorders necessarily dictate totally different treatment variables. For example, whether a language disorder is thought to be due to mental retardation or some unexplained environmental events may not be critical in shaping specific verbal responses in a group of clients.

It is clear that systematic replication across clients and disorders will help reduce unnecessary diversity in treatment techniques. If there are a few core techniques whose limited variations can help treat a variety of communicative disorders, so much the better. Economy in treatment procedures, which does not do any injustice to individual differences, can be a highly desirable outcome of systematic replication.

Conditions Necessary for Systematic Replications

Systematic replications are possible within a discipline only when that discipline meets certain criteria. The treatment techniques must be specific and well researched through experimental methods and direct replications. Procedures for measuring dependent as well as independent variables must be well developed. The dependent variables must be conceptualized on empirical (not just logical or theoretical) grounds, and they may be defined in such a way that reliable observations are possible. In addition, the treatment outcome criteria must be measurement-oriented. Finally, a strong experimental tradition should be a part of the history of the discipline.

Unfortunately, carefully planned and extensively conducted systematic replications are practically nonexistent in speech–language pathology because many of these criteria are not met by the profession. As noted before, direct replication follows experimental analysis of treatment procedures, which in turn leads to systematic replication. Unfortunately, treatment techniques in speech–language pathology are generally not subjected to experimental analysis. They are often vague and riddled with controversies. For the most part, treatment techniques are justified on the basis of clinical judgment, speculative theories and presumptions, liberal recommendations coming from nonclinical disciplines, well-recognized authorities, subjective preferences, tradition, dated training, and personal experience not supported by objective evaluations.

There is very little agreement on the dependent variables and their measurement procedures. As we shall see in Chapter 11, most of the dependent variables are conceptualized on logical, topographical, and speculative grounds. For example, what are the dependent variables in the case of language behaviors? Transformational grammar? Innate grammatical competence? Knowledge of language structures? Semantic notions? Pragmatic rules? Response classes? And, how any one of these can be measured? When there is so much controversy about the dependent variables, and the independent variables are nothing more than speculative opinions, experimental analysis becomes very difficult.

In the experimental evaluation of treatment, outcome must be specified in terms of some objective criteria that can be used by other investigators as well. If the few treatment evaluation studies that are done do not report their treatment evaluation procedures in objective terms, other investigators cannot replicate those studies. The questions are these: How did a clinician determine that a given treatment procedure was effective? What magnitude of change in the clients' problem behaviors were required before assuming that the treatment was effective? Was it a statistical or clinical criterion? Did the investigator adopt generalization or maintenance of the target behaviors as the criterion, or both? Obviously, answers to questions such as these are important in treatment evaluations and their replications.

One may think that different clinicians should agree upon the evaluative criteria so that the same criterion or criteria can be used by investigators. However, agreement among investigators is not the issue. Whether some specified criterion is described in operational terms at all is the issue. Such a criterion can be used in evaluating treatment effectiveness, regardless of agreement among investigators.

A discipline that does not have a strong tradition of experimental evaluation of its practices cannot even begin direct or systematic replications. Systematic replications are a sure sign of the advanced scientific status of a clinical profession. However, in order to achieve such a status, the entire membership of a profession need not agree upon their theoretical orientations or treatment biases. It is true that if the members of a profession achieve general agreement upon the dependent and independent variables and their measurement procedures, the profession is likely to make a rapid progress. Nevertheless, diversity of approaches, by itself, is not a hindrance to scientific progress. The hindrance is a lack of appreciation of the philosophy and methodology of science. What is crucially needed in order to achieve scientific progress is a commitment on the part of investigators to the experimental methodology of natural sciences. When such a commitment is made, the progress may still be slow, but it is inevitable. In the long run, it does not matter what theoretical orientation one takes. Some orientations may prove to be valid and others not so valid; many will be in between. Because science is a self-corrective method, things will be sorted out in the process of experimental research. However, what matters is whether one finds a way to experimental verifications and direct and systematic replications or whether one is satisfied with self-generated or other person-generated theoretical pronouncements.

FAILED REPLICATIONS: SOURCES OF TREATMENT MODIFICATIONS

A functional relation found in experimental research—whether in basic or treatment research—may or may not be replicated. Several reasons can account for such failed replications. When an investigator fails to replicate his or her own previous findings, the first question to consider is the reliability of the original findings. It is possible that the functional relation found in the original study was mistaken in that extraneous variables, not the manipulated independent variables, were responsible for changes in the dependent variables.

As you recall, this is the question of internal validity. Findings of questionable internal validity are not replicable, but typically one does not know this until an effort to replicate has failed.

On the other hand, a study may have had good internal validity in that the external variables were ruled out and the results obtained were valid in the case of the original subjects or clients. Direct replication of such a study across subjects may still fail. Such failures suggest a more complex situation than those involving questionable internal validity. Failures of this kind are both challenging and interesting. In clinical treatment research, those failures can be a valuable source of treatment modifications that suit individual clients.

When a well-researched treatment procedure cannot be replicated across clients, several possibilities must be considered. Perhaps important differences in the subject or client characteristics across the original and the replication series can account for a lack of replication. The clients in the replication series may be thought of as belonging to the same diagnostic category as those in the original study, but in reality they may form a subcategory. For example, "language handicapped children" may not be a homogeneous group in spite of commonly observed language problems. The children who show the same type of language disorder may be different in certain important characteristics in terms of past learning experiences, intelligence, or other variables. The importance of some of these variables may not have been apparent to the investigator. In essence, all language disordered clients may not benefit from the same treatment procedure. Similarly, all stutterers or aphasic patients may not react the same way to a treatment procedure known to be effective with *some* of them.

In systematic replication, the investigator takes careful note of client differences, since establishing generality across different kinds of clients is one of the goals in this type of replication. In direct replication, on the other hand, the investigator tries to have clients who are similar to those in the original study, but this objective may not have been realized in a particular replication. When the replication fails, one must look for possible differences in clients' background variables or the special characteristics of the disorder exhibited by them. In such cases, a modification in the technique or a totally different technique may be necessary. Aphasic patients in a replication study may have additional health problems that were not present in the patients of the original study. Stutterers in the replication series may have had marked breathing abnormalities associated with their stutterings, and this may render a pure syllable prolongation approach not as useful as with stutterers not having those abnormalities. A modified breathing component may prove effective either alone or in combination with syllable prolongation. The researcher may then pursue this question and eventually offer suggestions regarding differential treatment of stutterers or aphasic patients depending upon their unique characteristics.

The source or sources of failure to replicate in a systematic replication series can be more obvious than in a direct replication series. The investigator knows the differences between the subjects in the original study and those in the replication, since such differences are built into a replicative study. A treatment procedure known to be effective with children exhibiting an articulation disorder may be evaluated with adult clients. Or, a technique known to be effective with language disordered children may be tried with those showing an articulation disorder. There is no guarantee, however, that the known difference is the source of failure when it occurs. Failure with adults of a procedure known to be effective with children does not necessarily mean that age is the critical variable. Some unknown variable or variables may be responsible for the failure.

The influence of unknown variables can be suspected when replicative efforts are continued in spite of an initial failure and suddenly a success emerges, though the subjects showed the same difference as in the earlier series. For instance, following a failure to replicate the study with clients older than those in the original study, an investigator may be able to replicate the results in a subsequent effort, also involving older subject. This would then suggest that age may not have been the reason for the initial failure and that there are other unsuspected variables that must be studied. An unsuspected difference in the family background of subjects or hereditary differences may account for the initial failure.

Generally speaking, it is the success that must be replicated, but a single failure may also be replicated when there is reason to believe that the original findings were strong and reliable and that the initial replication may have failed because of some flaw in the study. A second failure, however, may convince the investigator that additional efforts are not worthwhile. In clinical treatment evaluations, attempts to repeatedly replicate failed treatments may be unethical as well.

What is done when a failure is considered genuine may depend on the inclinations of the investigator. Personal viewpoints seem to have a strong influence on the course of action taken in such situations. If the investigator still believes that the overall approach evaluated in the original study is valid, he or she may proceed to modify the procedure. This modified technique then goes through the initial experimental evaluations, followed by its own direct and systematic replications. However, if the investigator thinks that the technique was not all that strong anyway, then it is unlikely that attempts to improve it by specific modifications will be made. The reality of the research world is that replications are done to support as well as refute certain existing practices. When replications done to refute a given approach succeed in the refutation, the investigator is likely to stop, although those who believe in its success may redouble their efforts.

In essence, failed replications are full of good lessons. They point out possible exceptions to a general rule. Clinically, failed replications suggest limitations of generally effective treatment procedures. Such exceptions are important in science, since the scientist is interested in identifying the limits of known functional relations. Exceptions are equally important for clinicians, since their philosophy and methodology are based upon individual uniqueness as well as human generalities. The instant a generally effective treatment procedure fails with a given client, the clinician has made an empirical contact with individual uniqueness. A responsible clinician then may think that the best course of action is to modify the procedure to suit the individual or evaluate a totally new approach that may prove more successful. In this way, when the message of failed replication is heeded, a clinical science moves ahead.

TREATMENT VARIABLES AND TREATMENT PACKAGES

As we noted in our discussion of the interactional design strategy, most treatment procedures are technically packages of different treatment components. It is not uncommon to program multiple target behaviors that are taught with the help of multiple treatment components. A treatment package may be more successful in treating such complex disorders as stuttering or apraxia. In the treatment of stuttering, for example, such components as modified airflow, gentle phonatory onset, rate reduction through stretched syllables, and relaxed movements of the articulators are all a part of several treatment packages. In essence, when a disorder includes different classes of problem behaviors, different treatment components may be necessary to handle them. There is one method of developing treatment packages and another method of verifying existing packages. Both have implications for replications.

In the strategy of *developing* a treatment package, the clinician first individually tests each of the components to be included in a package and then replicates them separately in direct as well as systematic series. For example, if modified airflow, rate reduction, and gentle phonatory onset are to be included in a stuttering treatment package, then the independent effects of each of these components must be evaluated experimentally and replicated appropriately. When it is known that the three components are effective by themselves, they may be combined into a package and the total package can then be applied to clients. The process of combining treatment packages may also involve an analysis of the interactional effects of two or more components. With interactional analysis, only those components that yield the best possible results in combination may be included in the package. The total package itself then goes through direct and systematic replications. The direct replication of a treatment package with clients who fall into a single diagnostic category but showing multiple problem behaviors is sometimes described as *clinical replication* (Barlow & Hersen, 1984).

In practice, however, the ideal of independent evaluation of components that are then combined into treatment packages is rarely achieved. Many of the stuttering treatment packages, for example, have not been experimentally evaluated either in total or in terms of individual components. Some may have been evaluated in an uncontrolled series with the one group pretest–posttest design or case studies. Often, clinicians start with a treatment package the components of which are selected on theoretical grounds or clinical traditions. The philosophy of eclecticism, which has been so popular in speech–language pathology, has also encouraged the use of untested components in treatment packages. Typically, though, the philosophy of eclecticism has been justified on the basis of common-sense idea that one selects what is good from every viewpoint. Unfortunately, the justification requires more than common sense, which is to say that we need experimental evidence. Such evidence has been woefully lacking. As a result, the treatment packages may contain components whose effects are unknown, minimal, nonexistent, or even detrimental.

The method of *verifying* an already existing treatment package is to break it down into its components and experimentally evaluate each of the components for its independent effect. The components are then subjected to direct and systematic replications, and the components that prove effective are combined into a treatment package. In this process, the interactive effects of two or more components can also be determined. The final package that emerges through this kind of research may be different from the one that has been practiced by clinicians, because some of the components that proved useless will not have been included in the package.

The proliferation of untested treatment packages creates a dilemma for the practicing clinician who is not able to evaluate systematically the effectiveness of those that need to be used. It behooves those who advocate the use of treatment packages to verify the effectiveness of independent components in isolation and in combination. The total package is then applied to a group of well-defined clients with multiple problems. Additional direct and systematic replications, when successful, enhance the generality of the treatment packages.

Economy of clinical practice is enhanced when a clinician does not use all of the components of a widely recognized but experimentally untested treatment package. The do-everything-possible strategy is considered the safest because if some components fail, others may ensure success. But this strategy also encourages superstitious therapeutic practices. Therefore, an alternative, which may not be as safe the standard practice, is purposefully to eliminate some of the components and see what happens. If the clients improve, there will be no assurance that the treatment components used were indeed responsible for the improvement. Nevertheless, that the omitted components were indeed unnecessary will be loud and clear. In such informal evaluations, the clinician must make sure that the dependent variables are carefully monitored in every treatment session. Systematic measurement of the target behaviors will help clinicians make decisions regarding dropping the components when they prove ineffective, or when the data warrant, adding additional components. Constant monitoring of the target behaviors will help make those decisions at the earliest possible time so that the clients do not continue to receive ineffective treatment.

HOMO- AND HETEROGENEITY OF SUBJECTS

The issue of homo- and heterogeneity of subjects is relevant to animal as well as human, and to basic as well as clinical, research. Within a single study, whether the subjects were homogeneous or heterogeneous can make a difference in terms of both internal validity and generality. Typically, investigators strive to have either homo- or heterogeneous subjects, depending upon the research design philosophies and the purposes of the experiment.

Within the philosophy of group designs, heterogeneous samples are considered ideal because such samples are expected to represent the necessarily heterogeneous population. Only when this is not practical would an investigator think of using some homogeneous subjects, hoping to show that a given variable has an effect in the case of individuals with known (and homogeneous) characteristics. Within the single-subject strategy, investigators usually try to select homogeneous subjects. However, the single-subject methodology does not pose serious problems when heterogeneous subjects are used because the data analysis is subject-specific. Even so, heterogeneous subjects may not be preferable because if the results are different across subjects, the investigator does not know why.

When the purpose of an experiment is systematic replication across subjects, one would, of course, select subjects who are in some specified way different from those in the original study. The tactic is to select homogeneous subjects who are heterogeneous relative to those in the original study.

As noted earlier, homogeneity is more easily achieved in laboratory experiments involving animal subjects. We also noted that in human research and especially in clinical research, homogeneity of subjects is a strongly wished-for, but rarely achieved, goal of clinical researchers. In this section, we shall take a critical look at this concept, because so many clinical researchers agonize over it.

There is no doubt that homogeneity of subjects would make the life of the clinical researcher so much easier. If all children with language disorders were the same, the problem of replication would at worst be a minor one. If all stutterers were the same, then a single effective treatment would be sufficient and the burden of replication would be pleasantly light. However, people are just not as homogeneous as the methodology of research requires them to be. People are different, and they don't seem to care about the clinical researchers' pressing problem! Therefore, instead of searching for homogeneous subjects that may not exist, it may be prudent to consider heterogeneity as the fact of life and design studies accordingly. In essence, people cannot be changed, but research tactics can be.

The basic problem is that the concept of homogeneity is difficult to define. When are clients homogeneous? Is it when they are of the same age? (Do all children of the same age behave the same?) When they are of the same social status? (Do people within the same social status necessarily behave the same?) When they come from similar family background? (Do the members of a family always behave the same?) When they have similar intelligence? (Do people with similar IQ's behave the same?) When they have the same educational background? (Does a four-year college education create similar educational background?) When they all have suffered the disorder for the same duration? (Does two years of stuttering make some individuals the same compared with four years of stuttering?)

A set of converse questions can also be asked. Are there no behavioral patterns that are similar across age-groups? Do people with different social strata ever share common behavioral patterns? Do the members of the same family—let alone those with "similar family backgrounds"—behave differently? Do people with different levels of intelligence ever behave similarly? Do people with the same level of education behave differently? Do clients with the same disorder, the same level of severity, and the same duration of history ever behave differently?

The questions raised here are not just rhetoric. The point is that there are no fixed answers to those questions. A bias one way or the other is not implied. In case of given individuals, the answer to any one question may be positive or negative. What is suggested here is that the goal of homogeneity, either in an original series of experimental evaluation or in direct and systematic replications, should not stultify research. If the available clients are somewhat different, then the investigator should carefully describe the differences among them and offer results separately for the individuals. As long as the investigator does not feel compelled to offer group means that mask individual differences, there is no major problem with individual differences in reactivity to treatment variables. An ensuing analysis of reasons for variability may be required, but the data generated by the study will be just as valuable. It is better to do research with differing clients than to wait for homogeneous subjects.

The foregoing discussion suggests that there are significant subject selection problems in conducting direct and systematic replications. Besides, research strategies themselves make replications more or less difficult. Generally speaking, the group design strategy, which is difficult to employ in clinical treatment research, is also difficult to use in replication studies. The required number of subjects may not be realized for a series of direct and systematic replications. The single-subject strategy, on the other hand, has encouraged replications of treatment techniques in a variety of behavior disorders. In the treatment of language, articulation, and fluency disorders, the single-subject studies of behavioral treatment techniques have provided impressive replicative evidence. Comparable evidence has not emerged from the group design strategy. Every time a clinician uses a treatment procedure under controlled conditions with one or few clients, the cause of replication is advanced. This is made possible by the clinically practical single-subject strategy. ■

S T U D Y G U I D E

1 Why should a clinician be concerned with the generality of clinical and experimental data?

2 What kinds of generality are not established by a group design study even when the investigator is able to draw and assign subjects randomly?

3 What is the method of establishing generality of research findings?

4 What is direct replication?

5 Suppose that you have just completed a study in which you evaluated a particular method of teaching correct production of speech sounds to 5-year-old children who exhibit disorders of articulation in the absence of any other communicative disorders. Now you wish to do a direct replication study. How would you do it? You may make up whatever information you need to answer this question.

6 What is considered to be the safest initial direct replication strategy? Why?

7 Define systematic replication.

8 Suppose that you have completed a study in which you experimentally evaluated the effects of a treatment program designed to teach morphological features to mentally retarded 5-year-old children. Now you plan to do a systematic replication study. How would you do it? Specify the variables that will be the same as in the original study as well as those that will be different. Use hypothetical information.

9 What are the different parameters of systematic replication in clinical research?

10 What conditions are necessary for conducting systematic replication?

11 What is the value of failed replications? Give an example from clinical research.

12 Distinguish the strategy used in developing a treatment package from that used in verifying an existing package.

13 Assuming it is practical, what is gained by having homogeneous subjects in clinical research?

14 Critically evaluate the concepts of homogeneity and heterogeneity of human subjects.

15 In what kind of replication are subjects selected who are heterogeneous relative to those in the original study?

CHAPTER 10

Comparative Evaluation of Design Strategies

■ Research questions and investigative strategies, 301

■ Advantages and disadvantages of design strategies, 310

■ Problems common to design strategies, 313

■ Philosophic considerations in evaluation, 315

■ The investigator in design selection process, 315

■ The final criterion: Soundness of data, 316

■ Chapter summary, 317

■ Study guide, 321

n Chapters 7 and 8, I described two major approaches to designing experimental research: the group and the single-subject strategies. In this chapter, I shall discuss the strengths and weaknesses of the two approaches. The purpose of this chapter is to help student researchers select appropriate methodological strategies for investigating a variety of research questions.

A research strategy is appropriate, or not, only from the standpoint of a given investigation. Every design with a sound structure has its place in scientific research. However, a design that is perfectly suited to one kind of investigation may be somewhat inappropriate to another kind; it may be totally wrong for another study. Therefore, the appropriateness of a design is judged in relation to the research question or questions the investigator seeks to answer.

Many research questions can be answered by two or more methods. In such cases, selection depends mostly on the training, experience, and philosophy of the investigator. Most investigators tend to use either the group or the single-subject strategy. When an investigator is inclined to use either of those strategies, the selection may depend upon practical considerations. For example, the number of subjects available for a study may determine whether one selects a single-subject interactional design or a factorial group design. If many subjects are available, the factorial design may be used. If only a few subjects are willing to participate, the single-subject interactional design may be selected.

RESEARCH QUESTIONS AND INVESTIGATIVE STRATEGIES

Despite the amount of attention we pay to *methods* of research, we must still keep in perspective that methods are subservient to research questions. It is possible to become fascinated by a method and try to find a problem that can be investigated with it. Such a search for a problem can be intolerably long. More typically, scientists first have research questions and then look for methods to answer them.

Problems or research questions fall into different types of investigations, which were considered in Chapter 4. The kind of question and the type of research together determine the strategy selected for the study. I shall describe 15 kinds of research questions and suggest appropriate strategies or designs to answer them. Of necessity, the questions described will be generic, not specific. It is not possible to describe all the kinds of research questions one can investigate. Therefore, this discussion will be illustrative only; I shall not try to list every correct design one could use in answering particular types of questions. As you read these pages, you may wish to think of other types of research questions and appropriate strategies to answer them.

1. What Factors May Have Contributed to This Effect?

This type of question is asked when the event under investigation has a history and the causes of the event have occurred in the past. The type of research done to answer this kind of question is ex post facto. Most case studies are of this type. The effect is directly observable, but the causes are not. The experimenter cannot manipulate the causes. The investigator makes a search of the factors that may have contributed to the effect under study. See *ex post facto* research in Chapter 4 for details.

Factors that may have contributed to an effect are widely investigated in clinical sciences. Questions about the causes of most disorders often fall into this category. Questions about what contributed to the onset of stuttering, language disorders, articulation problems, or voice difficulties in given clients are of serious clinical concern. These questions can be researched with either the group strategy or the single-subject strategy. Often, the history of a small number of clients or of single clients is investigated to determine if factors known to cause the effect were present. Whether it is a group or a single-subject study, it is better described as a case study, and it does not have an experimental design in the technical sense of that term.

2. Does a Treatment Seem to Work?

In clinical sciences, treatment procedures may be initially evaluated informally. A clinician may try a new procedure by carefully measuring the behaviors before and after treatment. If systematic changes are seen after treatment, it is considered possible that the treatment worked.

Obviously, evaluations of this kind lack appropriate controls. Extraneous variables are not ruled out. Therefore, the studies lack internal validity, and the clinician cannot assert that the treatment was indeed effective. Nevertheless, research of this type may be useful because many clinicians may be willing to try new ideas informally. Improvement in client behaviors, when documented systematically, may suggest that it is worthwhile to design a more controlled study to evaluate the treatment procedure.

Uncontrolled treatment studies can be more or less useful depending upon the thoroughness of measurement. Repeated and reliable pretreatment measures, measurement during treatment sessions, and posttreatment measures that show a convincing change in client behaviors help establish the value of case studies. Missing pretreatment measures, lack of measures during treatment, and small changes after treatment invalidate most studies of this kind.

Uncontrolled treatment studies can use either a single–subject or a group design. The one-group pretest-posttest design of the group strategy, or the *AB* design of the single-subject strategy, would be appropriate for this kind of research.

3. How Are the Dependent Variables Distributed in the Population?

This type of question is a part of normative research. The investigator is interested in determining the distribution of certain dependent variables in selected populations, such as children and adults. Studies designed to answer this kind of question are descriptive. They do not manipulate independent variables; instead, they describe the characteristics of their subjects in terms of selected dependent variables. See *normative research* in Chapter 4 for details.

The distribution of dependent variables is the main concern in many kinds of research questions. For example, what are the language characteristics of 3- and 4-year-old children? How many phonemes can children in different age levels produce correctly? Do 5-year-old children produce more dysfluencies than 3-year-old children? Any kind of research that attempts to establish norms would ask questions of this kind.

Questions of the distribution of dependent variables are investigated without experimental designs. Generally speaking, the methods come from the group design strategy because a large number of subjects, selected randomly, is needed to answer such questions. Typically, a large group divided into age levels is observed for relatively brief periods with limited response sampling. The observed characteristics of subjects in different age levels are described. However, such descriptions rarely pertain to individual subjects. The performance of individual subjects in groups or subgroups of subjects is averaged to obtain single scores that distinguish one group from the other. These studies seek inferential generality, and therefore the method includes statistical analyses of data.

4. What is the Differential Distribution of a Variable in a Population?

Questions concerning the *differential* distribution of a variable are researched in clinical sciences. The research type involved is a combination of ex post facto, normative, and standard-group comparison types. The investigator who is asking such questions as whether stutterers and nonstutterers differ in their personality, or whether persons with and without laryngectomy differ in their smoking histories, is trying to determine the differential distribution of certain variables in contrasting populations. Whenever clinical and nonclinical groups are compared on some variable that is *not* manipulated, we have the question of differential distribution of variables.

Questions of differential distribution of variables use the group methodology. No experimental designs are required to answer these questions, however; the methods are descriptive. The selected dependent variable is measured in groups that are different on some criterion, which is often a clinical diagnosis. The different values of the dependent variables in the two groups are statistically evaluated and reported. For example, it may be found that the scores on a test of intelligence are differentially distributed in misarticulating and normally speaking children.

5. What Are the Effects of an Independent Variable?

An investigator may simply ask, what happens when I manipulate this variable? What effects follow when a factor is introduced, removed, or reinstated? Questions of this kind attempt to find out the unknown, or not well understood, effects of independent variables. For example, one may ask, what happens when the auditory feedback for speech is presented to the speaker with a delay? What happens to the electroencephalographic patterns when meaningful linguistic stimuli are introduced? What are the effects on children's language of training mothers to read stories aloud? What are the effects of reducing the rate of speech in stutterers? Questions such as these concern the effects of selected independent variables. Evaluation of clinical treatment procedures involve this kind of questions.

The evaluation of the effects of independent variables requires the method of experimentation. Questions of the effects of independent variables can be investigated through either group designs or single-subject designs. In order to control for potential extraneous variables, the investigator must select one of the true experimental designs. Within the group strategy, the pretest–posttest control group design or the posttest-only control group design may be selected to investigate the effects of independent variables. Among the within-subjects designs, the two-group single-treatment counterbalanced design is appropriate. Among the time-series designs, a nonequivalent two-group design may be used with the understanding that there is no sampling equivalence of the groups. Within the single-subject strategy, an *ABA* reversal or withdrawal design would be appropriate. The *BAB* single-subject design may also be used along with *ABAB* reversal or withdrawal designs. Although they are used more frequently in answering clinically oriented questions, the *ABAB* and multiple baseline designs can also be used.

6. Is a Clinical Treatment Effective?

Questions of the effectiveness of clinical treatment procedures are similar to those concerning the effects of independent variables. Both fall within the scope of experimental research. However, questions of treatment effects are a part of clinical research. Therefore, in answering such questions, some investigators avoid certain designs that are appropriate to investigate the effects of independent variables within basic research.

Effects of treatment procedures can be assessed with either the group strategy or the single-subject strategy. The pretest–posttest control-group design or the posttest-only control group design can help evaluate the effects of single treatment variables. Among the within-subjects designs, the two-group single-treatment counterbalanced design can be used. One of the quasi-experimental designs, such as the nonequivalent two-group time-series design, can also be used, but with some loss of rigor because of the lack of randomization.

Among the single-subject designs, the *ABAB* reversal or withdrawal design; the multiple baseline design across subjects, settings, or behaviors; and the changing criterion design are all available for selection. If the investigator does not wish to neutralize the treatment effects, the multiple baseline and changing criterion designs are preferable. Of the two, the multiple baseline design is probably more powerful and versatile. If there is no serious concern about using reversal or withdrawal as a part of treatment evaluation, the *ABAB* design can produce the most convincing evidence.

7. Is One Treatment More Effective Than the Other?

The relative effects of two (or more) treatments become an issue when it is known that compared with no-treatment, all of them are effective to some degree. Is reinforcing fluency more or less effective than counseling stutterers for their emotional problems? Is modeling without client imitation more or less effective than modeling that requires client imitation? Is informative feedback on performance accuracy in articulation therapy more or less effective than reinforcement in the absence of feedback? Questions such as these attempt to find out if one treatment is better than the other.

Evaluation of the relative effects of treatment requires the experimental method. However, since most designs that can be used to answer the question of relative effects of two or more treatments do not necessarily rule out extraneous variables, investigators usually focus on the relative, not the absolute, effects. Within the group design strategy, the multigroup pretest–posttest design may be used. The number of groups is the same as the number of treatments that are evaluated. An extra group that does not receive treatment is needed if the absolute treatment effect is also of concern. Factorial designs such as the randomized blocks design and the completely randomized factorial design are also excellent means of evaluating the effects of multiple treatments.

The single-group time-series design with multiple treatments can also be used to determine if one treatment is more effective than the other. The within-subjects crossover design can answer the same kind of questions.

The *ABACA/ACABA* design and the alternating treatments design are the most frequently used single-subject strategies for evaluating the relative effects of two or more treatments.

8. Is There an Interaction Between Treatment Components?

Many treatment procedures contain different elements. Questions regarding their independent and interactive effects are often raised. Does muscular relaxation and reinforcement for correct pitch interact in the treatment of a voice disorder? Does reinforcement for correct production and punishment for incorrect production of phonemes in articulation therapy produce a cumulative effect? Is it more effective to combine stimulus pictures and objects in language therapy? Questions such as these are about interaction. Analysis of interaction also requires the experimental methodology. Selected elements of a treatment program are typically applied in isolation and in certain combinations to assess the independent and interactive effects of those elements.

The group design strategy offers the factorial design to answer questions about the interaction of treatment elements. Of the several factorial designs, the completely randomized factorial design is best suited for an analysis of interaction. In this design, the effects of more than one treatment or treatment elements can be studied. The other factorial design described in Chapter 7, the randomized blocks design, contains assigned variables and is more suitable for answering a different kind of interaction (see Question 9, described next).

In the single-subject strategy, the interactional design can help answer the same question. It is generally thought, however, that the factorial (group) designs are better than the single-subject interactional design. In a factorial design, multiple treatments are not confounded because different treatments or components are applied to different groups of subjects. But the possibility of confounding effects exists in the single-subject interactional design because it evaluates the effects of multiple treatments in the same clients.

9. Do Subject Variables Interact with Treatment Variables?

Interaction can exist not only between treatment variables but also between treatment and subject characteristics. The same treatment may have different effects in male and female subjects, high school and college graduates, urban and rural clients. A treatment may be more or less effective depending on the severity of the disorder treated. Such assigned variables (see Chapter 3) interact with treatment. Therefore, to establish the generality of findings, one must know who reacts in what way to the same treatment procedure. This type of research is experimental, since the treatment is always an active variable.

The randomized blocks design of the group (factorial) design strategy is considered best for analyzing the interaction between the subject variables and treatment. By juxtaposing subject characteristics and treatment variables, the design can assess the interaction between these two sets of variables. Within the single-subject approach, a particular design that can help answer this kind of question is lacking. The question is addressed through replications. In a series of single-subject designs, the investigator studies subjects of different characteristics and notes possible differences in the effects of treatment. Eventually, this approach will be able to accumulate enough data on interactions between subject variables and treatment. Many consider this a less precise approach than that of the factorial design.

10. Is One Treatment Preferred Over the Other?

Two or more treatments may be equally effective in treating a disorder, but clients may prefer one over the other. As long as the preferred method is effective, it may be better to select that over the other, less preferred, method. In the treatment of stuttering, for example, both verbal "no" and reinforcement of fluency skills may be equally effective. In this case, the subjects may prefer the reinforcement procedure. A knowledge of client preference as well as objective effects of treatment can be useful in clinical practice. This kind of research requires experimental methods.

The group design strategy does not offer a direct approach to study client preference of treatment. Client preferences can be assessed indirectly by differential dropout rates when different treatments are offered and by post hoc analysis in which the subjects are questioned about their preferences. However, these procedures do not permit an experimental analysis of client preferences. Within the single-subject strategy, the simultaneous treatments design offers a direct method for analyzing subject preferences. When different treatments are offered simultaneously to the same client, the client may seek one treatment more frequently than the other. This then gives a clearer picture of the client preference. However, a preferred technique may or may not be the most effective technique, as noted in Chapter 8.

11. What are the Most Effective Components of a Treatment Package?

When several treatment components are included in a package, one may wish to know which ones are more effective. The question concerns an experimental analysis of existing packages whose development has not been based on systematic research. In this case, the package is broken down into its components to find out which ones are more or less effective. Two or more components may then be evaluated in a particular study. This question is of interest regardless of potential interaction, although it is better analyzed in an interactional design. As already noted, many treatments of communicative disorders are packages of different treatment components. What is needed is a strategy to discard elements that are ineffective, improve those that are somewhat effective, and identify those that are most effective.

The factorial design of the group strategy is useful in determining the relative efficacy of treatment components. The completely randomized factorial design is especially useful. Different components are applied to different subjects in a factorial arrangement. In the same process, one can also analyze the interaction between the applied components. Of the single-subject designs, the interactional design can be used for the same purposes. The design can help determine the relative and interactive effects of treatment components. Other factors being equal, the group factorial designs are a better alternative to single-subject interactional design.

12. Can an Effective Treatment Package Be Developed?

This question concerns the *development* of a treatment package when no effective one exists. It is generally true that multiple treatment variables are more effective than single variables. However, when treatment variables are combined without a separate analysis of their independent effects, the resulting package may contain useless elements. The total package may continue to be used because of the overall effectiveness. A better approach is to test each component in separate studies and then combine only those that have produced effects in isolation.

Obviously, a treatment package cannot be developed in a single study. There is no single design to accomplish this task. The research aimed at developing treatment packages is done in two stages. In the first, the clinician performs several independent studies in which the isolated effects of specific components are evaluated. The components that produce effects are retained and those that do not are discarded. If it is found that a few components produce the maximum effects, those that produce less impressive effects may also be discarded. In the second stage of research, the few components that are most effective are combined into a treatment package. The independent and the interactive effects of the components of the package are then determined.

Any of the group or single-subject designs that help evaluate the effects of a treatment variable may be used in the first stage. Factorial group designs or single-subject interactional designs can be used in the second stage of research. However, for various practical reasons, single-subjects designs have proved to be more useful than group designs in developing treatment packages.

13. What is the Optimal Level of Treatment?

This question concerns the mechanics of arranging treatment sessions or the intensity of treatment. The question can be asked even about the most effective treatments. For example, assuming that a given treatment is effective, one can ask whether a 50-minute treatment session is more effective than a 30-minute session. Is therapy two times a week just as effective as therapy four times a week? The answers to such questions help arrange effective and economical schedules of treatment.

Questions about the optimal level of treatment are better answered within the single-subject strategy. Single-subject designs that permit parametric variations of treatment are best suited for answering questions of this kind. The same subjects may be exposed to the same treatment but with variations in the durations of sessions or the weekly frequency. Such variations are counterbalanced across subjects. A second choice would be the single-group time-series design with multiple temporary treatments. The multiple temporary treatments would consist of variations designed to determine the optimal level of treatment.

14. What is the Behavior of a Group? Can We Predict It?

Although I have emphasized the importance of studying individual subjects in a clinical science, it is sometimes necessary to ignore the behaviors of individual subjects and ask a question of behaviors shown by a group of persons. For example, a classroom teacher may wish to keep a group of children relatively quiet although every child may not necessarily be quiet all the time. Small variations in individual behaviors are ignored as long as the collective behavior of the group is acceptable. The speech and language clinician treating a group of children may face the similar situation.

Analysis and prediction of group behaviors is better accomplished by the group design strategy. Most group prediction studies are not experimental, however. A pollster who predicts the winner of an election is simply measuring and predicting group behavior without trying to change that behavior. On the other hand, some questions of group behaviors may involve experimentation. Scientific or professional organizations may wish not only to find out about some particular behaviors of a group of people, but also to change some of those behaviors. A speech and hearing organization, for example, may attempt to first find out how much people know about its services and then design an experimental publicity campaign to increase the amount of information people have. Of the group designs, the time-series designs with repeated measures before and after the experimental manipulations are especially helpful. Single-subject designs are not efficient in predicting group behaviors.

15. How Effective is the Treatment Across Individuals?

Clients or their families often wish to know the overall success rate of treatments they seek. They ask such questions as "how many stutterers generally improve under treatment?", "what is the success rate of articulation therapy?", "can aphasic patients be helped?", "what percentage of children receiving language therapy improve?", and "how many children with early language intervention will be able to attend regular educational programs?" Such questions attempt to predict treatment effects across large numbers of subjects. Differential predictions may be attempted on the basis of diagnostic categories, age levels, and other such variables. These questions are important because the clinical services are supported by those who seek them.

The overall effectiveness of treatment procedures is also better evaluated with group designs. Group designs with a relatively large number of treated and untreated individuals can answer that question more effectively than single-subject designs. However, with accumulated evidence, single-subject designs can eventually answer such questions as well. A review of replicated single-subject studies can help determine the percentages of clients who improve with treatment. Nevertheless, a well-conducted group design study with a relatively large sample can provide that information more expeditiously.

The 15 types of questions described so far are by no means exhaustive, but they do illustrate the relation between research questions and designs. Each question is answered by different kind of data, and each design generates its own kind of data. After having asked a question, the investigator must determine what kind of data will answer it and what kind of design will generate those data.

ADVANTAGES AND DISADVANTAGES OF DESIGN STRATEGIES

Throughout the book, the various advantages and disadvantages of the group and single-subject design strategies have been discussed in several contexts. Therefore, what follows is a summative evaluation of both the group and single-subject design strategies. I shall list the major advantages and disadvantages of each of these approaches.

Advantages of Group Designs

Group designs are more appropriate than the single-subject designs in terms of the following features:

1. Group designs are generally effective in assessing the distribution of dependent variables in a population.

2. The designs offer a means of evaluating the *differential* distribution of variables in defined populations (normal versus clinical groups).

3. Group designs are effective in the analysis of the relative effects of multiple treatments.

4. The group strategy offers useful methods for assessing the interaction between two or more treatment variables.

5. Group designs are the most effective in assessing the interaction between treatment and subject/client characteristics.

6. The group strategy is especially useful in determining and predicting group behaviors.

7. The strategy is effective in predicting treatment effects based on diagnostic categories.

8. Because group designs have definitive structures, the investigator need not make too many decisions in the process of implementing a study.

Some of the advantages just listed may be hard to realize in practice because they are based on the theory, not practice, of group design strategy. Especially, the advantages associated with clinical treatment evaluations may or may not be realized in practice. However, the advantages relative to group behaviors and predictions are realized relatively easily. The designs are best suited for investigating nonclinical and nontreatment-related issues in which the behavior of individual subjects is not of particular interest.

Disadvantages of Group Designs

Most of the disadvantages of the group design strategy stem from its practical limitations. These limitations are magnified in a clinical science in which the formation of large groups, especially multiple groups, is a formidable task. Other sources of limitation are conceptual, centering on the statistical theory and practice of the mean, the probability, the inferential statistics, averaging the results of individual subjects, and so on. We shall address some of these issues in a later section. In any case, the disadvantages of the group designs include the following features:

1. The group strategy is generally not practical in clinical sciences that emphasize the experimental method in treatment evaluation.

2. It is weak in evaluating treatment effects on individual subjects. Because it lacks logical generality, the clinician cannot extend the conclusions of a group study to individual clients.

3. It is relatively weak in empirical manipulations because of its excessive reliance on statistically significant changes in dependent variables. Instead of producing larger effects of the independent variables, the approach seeks more powerful statistical techniques that show that smaller effects are "significant."

4. The group strategy is generally inadequate in measuring dependent variables. The pre- and posttests are a poor substitute for the continuous measurements of dependent variables.

5. The group strategy is weak in the analysis of individual behaviors and their controlling variables.

6. The strategy is not productive in the development of treatment packages.

7. The group strategy is not suited for evaluating the optimal level of treatment.

8. The strategy is not effective in assessing the individual preference of treatment procedures.

9. Group designs are not flexible. They must usually be carried to their conclusion even when things go wrong during a study.

10. The group design strategy is not conducive to replications. Because of the practical problems, group design studies are not replicated as often as single-subject studies.

In evaluating the group design strategy, one must make a distinction between its theory and practice, especially in a clinical science. The group strategy cannot be evaluated only in light of its theoretical elegance.

Advantages of Single-Subject Designs

Single-subject designs are more effective than the group designs in terms of the following features:

1. Single-subject designs are better in the analysis of individual behaviors and their controlling variables.

2. They are more effective in the experimental assessment of the effects of single treatment variables on the behaviors of individual subjects.

3. Single-subject designs can produce data that are more useful from the standpoint of individual clients. They are high on logical generality.

4. Single-subject designs are generally more practical than group designs. They have the potential of being replicated more easily than the group designs.

5. The designs offer a chance to build treatment packages.

6. They can help determine the client preferences of treatment procedures when multiple treatments are equally effective.

7. The designs are effective in determining the optimal level of treatment.

8. The designs typically produce larger effects of the independent variables, including clinical treatment variables.

9. Single-subject designs offer more reliable and extensive measurement of the dependent variables, since the measurement is continuous within a design.

10. The designs are more flexible and allow modifications during the course of investigations.

Many of the advantages of the single-subject approach are phrased from the standpoint of a clinical science. The same advantages hold good when the research is basic.

Disadvantages of Single-Subject Designs

Compared with group designs, single-subject designs have the following disadvantages:

1. The single-subject strategy is less effective in predicting group behaviors.

2. The strategy cannot make statistical statements regarding the overall effectiveness of treatment programs across large numbers of clients.

3. Single-subject designs are not efficient in evaluating the interaction between treatment variables and client characteristics.

4. Within the single-subject approach, the assessment of multiple treatments can be troublesome.

5. The approach is relatively weak in its assessment of interaction between different treatment variables.

6. Single-subject designs require on-the-spot decisions at various stages of a study.

In the final analysis, the advantages and disadvantages must be placed in a philosophical perspective, which will be done later. Also, the advantages are weighed against the disadvantages in the context of a particular study and its purpose.

PROBLEMS COMMON TO DESIGN STRATEGIES

Some problems are common to both the group and the single-subject strategies. It is necessary to note them because problems common to research in general may sometimes be blamed on one or the other design strategy. Many problems are simply a part of the research process.

Inter- and Intra-subject Variability. All research designs must handle variability in the phenomenon they observe. Generally, variability is not a creation of research strategies but a creation of nature itself. A subject's behavior varies because the factors that affect that behavior vary. Different individuals vary because they are exposed to different factors or independent variables.

As we know, design strategies handle this variability in different ways, however. In the group design strategy, typically it is handled statistically; in single-subject strategy, experimentally.

Unexpected Change in the Control Mechanisms. In either strategy, the control condition, subjects, or behaviors should not change. But sometimes such changes are seen in both strategies. Within the group strategy, the control group may improve without treatment. Within the single-subject strategy, the behavior under a control condition may change. For example, a behavior in a multiple baseline may change before the treatment is applied to it.

Problems of change in the control mechanism suggest that either the conditions were not well controlled or the behaviors were correlated (not independent response classes). Other independent variables may have been active, or the treated and as yet untreated behaviors may be responses of a single class.

Generality. Generality is a common problem of research, but the proponents of group designs usually make it appear to be predominantly a problem of single-subject designs. Because group designs are supposed to draw random samples that represent the population, it is usually believed that they have generality. However, in using group experimental designs, investigators rarely draw random samples from *clinical* populations. Even if a random sample is drawn, inferential generality to the population may be achieved, but there is no assurance of other kinds of generality. For example, the clinician and setting generality would not be established by a group design study that had an adequate random sample.

Generality is not a problem of designs; rather, all designs have to face this problem. It is a problem that requires replication. To achieve generality, studies of both group and single-subject designs must be replicated. No strategy offers it automatically. In fact, the group strategy lacks logical generality by design and inferential generality by default. The single-subject strategy lacks inferential generality by design, but it does provide logical generality. Both strategies can demonstrate other kinds of generalities only through replications.

Slow Accumulation of Scientific Evidence. Scientific data, especially experimental data, accumulate at a slow rate. The rate is slower still in clinical sciences in which the variables are many and hard to control and ethical restrictions are justifiably stringent. It is often thought that group designs advance the rate of data accumulation whereas single-subject designs retard it. This is not true, since what takes time is replication. Whether an effect is initially demonstrated in two subjects or ten subjects is not as critical as is generally thought.

In behavioral research, single-subject designs have generated more experimental clinical data than have group designs. Because of their relevance to clinical work, which involves single or small groups of subjects, single-subject designs have been used in many more treatment evaluation studies than group designs.

Though scientific data generally tend to accumulate slowly, it is possible to accelerate the pace. Among other factors, practical methods of research, better training of clinicians in research, and better support for research can make a difference.

Problems of Implementation. Many problems of research are not those of design strategies but simply of the task of implementing research. It is a complex task, the implementation of which can go wrong at any time. Subjects may be hard to find and, once found, hard to retain until the end of the study. Needed instruments may be expensive, but once acquired, they do not seem to give notice before they break down. These and many other problems of implementing research studies are common features of research.

PHILOSOPHIC CONSIDERATIONS IN EVALUATION

In the comparative evaluation of design strategies, one cannot ignore the philosophical considerations that created some of the differences between the group and the single-subject approaches. Many of the procedural differences grew out of different conceptual approaches. Investigators also operate on the bases of these differing conceptual approaches.

As noted elsewhere, the group design strategy is heavily influenced by the logic and the procedures of statistics. Statistical reasoning treats individual differences and variability as controllable mostly through methods of analysis, not experimentation. The behavior of the individual is of interest only as it contributes to the statistically stable measure, such as the mean. Theoretically, the group design approach tries to build a science of behavior by observing many subjects in single studies.

The single-subject strategy, on the other hand, was influenced heavily by the tradition of experimentation, not statistical analysis of data. It treats individual differences and variability as experimentally controllable phenomena. The behavior of the individual is of primary concern. The approach considers the statistically stable mean a creation of methods of analysis. Therefore, the mean is not considered an empirical value. Theoretically and practically, the single-subject approach starts with one or a few individuals, studies them, draws conclusions, and extends those conclusions only to similar individuals, if at all. This approach also tries to build a science of behavior by observing many individuals, but few in given studies.

As I have pointed out in other contexts, the two major problems of the group design strategy are (1) the gap between its theory and practice and (2) its limited relevance to a clinical science. Except in nonexperimental research (such as surveys), the method does not work in the way proposed by the theory. As a result, the group design approach lacks its greatest purported strength.

THE INVESTIGATOR IN THE DESIGN SELECTION PROCESS

One of the themes of this book is that science is both a public and a personal matter. Many scientific decisions are made for objective and personal reasons. Many other decisions are also made for practical reasons. There is nothing good or bad about these reasons; that is simply the way it is. Also, there seems to be no other way, because scientists are people and science is what these people do.

All responsible scientists first consider what they think are the objective bases of selecting a design. The investigators first determine the nature of the question asked and what kind of data will answer it. Then, a design that will produce relevant data in a reasonably unambiguous manner is selected. Once the method has been selected, scientists try to use it as precisely and thoroughly as they can.

Those objective reasons are not entirely free from personal reasons, however. Personal reasons are nothing but the past training and experience of the investigator. They are not necessarily subjective, in the prejudicial sense of the word. An excellent design choice is as subjective as a poor choice; both are partly determined by the scientist's training and experience. Generally speaking, those who are trained in a particular tradition of research try to make the best possible decision within that tradition. Sometimes, scientists reject the tradition of research in which they were trained. In such cases, the scientists are said to "adopt a different tradition." This happens because their experience has taught them a different lesson. When scientific behavior itself becomes a subject matter of scientific analysis, these reasons will be objective in the same sense that any other behavioral phenomenon is objective.

Finally, the selection of a design is also partly a matter of practical exigencies. The investigator may know very well that an elegant factorial design with multiple cells is the best design to analyze the interaction between treatment variables, but not having enough clients, may settle for the less efficient single-subject interactional design. Another investigator may select a single-group experimental design because of a preference for avoiding a control group to which the treatment must be denied or postponed. Practical exigencies seem to play a greater role in clinical treatment research than in basic laboratory research. Availability of clients, the need to offer treatment as promptly as possible, and other ethical considerations create a host of exigencies for the clinical investigator.

THE FINAL CRITERION: SOUNDNESS OF DATA

In the evaluation and selection of a design, it is better to keep in perspective that after all, a design is only a means of producing data. A method is as good as the data it generates. As pointed out by Sidman (1960), though the type and the quality of data depend upon the method used, sound data can stand by themselves. Bad methods may not produce sound data, but sound data must be accepted regardless of the methodological biases one may hold.

The soundness of data must be judged in a broader context and no objective rules are available to make this judgment. Even the original investigator's judgment regarding the importance of his or her data cannot always be trusted (Sidman, 1960). Data rejected by the investigator may be important or may prove to be important in light of evidence that may come later. Data hailed as important may be worthless or may prove to be irrelevant later. Methodological or theoretical faddishness may make poor data look good as long as that faddishness lasts. Relevant data that contradict faddish trends of the times may be considered irrelevant.

The value of given data can and must be judged regardless of the hypothesis they are supposed to support or refudiate. A set of data may not have served the purposes of an investigator, but it may still be sound. The data generated by a particular study may have failed to confirm a pet hypothesis or forced the acceptance of an unfavored one. Data that were not sought in a study may have emerged accidentally, and those that were sought may not have emerged. None of these contingencies are important in evaluating the importance of data.

Another consideration in the evaluation of data is the methodological soundness of studies, which can be determined regardless of theoretical or personal biases (Sidman, 1960). Data that are generated by acceptable methods of observation and experimentation must be welcomed even if the data contradict one's own preconceptions. Strong and unambiguous effects of independent variables demonstrated under controlled conditions must be accepted regardless of theoretical or personal points of view. Data that resolve contradictions, shed light on poorly understood phenomena, clarify relations between events, and show patterns in seemingly chaotic happenings are always important. Similarly, data that show effective treatment of disorders, methods of solving practical problems, and effective ways of studying a difficult phenomenon are valuable. As Sidman (1980) has pointed out, it is the cumulative development of a science that eventually determines the importance and soundness of data.

CHAPTER SUMMARY

In evaluating designs and design strategies, the clinician should consider the type of research question, applicability to clinical science, and soundness of data. Since a design is a strategy for answering a certain research question, the first important consideration is whether a particular design will indeed answer the question proposed for an investigation. Table 10-1 summarizes the major research questions and design options.

Several designs may be able to answer the same research questions. In such cases, selection may be based on applicability and the investigator's expertise. Some designs may be more applicable than others. In clinical treatment evaluation, a strict adherence to the requirement of sampling equivalence is not practical. Therefore, the applicability of group designs in treatment evaluation research is limited. When they are used in clinical research, group designs almost always involve major compromises in achieving sampling equivalence.

TABLE 10-1.

Comparative summary of design options.

Research Questions	Design Options		Comments
	Group	**Single-Subject**	
What may have caused this effect?	Case study	Case study	Not experimental; no controls
Does a treatment seem to work?	One-group pretest–posttest design	*AB* design	Uncontrolled treatment evaluations; similar to routine treatment, but more systematic
How are selected behaviors distributed in certain populations?	Uses the group method; no particular design; longitudinal or cross-sectional method	None available; philosophically unat-tractive questions	This type of research is based on the assumption that sta-tistical average is the norm
What is the differential distribution of selected variables?	Uses the group method; no particular design; descriptive studies	None available; unattractive because of its nonexperimen-tal approach	"Normal" versus "clinical" group comparisons involve this type of questions
What are the effects of an independent variable?	Pretest–posttest control group design; post-test-only control group design; within-subjects and time-series designs	*ABA* reversal or with-drawal design; *BAB* design; *ABAB*, multiple baseline, and changing criterion design	Controlled design is needed; both strategies offer designs; consider the strategic and design-specific limitations
Is a clinical treatment effective?	Pretest–posttest control group design; posttest-only control group design; within-subjects and time-series designs	*ABA* reversal or with-drawal design; *BAB* design; *ABAB*, multiple baseline, and changing criterion design	Controlled design is needed; both strategies offer designs; consider the strategic and design-specific limitations
Is one treatment more effective than another?	Multigroup pretest–posttest design; factorial designs; crossover design; time-series designs	*ABACA/ACABA* design; alternating treat-ments design	Only relative effects are frequently assessed; control groups or conditions may be added; group designs are somewhat better
Is there an interaction between treatment components?	Completely randomized factorial design	Interactional design	Group strategy is better; multiple treatment inter-ference in the single-subject design

TABLE 10-1 (continued).

Research Questions	Design Options		Comments
	Group	Single-Subject	
Do some clients benefit more than other clients from the same treatment?	Randomized blocks design	An efficient design is not available	Group strategy can isolate an interaction between assigned variables and treatment
Do clients prefer one treatment over the other?	An efficient design is not available	Simultaneous treatments design	Preference, not necessarily effectiveness, is analyzed
What are the most effective components of a treatment package?	Completely randomized factorial design	Interactional design	Relative as well as interactive effects are analyzed
Can an effective treatment package be developed?	Any controlled design to begin with, and then one of the factorial designs	Any controlled design to begin with, and then the interactional design	This kind of research requires a two-stage evaluation of independent components and their interactions
What is the optimal level of treatment?	An efficient design is not available except for the single-group time-series design with multiple temporary designs	Most single-subject designs; parametric variations of treatment may be introduced in successive stages of treatment	Single-subject approach is preferable because of its flexibility
How do certain groups behave?	Time-series designs with repeated measures before and after treatment	An effective design is not available; handled through replications	Group strategy is useful in describing as well as predicting group behaviors
How effective is the treatment across clients?	Any well-controlled group design	An efficient design is not available; handled through replications	Group designs, though better in this respect, are not efficient in evaluating treatments in the first place

Generally speaking, group designs are more effective than single-subject designs in determining the distribution of dependent variables in samples of subjects, group trends and characteristics, the differences between clinical and nonclinical groups, interaction between treatment variables, and interaction between treatment and subject variables. Group designs are also effective in predicting treatment effects based on diagnostic categories. Finally, the designs are well-structured, so that the need to make on-line decisions is minimal.

The disadvantages of group designs include limited applications in clinical treatment evaluation, lack of logical generality, weak empirical manipulations, inadequate measurement of dependent variables, insensitivity to individual uniqueness, and rigidity of experimental conditions. Also, group designs are not able to evaluate optimum levels of treatment or client preferences for treatment procedures when multiple procedures are equally effective. Finally, group designs are not conducive to direct or systematic replications.

The advantages of single-subject designs include their sensitivity to individual behaviors and uniqueness, appropriateness to treatment evaluations, high logical generality, practicality, replicability, reliable measurement of dependent variables, large magnitude of treatment effects, and flexibility. Also, the designs help build treatment packages, determine client preferences for treatment procedures, and help establish optimum levels of treatment.

The disadvantages of single-subject designs include their limited usefulness in predicting group behaviors and performance of many clients under given treatments. They are less effective than group designs in evaluating the interaction between multiple treatments or between treatment and client characteristics. Also, they require on-the-spot decisions.

Problems such as inter- and intrasubject variability, unexpected changes in the control mechanisms, problems in achieving generality, slow accumulation of scientific data, and practical problems of implementation are common to both design strategies.

The final criterion in the selection of design strategies is the soundness of data. Procedure that produce sound data are always acceptable. ■

S T U D Y **G U I D E**

In answering questions 1 through 11, make sure you (1) identify the type of research, (2) specify the type of design (group or single-subject), (3) describe the basic elements of the procedure, and (4) justify the selection of the design. You must make up such needed information as the age of the subjects, the kind of disorder, sample size, and severity of the disorder.

1 Design a study in which you would investigate the potential independent variables of conductive hearing loss in a group of school-age children.

2 Suppose you wish to find out the stages in which children acquire the passive sentence forms. Design a study that would have a local but adequate sample. Use hypothetical information regarding the size of the population.

3 Compared with normally hearing persons, how frequently do hearing impaired adults initiate conversation in a group? Design a study to answer this question.

4 Design two studies in which the effects of an independent variable are evaluated under controlled conditions. In the first study, the temporary effect of a variable on some aspect of speech, language, or hearing will be evaluated. For example, the effects of white noise or delayed auditory feedback on speech may be temporary. In the other study, the relatively permanent effect on some aspect of speech–language behavior will be evaluated. The effects of treatment or teaching procedures are of this kind.

5 You wish to find out if one teaching–treatment method is more effective than the other. From your study of your specialty, select two potential treatment procedures and design a study to evaluate their relative effects to determine if one of them is more effective than the other.

6 Find a treatment procedure that contains at least two dissimilar elements. Then, design a study in which you would determine the interactive effects of the two selected components. In this case, design both a single-subject study and a group design study.

7 You suspect that the social class of your clients influences the outcome of language treatment. Design a study to investigate this possibility.

8 Find two equally effective treatment procedures for a given disorder. Then, design a study in which you would determine if selected clients prefer one over the other procedure.

(continued next page)

Study Guide *(continued)*

9 Suppose you wish to find out if one of the components of a treatment package is more effective than the other. Find a treatment package used in your field and select two of its components. Design a study to find out the relative effects of the two.

10 Design a study in which you would evaluate the optimum level of a selected treatment procedure. Let your independent variable be either the duration of treatment sessions or their weekly frequency.

11 Suppose you have repeatedly faced parents of language handicapped children who ask you whether language therapy for these children will increase their chances of completing high school. Assuming an answer is not available, how would you design a study to find out?

12 Summarize the advantages and disadvantages of the group design strategy.

13 Summarize the advantages and disadvantages of the single-subject strategy.

14 What kinds of problems are common to different design strategies?

15 Specify why the soundness of data is an important criterion in the evaluation of design strategies.

■ C H A P T E R   **11**

Designs Versus Paradigms in Research

■ Limitations of exclusively methodological approaches, 324

■ Research methods and subject matters, 324

■ Philosophy as methodology, 326

■ Philosophy of subject matters, 327

■ Philosophy of the science of speech and language, 329

■ Philosophical ways of handling methodological problems, 339

■ The interplay between philosophy and methodology, 342

■ Study guide, 343

G enerally speaking, graduate courses on research teach how to do research. Naturally, the information presented is about the methods and procedures of conducting research investigations. Textbooks and articles on research are also typically concerned with the methodology of research.

Methodology, however, is only a part of research. Two other parts of research are equally important: knowledge of the subject matter and its philosophy. It is important to understand what to investigate and why it is important to investigate it, as well as how to investigate it. It is not clear why, in discussions of research, the knowledge and philosophy of subject matters do not receive the kind of attention they deserve. Many writers tend to pay exclusive attention to the methods of research and ignore the questions of the conceptual as well as philosophical bases of research.

LIMITATIONS OF EXCLUSIVELY METHODOLOGICAL APPROACHES

It is important to know how research is done. The methods and procedures by which research questions are investigated constitute a large body of technical information. Methodology can be defined as the study of how to do research. How to observe, measure, and record a phenomenon; how to fit research questions to research methods; how to set up conditions in such a way that a cause–effect relation is revealed; how to manipulate independent variables; and how to make sure that unwanted variables do not influence the results are all a part of methodology. As such, methodology tells a researcher *how* to investigate when he or she knows *what* to investigate.

However, methodology does not tell what to investigate. A thorough study of the methods of research may still leave the investigator with nothing to investigate. Knowledge of the group and single-subject designs or of the various statistical techniques will not necessarily suggest what questions to investigate. The knowledge of research designs is useless without a worthwhile question that can be answered by those designs.

An important point about research methods is that they are secondary to the subject matter and its philosophy. In many ways, the nature of a subject matter and its philosophy shape methodologies. Meaningful studies can be designed only when an investigator has a critical understanding of the subject matter, its philosophy, and the concepts and methods of research.

RESEARCH METHODS AND SUBJECT MATTERS

To a certain extent, methods are independent of subject matters. It was pointed out in Chapter 3 that the methods of science are independent of any subject matter. Investigators can borrow methods from science as long as those methods are applicable to a given subject matter. A subject matter that successfully applies the methods of science will be regarded as a branch of science. However, the methods of science do not constitute a closed set. It is an open and dynamic set shaped by the nature of different disciplines that have used the basic scientific approach in studying common as well as unique problems. New methods are added to the set by different disciplines. As long as the methods do not violate the basic logic and approach of science, such additions enrich scientific methodology.

The fact that most methods of science are independent of subject matters does not suggest that an understanding of the methods alone will lead to meaningful research in given subject matters. A thorough knowledge of the subject matter is necessary to enable applications of the methods in answering significant questions. Theoretically, the independence of methods and subject matters may suggest that students can learn how to do research independently of their subject matters. They can combine this information on research methods with their knowledge of the subject matter acquired independently. In practice, however, this may not be the best strategy for learning how to do research.

The way many graduate students are asked to study research methods suggests that it may not be important to understand what to investigate and how to investigate in the same context. Graduate courses on research methods, often taken in departments outside students' major disciplines, offer "methods" as independent not only of the "contents" of research but also of all philosophical concerns. Because of the highly prevalent notion that statistics is research designs, more and more students in a variety of social, behavioral, and health-related disciplines are asked to take courses on statistics that count as courses on research designs. Students from different disciplines take these courses with the implied assumption that information on research can be acquired with no philosophical concerns relative to their subject matter. Many students, however, are not able to integrate the subject matter with research methodology offered in a content-neutral manner. They are also not able to understand the philosophical issues relative to their subject matter. A knowledge of analysis of variance or specific group or single-subject designs does not necessarily make a student a competent researcher.

An exclusive concern with methodology leaves the student with no philosophical sophistication needed to do research. Therefore, in this chapter, I will address some of the philosophical issues that play a major role in the research process.

At the very outset, I wish to make a few points clear. An examination of philosophical issues inevitably raises questions about personal biases and viewpoints. Also, such an examination raises the question of what kinds of research (unrelated to methodology) are more or less valuable. The discussion can raise unsettling questions about one's own philosophy, which is, from the standpoint of a researcher, an inclination to investigate certain kinds of questions with certain types of methods. Perhaps partly because of this reason, authors typically shy away from philosophical issues and stay close to methodology.

Methodological questions have relatively straightforward answers. Although different tactics can be used to investigate a certain problem, some are clearly more appropriate than others, and some are undoubtedly wrong. However, philosophical issues are not as easily resolved as methodological issues. Therefore, I fully realize that the *philosophical questions to be discussed in this chapter do not have right or wrong answers.* The sole purpose of this chapter is to draw attention to a neglected aspect of research. I do take certain philosophical positions relative to the issues to be discussed, and surely (and I believe appropriately) they will be clear in the discussion as one of the different viewpoints.

Another point that must be made at the very beginning is that both methodology and philosophy are important. There is no suggestion here that philosophical considerations should supersede methodological considerations. The main emphasis is on giving philosophical issues the attention they deserve. In the best tradition of research, both methodology and philosophy play a significant role. They influence each other and help each other evolve. At a more advanced stage, there is a productive interplay between the philosophy and methodology of a subject matter. I shall return to this point later.

PHILOSOPHY AS METHODOLOGY

It is appropriate to contrast philosophy with methodology as I have done earlier in the chapter, but probably a more significant factor about philosophy is that it can have very direct consequences for methodology. In many respects, the philosophy of a subject matter is also its methodology. In this section, we shall explore this idea and then return to the question of interplay between philosophy and methodology.

Very few, if any, disciplines have a single philosophy. Different philosophical approaches coexist in many disciplines. In other words, disciplines are likely to have different *paradigms.* Paradigms are conceptual frameworks that include certain basic assumptions about a discipline. Such assumptions dictate the nature of questions asked and the methods used to answer them. Philosophical or paradigmatic variations within a discipline create a number of issues relative to methodology. In our discussion, we shall focus upon (1) the philosophy of subject matters, (2) the philosophy of the science of speech and language, (3) the philosophical ways of handling methodological problems, and (4) the interplay between philosophy and methodology.

Philosophy of Subject Matters

The philosophy of a subject matter is different from the "contents" of that subject matter. For example, the kinds of questions researched and the knowledge generated in different disciplines constitute their respective subject matters. However, an overall philosophy of a subject matter is a broader viewpoint of what that subject matter has been and what it ought to be. The philosophy of a subject matter is a conceptual evaluation of the methods, the questions, the theories, the social applications, and the overall implications of that subject matter. Such a philosophy does not necessarily evaluate the empirical findings found in a discipline; that is the stuff the subject matter is made of. It does not directly evaluate particular designs, methods, or modes of data analysis. Instead, the philosophy concerns itself with the way the subject matter and its methods have been conceptualized, the approaches taken to the issues of methodology, the strengths and the limitations of those concepts and methods, and the overall significance of the knowledge generated within the discipline.

When a discipline is also an applied profession, additional philosophical considerations emerge. Among the questions a clinical profession attempts to answer are these: Can the discipline solve its problems? Does it address the concerns from a philosophical perspective that seems to take the discipline forward? Is the discipline taking a methodological posture that seems consistent with its applied objectives? Is it encouraging appropriate considerations of ethical issues? In essence, the philosophy of an applied discipline asks and evaluates a generic question: is the profession able to meet its scientific and social challenges in an efficient and responsible manner?

It is obvious that philosophical concerns of the kind described here are not totally independent of the subject matter and its methodology. In fact, questions of philosophy can be answered only in the context of a particular discipline, its methods, and their outcome.

The philosophy of a subject matter is not a discussion of vague and irrelevant issues. Contrary to the popular notion, philosophy is concerned with conceptual as well as practical issues. There is nothing more practical than an evaluation of the degree to which a profession has achieved its scientific and applied objectives. Such an evaluation is a philosophical venture. A serious examination of the philosophy of a subject matter and its conceptual frameworks can suggest better ways of reconceptualizing the issues or even the entire subject matter in such a way that the practical challenges are met.

When a discipline reaches a certain stage of sophistication and advanced knowledge, philosophical issues become clear and often pressing. The question of life and death, certainly one of the most profound of the philosophical issues, became quite pressing when medical technology advanced to the stage where life, as defined in a technical and legal sense, could be sustained through artificial means. On the other hand, if individuals belonging to a discipline are sensitive to philosophical issues from the beginning, then it is quite possible that certain faulty conceptual as well as methodological postures can be avoided.

Philosophies of a subject matter have a profound influence on the kinds of research done in a subject matter and on how that research is done. Different philosophies within a discipline direct researchers' attention to different kinds of questions and methodologies. As a result, different "traditions" of research emerge. Eventually, viewpoints or theories of varying degrees of similarity and contrast result from such differences in research traditions.

Natural sciences are bound by some common assumptions about natural phenomena. As we noted in Chapter 3, natural scientists believe that events are caused (determinism) and that causal relations between events can be discovered. Scientists also believe that some form of sensory observation is necessary for a thorough study of a phenomenon (empiricism). Also, natural sciences have certain common philosophical assumptions about their methods. Most natural sciences have a commitment to experimental methodology. They have a strong tradition of experimental research. As a result, there is a large body of replicated knowledge. Natural scientists also believe that variability is mostly extrinsic and therefore subject to experimental control. This philosophical assumption may have done more than anything else to successfully control and alter the variables dealt with in natural sciences. It also shows how a philosophical assumption dictates a certain methodology.

In natural sciences, there is a long tradition of empirical research as opposed to logical speculation. This may also be partly due to the philosophy of natural sciences, which drives the scientists out of their armchairs and into their laboratories. The philosophy of natural sciences insists that empirical investigation is the best method of producing knowledge. One must find out through experimentation. Speculation can serve a purpose only when it leads to experimentation.

The philosophy of science makes a distinction between scholarship and scholasticism. Scholarship is the product of informed, authoritative, and evaluative awareness of the existing knowledge in a given subject matter. Scholarship is needed and valued in sciences, art, literature, and the professions. Scholasticism, on the other hand, is a *method* of generating knowledge that does not necessarily use observational and experimental methodology. It relies on authorities, traditions, ancient sources, and logic. Natural sciences have moved away from scholasticism, which is good at generating controversies but inefficient in producing empirically validated knowledge. Unfortunately, some of the lesser developed sciences have not been especially successful in rejecting scholasticism and moving on to the realm of empirically verified knowledge based on observation and experimentation.

Philosophy of the Science of Speech and Language

A philosophy of the *science* of speech and language should have emerged before a philosophy of clinical intervention in speech and language disorders. However, the sequence of development within our field has been the other way around. The field started as a profession and then slowly began to move in the direction of scientific study. It is probably accurate to say that failures and inadequacies in the practice of the profession have prompted us to become more and more scientific. Therefore, it is not clear whether we have a dominant philosophy of the science of speech and language, and if we do, what it is.

When a subject matter starts as a profession, it is very likely to borrow philosophies from fields considered relevant. There were probably three major sources of influence in this regard: medicine, education, and behavioral and social sciences. Most of the early clinical conceptual models were influenced by medicine. Medical concepts such as symptomatology, diagnosis and differential diagnosis, etiology, prognosis, and functional–organic distinction were all influential in speech–language pathology.

Much of the training and practice model of speech–language pathologists was influenced by schools of education. Largely because the public schools provided most of the jobs, the philosophy of education has had a large influence on the way the profession was conceptualized and the clinicians educated. Most speech–language pathologists were and still are asked to take several courses in the departments of education with the idea that both the science and the profession of speech and language have something to gain from such courses. Possibly, this approach had some negative impact on the development of speech and language as a science.

The behavioral and social science influences on our field of study are probably due to two disciplines: psychology and linguistics. The early influence was from psychology, which probably had a more favorable impact on audiology than it did on speech pathology. Experiments in sensory psychology, especially auditory sensations and perceptions, had a tremendous impact on the new science of audiology. Initially, the branch of psychology that tended to influence speech pathology was not experimental, but clinical. The clinical psychology of the time was mostly Freudian in its orientation. Psychodynamics and psychodiagnosis were and have been the dominant themes of clinical psychology. These themes blended well with the medical philosophy of finding an internal cause and treating it; the only difference was that the cause happened to be in the mind of the client (such as the bad self-image of a stutterer).

Subsequently, another kind of psychology, applied behavior analysis, began to influence speech–language pathology. Techniques of behavior change began to be used in the modification of speech, language, fluency, and voice disorders. However, this influence, even today, is strictly methodological.

The parent of behavior modification, which is radical behaviorism, has had very little impact on the way the behavioral principles are applied in speech–language pathology. In other words, there is some appreciation of methodology of behavior change but not of the philosophy of that change (behaviorism). Consequently, the application of behavioral technology within the field of speech and language pathology has been devoid of philosophical strengths. Behavioral methodology is often grafted onto the incongruent philosophies of cognitivism and nativism, whose major sources of influence have been linguistics and psycholinguistics.

The discipline of linguistics did not exert much influence until the entry of speech–language pathologists into the realm of language and its disorders. At the time when language clinicians began to be involved with language disorders, Chomsky's (1957) generative transformational grammar dominated linguistics. The same philosophical approach, with its purely structural orientation and a tendency toward nativism was borrowed by speech–language pathologists. This philosophical approach encouraged speculative writing, which has been flourishing ever since. Contrary to what one might expect, experimental research on the treatment of language did not come from speech–language pathologists. Instead, it came from behavioral psychologists who did not share Chomsky's philosophy of nativism and rationalism. Nor did the behaviorists share Chomsky's nonexperimental approach to studying language.

The observation that a philosophy either encourages or discourages certain kinds of research is clearly demonstrated in the case of language. Structurally oriented linguistics encourages normative and descriptive research. The presumed independent variables are often not susceptible to experimental manipulations. Innate structures, cognitive notions, knowledge of the universal grammar, and grammatical competence are not experimentally manipulable independent variables, though they figure importantly in linguistic theories of language. On the other hand, environmental contingencies that are supposed to control language within the behavioral philosophy encourage or even require experimental methodology. Experimental research on language and language treatment has typically been the product of behaviorism, whereas descriptive, normative, and predominantly theoretical writing has been the product of the linguistically oriented approach.

If the contemporary scene of speech–language sciences and disorders does not permit definitive statements about a philosophy, that is probably because we have not been philosophicalally aware as a discipline. There have been no systematic attempts at creating a unifying philosophy of research and clinical practice. The "science" in the profession has followed a certain subject-matters-are-science approach. Anatomy and physiology and acoustics are typically considered under speech science, whereas the study of articulation or fluency disorders is "clinical." Offended by this approach, some who studied language simply renamed their subject matter "language science," with very few consequences.

In the area of treatment and application, eclecticism has prevailed. Within the best tradition of eclecticism, one is supposed to select what is valid from different approaches. Validity is determined on the basis of controlled, replicated evidence. In practice, however, eclecticism has meant borrowing from different sources with no regard for philosophical or paradigmatic differences. Such borrowings have been based simply upon subjective opinions and feelings. The most distressing thing about this trend is that the prevailing approaches from which clinicians chose were also based on unsupported opinions.

When the basic study of a subject matter and its clinical activities are influenced by contradictory philosophies, then that subject not only lacks a unifying philosophy but is also riddled with controversies. This has been a major problem in the areas of language and, more recently, phonology. While the basic analyses of language and phonological aspects have been based mostly on structural properties, remedial approaches have necessarily looked elsewhere for help. Behavioral and other approaches that are not necessarily congruent with purely structural approaches have influenced remedial efforts and research. Consequently, conceptual inconsistencies and philosophical problems have resulted.

In its efforts to establish a philosophical base, a new discipline must consider several factors, some of which will now be addressed.

The Dependent Variables

It is generally true that research consists of a search for the independent variables that created the effects under study. Typically, we know the effects but need to find the causes. Therefore, much scientific discussion centers on independent variables (causes), not dependent variables (effects). Nonetheless, the neglected question of the dependent variables is important.

The question of the dependent variables is none other than the all-important question of what it is that we are trying to study. A scientific study starts with an observed effect, but the scientist may face two problems to begin with. The first problem, which is generally appreciated, is that the effect may not have been understood fully. In the study of stuttering, the analogy of the six blind men trying to explore an elephant is often used to describe the problem of each investigator seeing only a part of a large effect. When the totality of an effect is not understood, descriptions, explanations, and theories of that effect will be inadequate. In the course of a causal search, more may be understood about the effect itself. Descriptions and explanations of the effect will be modified as more is learned about the nature of the effect.

The second problem is not as well appreciated as the first. A serious problem with the dependent variable can arise when its conceptualization is inadequate, is mistaken, or does not allow experimentation. It is well known that a science makes significant progress when its dependent variables are firmly and clearly established. This simply means that when we are sure of what we are studying, we may be better able to explain it through experimental research. Obviously, experiments on vague effects may not isolate specific causes. Physical sciences have made great strides partly because of their more definitive dependent variables.

The problem with the dependent variables used in speech–language sciences and pathology are basically conceptual and philosophical. We face methodological problems largely because of these conceptual and philosophical problems. Obviously, whether the dependent variables we study are inadequate or mistaken depends upon particular points of view, but whether the variables are experimentally accessible can be better argued or illustrated.

Many controversies about language have resulted from the confusion regarding the dependent variables themselves. The so-called grammatical, semantic, and pragmatic "revolutions" in linguistics that have affected speech–language pathologists are, for the most part, a debate about the dependent variables. The single most critical question to these controversies is this: What is language? As the answers have differed, so have the dependent variables: Is language the innate knowledge of the rules of universal grammar, as Chomsky claimed? Is language simply grammar, as is also claimed by the generative linguists? Is language semantic notions, as is claimed by generative semanticists? Is language pragmatic structures or notions or rules? Is language the use of those pragmatic rules? Is language cognitive structures, as is claimed by other scientists? Is language an unobservable mental system, or is it the observable production of whatever it is supposed to be? Is language a type of behavior? Is it similar to other kinds of behaviors, or is it special? These are only a sampling of questions asked in the study of language, and as can be seen, they are not about the causes but the effects being studied. In essence, we have been wondering about the dependent variables themselves.

The way a dependent variable is conceptualized can make it more or less susceptible to an analysis of cause–effect relations. In other words, the philosophy of the dependent variable will determine to a large extent what kinds of methodology will be used and, in turn, what kinds of knowledge it will generate.

When the effects are supposed to lie in a realm not accessible to observation, the causes also tend to be hypothesized to exist within that unobservable realm. If the dependent variable is a mental system, then its independent variable is typically thought to exist within the same mental domain. It need not necessarily be that way, but those who postulate internal effects also tend to explain them on the basis of internal causes. Then, neither the effect nor the cause is observable. Science requires, however, that both the effect and the cause be observable; but on a temporary basis, scientists can tolerate the idea of causes that have been postulated but not yet demonstrated. There is then an expectation that such a demonstration is forthcoming. But scientists may not have much patience with effects that are not observed and perhaps cannot be observed. In such cases, scientists do not see anything to be explained. Mental rules, cognitive structures, innate systems, and such other internal dependent variables fall into this category.

The same situation exists in phonology. The real dependent variables, it is argued, are not the production of particular phonemes, but the knowledge of the speech sound system. Phonological rules, which are extracted from behavioral regularities, are considered the essence of phonological behaviors. The dependent variables are once again unobservable.

The question of the dependent variable has also plagued the field of stuttering. The multitudinous definitions of stuttering reflect nothing but a controversy (or confusion) about the dependent variable. Stuttering is variously defined as role conflict, avoidance behavior, prosodic defect, phonatory problem, laryngeal aberrations, incoordination between neuromotor systems, auditory perceptual defect, production of certain kinds of dysfluencies, or production of all kinds of dysfluencies at a certain frequency level, just to name a few. When investigators within a discipline do not agree on the nature of the effect, there can be little agreement on its causes.

In a clinical discipline, controversies concerning the dependent variables are carried into treatment. Such controversies make it difficult to conduct research on treatment effects. When certain treatment effects on controversial dependent variables are evaluated, the clinician does not know which dependent variables change under what treatment conditions. Such treatment evaluation studies are also not easily replicated.

Empirical specification of a dependent variable is essential for successful treatment of a disorder by different clinicians. If clinicians are researching and treating different dependent variables, there can be very little unambiguous communication between them. In the case of stuttering, for example, the clinician who is correcting the prosodic defect may not be doing the same thing as the one who is trying to reduce the avoidance behaviors. Success rates of treatment procedures also vary tremendously, not necessarily because stutterers are heterogeneous, but simply because different dependent variables are involved.

From the standpoint of the philosophy of science (not that of subject matter), the dependent variables must at least be observable in some empirical sense. Effects that do not generate empirical consequences cannot be observed or explained. Scientists, like every one else, do not try to solve problems that do not exist. Unobservable dependent variables are especially a luxury for the clinician who must stay close to empirical data. Dependent variables in the area of language, speech, fluency, and voice must be empirically real. There is no assurance that such variables as the rules of universal grammar and knowledge of phonological systems are simply not inferred entities. There is even no assurance that grammatical categories, semantic notions, and pragmatic rules are separate and independent behaviors.

Questionable dependent variables pose another danger to the researcher and the clinician. It is easy to confuse those dependent variables with independent variables. Is knowledge of the rules of universal grammar a dependent variable or an independent variable? In other words, is it part of the language or is it the cause of language? It can be either, depending on whose writing you are reading. In the Chomsky-type theory, knowledge of the rules is sometimes the dependent variable and at other times the independent variable. Similar confusions exist in phonological and pragmatic analyses.

Sometimes a confusion between dependent and independent variables can exist even when the status of a given variable as being dependent is very clear. This problem exists in stuttering research concerned with various neurophysiological activities of stutterers. For example, is the slow phonatory reaction time in stutterers a dependent variable or an independent variable? In other words, when stutterers take more time to say what they are asked to say, do we observe a part of stuttering or do we observe a cause of stuttering? Is the observed excessive tension in the laryngeal muscle during stuttering a part or a cause of stuttering?

It is not suggested here that all researchers should agree on certain dependent variables so they can make collective progress. Such a prescriptive suggestion is not acceptable to scientists since it is likely to inhibit creativity. What is suggested here is that we pay attention to some fundamental philosophical issues when considering, advocating, and researching certain dependent variables. At the least, in formulating their dependent variables, investigators must address questions such as these: Are the dependent variables observable? Do they have empirical validity? Do they have more than speculative substance to them? Do they encourage experimental research? As can be seen, these questions do not stem from a particular viewpoint of the subject matter, but rather from the philosophy of science itself.

The Philosophy of Measurement

It was noted briefly in Chapter 5 that measurement philosophies are a part of the subject matter. Such philosophies can have significant impact on the kinds of research done in a given subject matter. The point is that the philosophy of measurement is itself a part of methodology used in many investigations and that those philosophies are intricately connected with the conceptualizations of the dependent as well as the independent variables.

The two interrelated questions relative to the philosophy of measurement concern what is measured and how it is measured. Both dependent and independent variables are measured in research, but it is the measurement of the dependent variable that can pose significant problems. It is obvious that the measurement of any variable depends upon the way it is conceptualized. In the case of dependent variables, some can be measured directly, others only indirectly, and some not at all.

Social and psychological sciences have devised a variety of indirect measures of their dependent variables, largely because of the prevailing tendency to hypothesize dependent variables that are not directly observable and hence not measurable. Elaborately developed rating scales; personality inventories; and interest, attitude, and opinion questionnaires illustrate a complex set of measures analyzed through an equally complex set of statistical techniques. Unfortunately, the scientific return on such complex activities is usually poor because the nature of the dependent variable thus measured is not at all clear. It is one thing to measure the number of times a college student visits the library over a period of time, and an entirely different thing to measure what the student says or indicates on a questionnaire about the same behavior. The dependent variable, in this case the frequency with which he or she visits the library, is perfectly observable, although not without some inconvenience on the part of the researcher. The short-cut often taken is to simply ask persons about a particular behavior and treat their verbal statements as the measure of the dependent variable.

In communicative disorders, indirect measures have been used frequently. Instead of measuring stuttering directly, it may be measured through a rating scale. Experts may be asked to judge whether a person is a mild, moderate, or severe stutterer. Different judges' ratings may be averaged to derive a single rating on a given client. The rate of speech has sometimes been used as a measure, not of rate itself but of stuttering, on the assumption that slower rate is indicative of stuttering. If one wonders why stuttering could not be measured directly, the answer lies in the way stuttering was conceptualized. Evidently, to some investigators, stuttering is not a dependent variable that can be observed and measured in terms of *real numbers*. When stuttering is conceptualized in terms of bad self-image, it is difficult to count it in terms of real mathematical units. Some indirect number systems that give the impression it is being measured will have to be devised.

It is probably better to have dependent variables that permit at least indirect measures than to have those that do not permit any measurement at all. Many of the variables that figure in the linguistic analysis of language and phonology can hardly be measured. It is not clear how one measures the knowledge of the grammatical or phonological rule system. In such cases, observable behaviors are measured and their patterns established. Patterns of correct and incorrect responses are thought to reflect the underlying knowledge systems. Such knowledge systems are then thought to have been measured indirectly. In this case, measurement is by inference, which is a highly questionable scientific practice indeed.

It appears as though the philosophy of the subject matter of speech and language pathology considers direct measures of behaviors either not adequate or not valid. The prevailing practice of measurement by inference in communicative disorders suggests that somehow counting the production of various language responses in terms of real numbers and percentages is either unimportant, invalid, or both. There is probably a prevailing opinion that directly observable dependent variables are superficial and that in-the-head, inferred variables are complex and scientifically more valuable.

In summary, one can measure only what one thinks is important to measure, and what one thinks is important is a matter of the philosophy one adopts regarding the subject matter. Once again, it is possible to think of some conditions of measurement purely from the philosophy of science. It is preferable to measure the dependent variable as directly as possible. It is also preferable to measure the variable in terms of real numbers and not with a simulated system of "numbers" that need nonmathematical definitions (see Chapter 5 for details). It is certainly best to avoid measurement by inference, whose inevitable effect is unchecked speculation.

The Locus of the Independent Variables

Another philosophical factor that profoundly affects the methodology of research and writing in a given discipline is the manner in which the independent variables are conceptualized. It may be recalled that in order to establish cause–effect relations, independent variables are manipulated by the experimenter under controlled conditions. The cause of a certain event may be discovered accidentally, in which case the influence of prior conceptualization may not have played a critical role. In fact, prior conceptualization can sometimes delay accidental discoveries by making the scientist less observant of unsuspected relations. In any case, what we are concerned with in this section is the interrelation between two questions regarding independent variables: what they are and where they are located within the operating philosophy of a given discipline.

Systematic thinking about the nature of causes and the philosophy of causation has a long history, because this is the stuff science is made of. As we noted in Chapter 3, most dependent variables have a chain of causes, which can be analyzed at different levels. An aphasic patient's speech problem may have been caused by brain damage, but the brain damage is also an effect of some other cause such as a head injury or a stroke. The head injury and stroke have their respective causes, and so forth. In this chain of events, a particular event and its cause may be the focus of analysis at a given time, but it is important to remember that there is a larger picture of more complex and interrelated events.

In the case of communicative behaviors and their disorders, causes are complex and perhaps involve multiple chains of events. But more importantly, the causes are often historical. By the time a clinician sees a child who has a language disorder or other disorder of communication, the independent variables will already have occurred. That is why in clinical sciences, a retrospective search for causes through the method of case history is so commonly employed. As we noted in Chapter 4, such ex post facto studies are done with the hope of uncovering past causes of current effects.

Uncovering the past causes of current effects has many pitfalls. We can never be sure that the event identified as the cause in a historical record was indeed the cause of the effect under study. Because the experimenter is not able to manipulate the suspected independent variable under controlled conditions, the cause–effect relation remains correlative and somewhat speculative.

The search for a cause that is still in the "system" has been probably prompted by the medical model. A virus or a bacterium or a lesion may be found in the body while still the disease is current. In this sense, the past cause is still active and observable, and in many cases that cause can be removed, killed, or neutralized in some manner. In the case of communicative and other behavior disorders, causes that are "sitting" in the system are not encountered frequently. Even when they are, they are confounded with events in the life of the client. Factors such as a cleft palate, mental retardation, and brain damage are often suggested as the causes of certain communicative disorders. Such causes are comparable to the causes found in medical diagnosis. While this may be true to a certain extent, the resulting effect is not entirely the product of those causes. In most cases, environmental events interact with those causes and produce a more complex effect on communication. This point is illustrated by the fact that a surgical repair of the cleft will still leave the need for speech modifications intact. People with similar organic conditions may have vastly different behaviors or behavior potentials.

The nature of the independent variables we deal with in communicative disorders are complex because some of them are relations between events. Such relations are transitory. They have occurred in the past and they often produce effects that accumulate over time. In this process, many variables come together to produce the eventual, magnified effect called a disorder that the clinician sees all at once and often after a lapse of time. If one suspects a certain pattern of parent–child interaction as the cause of stuttering in young children, then those interactions are simultaneously transitory, historical, cumulative, and interactive. Tracking such cause–effect relations is one of the most challenging tasks we face.

The locus of the independent variables is a question that has not received much direct attention, but it has been debated in an indirect manner. The question, phrased in nontechnical terms, is this: Where are the independent variables located? Where do we look for them? Some tend to look for them in the genetic mechanism of individuals, whereas others look for them in the dynamics of the neurophysiological systems involved in the production of speech. Still other investigators look for the causes in the environmental events that may be responsible for the effects under study. At a more complex level of analysis, interaction between some of these variables may be the target of study. In their wiser moments, all investigators know that probably everyone is doing an equally necessary and valid job in constructing a total picture of the causes as well as their effects.

The philosophy of the locus of the independent variable one adopts has a significant impact upon his or her methodology of research. Of course, the philosophy has an initial impact on the kinds of causes looked for: genetic, neurophysiological, environmental, interactive, and so on. The kinds of causes thought of will influence the methods used to track them down.

If the causes looked for are within the genetic and neurophysiological mechanisms, then the methodology is mostly nonexperimental. Genetic studies of human behaviors and disorders are retrospective, and they make the best effort at reconstructing the events so that a pattern emerges. The patterns may suggest different possibilities of inheritance or potential genetic mechanisms at work. Investigations of neurophysiological mechanisms are examinations of existing structural variables and functional (working) dynamics. Such investigations are typically comparative in terms of the structures and dynamics found in individuals with a given effect as against those without the effect. In other words, the method is mostly that of standard-group comparison. Observed structural and dynamic differences may then be related to the existing effect in one population and its absence in the other. Stutterers, for example, may be found to be slower than nonstutterers in their muscular or vocal reaction times. The stutterers and nonstutterers may be different in their reactions to certain central auditory stimulus materials.

When independent variables have an internal locus, analysis concerns what happens internally when an observable response is made. For example, when it is proposed that some fault in the phonatory or auditory system is responsible for stuttering, the fault, which is the independent variable, will not have been observed. It will have been inferred from a dependent variable (stutterers' responses that are different from those of nonstutterers). Similar problems exist with such proposed independent variables as grammatical competence, knowledge of the rules of grammar or phonology, cognitive structures, and pragmatic rules or notions. The nature of these independent variables is such that they do not allow direct experimentation, and hence they have to be inferred from dependent variables (client responses of one kind or another). This comment is not necessarily a reflection on the validity of those inferred independent variables. A knowledge of phonological rules may indeed underlie articulatory productions, both normal and deviant. But the method used to analyze that knowledge has its limitations, which are not often appreciated.

Independent variables that have external locus can be investigated with experimental methods. Those independent variables can be controlled by the investigator. Opportunities for direct experimentation in themselves do not validate the proposed independent variables, but they are also opportunities for self-correction. Various environmental reinforcement, punishment, and other kinds of contingencies are more susceptible to experimental analysis than are genetic or neurophysiological independent variables. Indeed, most of the experimental research in speech–language pathology consists of independent variables of external locus. Controlled treatment research in the areas of articulation, language, fluency, and voice disorders have necessarily manipulated independent variables in the form of various stimuli and response consequences.

The question of the locus of the independent variables is also related to the issue of variability discussed in Chapter 6. The assumption of intrinsic variability is the same as the assumption of internal locus of independent variables, and the assumption of extrinsic variability is the same as that of the external locus of independent variables. These philosophical positions have similar methodological implications. The notions of intrinsic variability and internal locus of independent variables are hard to adapt to the experimental methodology.

Philosophical Ways of Handling Methodological Problems

Generally, and often appropriately, investigators think of methodological solutions to methodological problems. However, philosophical solutions to methodological problems do exist. An investigator must at least be aware of such solutions, even if he or she rejects them after due consideration. There are several ways of handling methodological problems from the standpoint of philosophy. A few illustrations will serve to make this point.

When we say that a methodological problem is handled philosophically, we do not mean that somehow the need to design a procedure is bypassed. We mean only that the problem is approached from a different philosophical, rather than methodological, perspective. Instead of adding another procedural component to the methodology, the investigator reconceptualizes either the dependent or the independent variable or some aspect of the experimental control. The new perspective may lead to new methods.

Intersubject Variability

As we noted in Chapter 6, intersubject variability poses a significant methodological problem in most animal and human research. This problem is handled with relative ease in animals by controlling their genetic as well as environmental history. Obviously, such tight control cannot be achieved with human subjects. Therefore, human intersubject variability must be handled differently.

Intersubject variability can be handled either methodologically or philosophically. Statisticians have historically offered methodological solutions to the problem of intersubject variability. When a given sample of subjects shows unacceptable amounts of intersubject variability, the investigator is advised to increase the sample size. The assumption is that the greater the number of subjects, the higher the chances of neutralizing the effects of variability, because the opposing directions of variability within large groups may cancel each other.

A related methodological solution to intersubject variability is the use of statistical procedures of analysis. Bypassing the variability within the group, one can analyze the results through such techniques as the analysis of variance and still be able to draw some conclusions regarding the effect of independent variables on dependent variables. To be sure, within-group variability affects the analysis, but having more subjects will make it possible to tease out the effects in spite of background variability.

There are two philosophical ways of handling intersubject variability. First, variability is not treated as an unwanted or interfering problem. Within this philosophy, intersubject variability is not a problem that needs bypassing techniques. This position also holds that statistical methods of handling variability are not effective. Those methods leave variability untouched and in fact magnify it by increasing the number of subjects. Variability, on the other hand, is thought of as a matter of exerting greater control over the extraneous variables that are responsible for that variability. Instead of leaving the variability intact and finding methods of analysis that would still show the effects of independent variables, the investigator may take extra steps to control the conditions of the experiment so that the variability across (and within) subjects is reduced. Behavioral research has shown that variability is often the result of poorly controlled experimental conditions.

Second, variability itself may be the subject of experimental analysis. Within this philosophical viewpoint, questions about why individuals differ are considered worthy of research. This approach may need new methods, but only after such a philosophical shift.

Integrity of Dependent Variables

As we know, the kinds of dependent variables selected for study are often a matter of the philosophy of a given subject matter. A problem that has plagued investigators in psychological and social research is the reactivity of the dependent variable (see chapter 6). Reactive dependent variables are those that change simply because they are measured. Such changes then confound the effects of the independent variables. Since the dependent variables must be measured before the independent variable is introduced, reactivity can pose significant problems.

We noted in Chapter 7 that Solomon had devised a methodological solution to the methodological problem of measurement effects on dependent variables. His four-group design, considered one of the most complex and ideal of the group designs, makes it possible to identify the presence and the magnitude of reactivity. He simply increased the number of groups in a design so that the effect of the independent variable could be tested with and without pretesting. This is an excellent illustration of methodological handling of a methodological problem.

A philosophical approach to the same problem would prompt serious thinking about the integrity of the dependent variable under study. Perhaps the dependent variables must be reconceptualized. Possibly, attitudes and opinions that are notoriously reactive are not solid dependent variables. Such unctuous dependent variables may suggest that at best they are indirect measures of whatever is measured. Perhaps there is a more direct way of measuring what the reactive variable is supposed to measure. Such a philosophical approach asks some basic questions, like What is it that we wish to change? In other words, what is the true dependent variable? Is it a person's response to a questionnaire, or is it the actual behavior under some specified conditions? Can we measure the behavior more directly than by accepting an indirect measure of it from what the person says about it?

A reconceptualization of "attitudes," for example, would show that they are a surrogate for real behaviors and that the only practical reason to measure them is the difficulty in measuring those real behaviors. However, it is not impossible to measure the real behaviors for which the attitudes are a surrogate. A philosophical shift, then, would suggest that instead of a four-group design to handle reactivity, one might measure dependent variables that have some degree of integrity.

Reconceptualization of dependent variables is perhaps the most important method of handling a methodological problem from a philosophical standpoint. The very first question an investigator should ask about a research problem is the integrity of the dependent variable. It should be measurable in a reliable and valid manner. When there is no reasonable assurance of this, the investigator must consider other dependent variables. Generally speaking, if a dependent variable has to be measured only indirectly and without its actual occurrence, then a reconceptualization must at least be considered. Such dependent variables are abundant in speech–language pathology.

The Magnitude of Change in the Dependent Variable

How much of an effect the independent variable must produce in order to suggest a cause–effect relation is a significant problem in research. The problem is compounded by inter- and intrasubject variability. Under an experimental condition, the dependent variable must change more than it typically does on its own. How much more it should change has always been a difficult question, which has traditionally been approached from a methodological standpoint.

The methodological approach is to use statistical methods of analysis that, depending upon the sample size, require relatively small amounts of change in the dependent variable. Statistical significance is the measure of the effect of the independent variable over and beyond chance variations in the dependent variable. An important factor related to statistical significance is the sample size. When the other variables are held constant, the larger the sample size, the smaller the magnitude of change (in the dependent variable) needed to conclude that the manipulated variable was indeed responsible for the change. In essence, in order to show an effect, the methodological approach recommends that a large number of subjects be used. Taking this recommendation seriously, social scientists have produced increasingly smaller effects with increasingly larger numbers of subjects.

A philosophical approach may not accept a methodological shortcut to this problem. Accordingly, there is no substitute for producing a large enough change needed to show that the independent variable did produce a change. Therefore, the only acceptable solution is to make the changes large enough to convince an observer without help from levels of statistical significance. This philosophy has gained additional strength in clinical sciences, where the effect of treatment procedures must be large enough to make a difference in the life of the clients. Statistical significance may or may not mean much in this respect. So the philosophical solution, which of course is no solution at all from the critics' standpoint, is to produce large effects after all.

The Interplay Between Philosophy and Methodology

We have so far considered how philosophical positions can influence methodological problems. However, methodology also has philosophical implications. Different methods shape different philosophies. Methods limited to naturalistic observations lead to different philosophies than those that involve experimentation. For example, pure normative research is likely to shape a philosophy of language that is very different from the philosophy that would emerge from experimental analysis of the language acquisition process. Questions such as what is language, and how and why is it acquired, are answered differently by investigators who merely observe it than by those who affect language by experimentation. In a more advanced stage of scientific research, there is a lively interplay between philosophy and methodology.

Although it was suggested earlier that philosophy can help resolve some of the methodological problems, it is not necessary to have a firm philosophy of the subject matter before one ventures into research. Also, in the beginning stage of a discipline, a commitment to a philosophy of a subject matter can be premature and can limit the kinds of questions asked or methods tried. In the absence of a philosophy of the subject matter, empirical scientists should simply adopt the philosophy of science. The basic philosophy of science can often be a better guide than premature philosophies of the subject matter. It can also suggest more fruitful questions for research than existing nonexperimental data, speculative theories, untested clinical procedures, and personal philosophies, which are often no more than pet notions.

In the context of behavior science, Skinner (1956) has stated that when he started his research career, he had no particular physiological, mentalistic, or conceptual model of behavior. He was committed to the methods and philosophy of the natural sciences. Behaviorism, which is the philosophy of his kind of behavior science, evolved as data evolved. As the philosophy evolved and began to be applied to various behavior disorders, new methodologies also evolved. Some of the experimental designs, including the multiple baseline design and the changing criterion design, were developed or modified in the applied contexts. However, in this endeavor, the applied researchers were guided by the philosophy of behaviorism.

A long tradition of research helps accumulate replicated data on the important questions pertaining to a given field of study. Whether this research is done with the philosophy of the subject matter or within the philosophy of science may not be crucial. Once an experimentally valid data base is created, philosophical implications begin to emerge. Those implications then guide further research. From this point on, methodology and philosophy influence each other.

When a given philosophy is not yet capable of suggesting appropriate methods, one should again follow the lead of the basic methods of science. Whenever possible, the experimental methodology should be preferred, since this method can pay larger dividends than any other. Cumulative experimental research can help shape a more useful philosophy of the subject matter and take both the subject matter and its philosophy to a level of development where new methods can be derived from that philosophy. One hopes that speech-language sciences and disorders will soon reach this level. ■

S T U D Y   **G U I D E**

1   In addition to a knowledge of methodology, what are the two other parts of research that you must be familiar with?

2   What are the limitations of a pure methodological approach to research?

3   Why should you be concerned with the philosophical issues relative to research?

4   How is a philosophy of a subject matter different from its "contents"?

5   What are some of the philosophical concerns of an applied (clinical) discipline?

6   What discipline seems to have had an early influence on the training of speech–language pathologists?

7   What are the two behavioral and social sciences that had an influence on the development of communicative disorders?

8   Specify the importance of dependent variables in developing a philosophical base for research.

(continued next page)

Study Guide *(continued)*

9 What are some of the problems associated with many of the dependent variables used in speech–language pathology? Give examples.

10 Specify the relation between the way a dependent variable is conceptualized and the method of measurement used to measure that variable. Give an example.

11 What do you mean by the *locus* of independent variables? How are the loci of such variables related to research methodology?

12 Which kind of locus is more susceptible to experimental methodology? Why? Illustrate your answer.

13 How is intersubject variability handled methodologically? How is it handled philosophically?

14 What is meant by "integrity of dependent variables"?

15 What is a methodological approach to handling the issue of the magnitude of the effects of independent variables? What is a philosophical approach?

■ P A R T **T H R E E**

Doing, Reporting, and Evaluating Research

■ C H A P T E R ⎯⎯⎯ **12**

How to Formulate Research Questions

■ Where are the research questions?, 347

■ How to formulate research questions, 348

■ Preparation of theses and dissertations, 359

■ Study guide, 361

One would think that it should be possible to tell a beginning graduate student how to do research and the student in turn should be able to follow the suggestions and complete a study. Unfortunately, telling someone how to do research is not easy and the effects not always predictable. Therefore, the author realizes the potential pitfalls in writing this and the other chapters in this final section of the book. Nonetheless, it is possible to offer a few suggestions that may help in the pursuit of knowledge.

Most graduate seminars on research methods and designs require the students to write a research proposal. Students are typically expected to suggest a research question and describe an appropriate method for investigating it. A majority of students probably do not find this to be an easy assignment. The very first question they face is simple but often debilitating: where do I start? Students will also quickly find out that answering one question will only make them qualified to face other questions.

As described in Chapter 2, research generally does not follow a fixed pattern that can be described. The formative process of research is a set of ever-changing contingencies. Therefore, the researcher should train himself or herself to become more sensitive to the changing contingencies in the process of research and keep learning in that process. In the beginning, this learning is difficult and full of uncertainties. Therefore, the difficulties faced by graduate students in writing a research proposal are both natural and inevitable.

Uncertainties in the research process are never totally diminished, no matter how experienced the investigator is. Therefore, students should hope to do their best, start the work as early as possible, and think that research is fun, but if it is not, think that it is going to be fun soon.

In this chapter, the emphasis will be on formulating research questions. Once a research question is formulated, the investigator thinks of the best method of studying it. The information on methods of study is the essence of many previous chapters. Therefore, the issue of selecting methods will be addressed only briefly in this chapter.

WHERE ARE THE RESEARCH QUESTIONS?

The first problem faced by the student is how to find a "topic" of research. This is essentially the problem of finding research questions. Research questions are sometimes literally found in some sources, and at other times they are formulated. A research paper, a textbook, a review article, or another researcher may suggest a problem that needs to be investigated. In this case, the student finds a research question. The student's own scholarship in a given area of investigation may lead him or her to think of a new question that must be answered. In this case, the student will have thought of an original idea, and the resulting question is a formulated one.

As long as the question is considered worthy of investigation, either a found or a formulated research question is acceptable. Nevertheless, it is better for students to learn the process of formulating research questions. The best way of learning to be independent researchers is to develop the ability to formulate research questions based on critical scholarship.

How to Formulate Research Questions

Research questions identify gaps in our knowledge about a phenomenon. Answers to those questions, when produced with appropriate methods, can be expected to fill those gaps. Research questions, when researched, may produce new information or extend the reliability and validity of known information. Research that produces new information is original, and that which verifies the results of earlier studies is replicative. Both kinds of research are valuable. However, from the standpoint of learning more about the research process, the student should think of a question that has not been answered, or not been answered appropriately. An exercise of this kind will teach the student more about research than an attempt to replicate a well-done study. In any case, the student needs to start looking for a problem to investigate, and there are several places to look.

Formulating research questions may be relatively easy or difficult depending upon the degree of knowledge and scholarship the student has in his or her field of study. Knowledge itself does not guarantee that research questions will be found, however. The student should read the literature critically, taking note of the kinds of research done, and the methods used. The student should judge how well the research has been done. At this point, it may be appropriate to give the student the bad news: no amount of "how to" suggestions will be able to replace careful and scholarly reviewing of the literature. But even before doing that, there are a few things the student should do. What follows is a series of interrelated steps the student should take in order to formulate a research problem and plan for an investigation.

Identify a Broad Area of Research

The first thing to do is find a broad area of investigation or a general topic. At this stage, the student may consider such areas as cleft palate, dysarthria, language acquisition, phonological disorders, treatment of stuttering, types of aphasia, or maintenance of treatment targets. It is better to select an area that is interesting; after all, the student will be spending much time on it.

Once an area or topic has been selected, the student should read or reread the basic information on it. It is often useful to read what is written on that topic in a recently published standard textbook. Even research that produces advanced information requires a command of the elementary information. For example, a student wishing to do a piece of research on language acquisition should have a good grasp of the basic textbook information on it.

Identify the Current Trends

The researcher should then proceed to find out the current trends on the topic. The research done in recent years must be carefully reviewed. There are no specific guidelines on what is recent and what is not; it depends upon the amount and the chronology of research in a given topic of investigation. Some topics have both a long history and a high level of research activity. Other topics have a long history but a low level of research activity. Still other topics have a recent history with a high density of studies. Finally, there are recent topics with sparse research studies on them.

Generally speaking, 7 to 10 years of research may be considered current or recent. There are many ways of finding the current trends, and the student must use most if not all of them. The basic task, however, is to search the literature to find both recent trends and a general topic of interest. A thorough and systematic literature search is essential in identifying current trends and possible topics for research.

Journals. First, the student must find the major journals that publish research articles on the selected topic. In communicative disorders, they include not only the journals published by the American Speech–Language–Hearing Association (ASHA), but also several others published by independent national and international publishing houses and other professional associations. Journals published in such related fields as medicine, psychology, linguistics, education, physics, biology, and acoustics, may also provide information from different perspectives that might suggest research questions. A list of major journals in which publications on speech, language, and hearing can be found is included in the Appendix.

Depending on the general area of investigation being considered, the student will have to focus upon certain kinds of journals. In the case of most topics in communicative disorders, the journals published by ASHA will serve as the primary source of information. It is generally preferable to first search the ASHA journals and then consider other journals. (The list of journals in the Appendix identifies the ASHA journals.) Additional information on specific disorders or topics can be found in specialty journals published by other publishing houses or professional organizations. Depending on the topic, for example, the *Journal of Fluency Disorders, Journal of Communication Disorders, Cleft Palate Journal, Brain and Language,* and *Neurology* may be useful. If the general area of investigation is language and language acquisition, some of the journals published in the fields of linguistics and psychology are likely to have relevant articles. If the topic researched is treatment of communicative disorders, such additional sources as *Journal of Applied Behavior Analysis, Behavior Modification, Behavior Therapy, Applied Psycholinguistics,* and *Mental Retardation* may be searched. International journals on speech, language, and hearing may also be considered.

In searching topics related to hearing, one must consult the ASHA journals as well as several other journals. A journal in which many audiologists publish their research studies is the *Journal of the Acoustic Society of America*. In addition, such journals as the *Annals of Otology, Rhinology and Laryngology, Audiology, Journal of Auditory Research* and the (journal of) *Academy of Rehabilitative Audiology* can be useful.

Most journals are published quarterly. This means that a given volume has four issues per year. Typically, the final issue of a volume contains an annual index. The ASHA journals have an author index, a subject index, and a title index. As an initial step, it is best to look into the final issues of selected volumes and go through the indexes to find the articles of interest.

Abstracts.   Another method of literature search is to use the abstracts, which help make a quick review of recent research. Most abstracts publish brief and nonevaluative summaries of research published in various sources, both national and international. Some specialized abstracts include such unpublished research as doctoral dissertations and master's theses.

The American Psychological Association (APA) publishes the *Psychological Abstracts*, which can be useful in literature search. They are a monthly publication of nonevaluative summaries of the world's literature on psychology and related subject matters. Articles are classified according to 16 subject-topic areas. Of particular interest to students in communicative disorders are the subtopics "Speech and Language" under "Communication Systems" and "Speech Therapy" under 'Treatment and Prevention".

Another major abstract service is offered by the University Microfilms International (UMI). UMI publishes *Dissertation Abstracts International*. It is a monthly publication of doctoral dissertations and master's theses accepted in North American Universities. Each monthly edition has two sections, bound separately. Section A abstracts dissertations and theses submitted in the humanities and social sciences. It includes such relevant fields as communication, education, language, and linguistics. Section B of each issue is devoted to sciences and engineering, including biological sciences, health sciences, and psychology.

Another publication of the Dissertation Abstracts International is the *Comprehensive Dissertation Index*. This may be especially useful to students because it lists dissertation and thesis research under the heading "Speech Pathology." Research on audition is included under this heading.

When the general topic of interest is medically related, the *Cumulated Index Medicus* may be useful. This is a monthly publication of the National Library of Medicine. It is a bibliography of the literature on biomedicine.

Another useful source of abstracts of research, which is no longer published, is the Deafness Speech and Hearing (dsh) Abstracts. These abstracts were published quarterly and contained entries under *Language, Hearing, Perception and Psychoacoustics*, and *Professional Affairs*. Unfortunately, dsh Abstracts ceased publication in 1985.

Finally, *Linguistics and Language Behavior Abstracts*, published quarterly by Sociological Abstracts, Inc., can be useful in searching literature on a variety of subjects including audiology, speech pathology, laryngology, neurology, otology, linguistics, and applied linguistics. It was originally published under the title *Language and Language Behavior Abstracts*.

Computerized Data Base Services. An efficient method of information retrieval is to use one of the several computerized data search services. Most of these services have bibliographies of published research on magnetic tapes. Some are interactive. That is, a student can first ask the system to list articles on a general topic and then narrow the field down to a specific area of investigation. Some entries are printed out right away, and additional entries are sent to the student by mail. Most computerized services save time, although the specificity of information on speech and hearing publications may be variable. Usually, you must pay a fee to hire one of these services. Typically, the student does the search with the help of an information specialist in the library. The student must plan the search well and make sure the terms to be used in the search are specific and are known to be a part of the data base. The reference librarian and information specialists at the university libraries will be able to help students with all aspects of information retrieval systems, including printed and computerized systems.

ERIC (Educational Resources Information Center) is a computerized data base service devoted to research in education. *Exceptional Child Education Resources* is a related service, and it can be combined with ERIC in the process of information retrieval. *Psychological Abstracts Information Services (PsychINFO)* offers data base search and retrieval of articles summarized in the printed abstracts and many others that are not in those abstracts.

Research publications in medicine, nursing, and health sciences are computerized by MEDLINE, which includes most of the printed information found in Cumulated Index Medicus. The original MEDLINE program was not especially helpful to students in communicative disorders. In recent years, the specificity with which research studies in communicative disorders are entered has been increased with additional terms and topic entries. It is possible to obtain a list of articles on specific topics such as language disorders or speech disorders, or, more specifically, stuttering or cleft palate. The system can also search for articles whose titles or abstracts contain specific terms such as *Dysfluency* or *Presbycusis*. The system can print out a bibliography as well as abstracts of articles. The interested student should read an excellent article by Reiner and Ludlow on MEDLINE published in the 1981 *ASHA*.

Any computerized data search helps the student in identifying articles published in various sources. The student then must go to those listed sources and read the articles. Most likely, the articles will be found in a variety of journals. In reading journal articles on the topic, the student should take note of the kinds of studies that are repeated. In a given period of time, several persons may have published on a particular topic, and the questions researched may be the same or similar. Should the student find this to have happened during the last few years, a recent trend may have been identified. In such cases, it is also necessary to find out why similar studies were repeated. It is possible that a controversy about the first one or two studies stimulated people with different viewpoints. This may have led to studies designed to produce contrary evidence. If this is the case, the research information will be controversial. The student may find it relatively easy to find a problem, because controversies are an excellent source of research questions.

Review articles are especially good sources for research questions. In a review article, the author has surveyed most of the published information on the topic and made a critical analysis of what is known and with what degree of generality, and what kinds of research needs to be done. The author has essentially pointed out the good and the bad about the research attempts in a particular area of investigation. A good review article points out both the methodological strengths and weaknesses of the past studies. Frequently, a well-written review article identifies several research questions for future investigations. One of those questions may be quite appropriately selected. Unfortunately, though, journals in speech, language, and hearing have not published many comprehensive review articles. Most of the psychology journals regularly publish review articles. One journal, *Psychological Review*, is devoted entirely to review articles.

Studies that are described as "exploratory" or "preliminary" may also be a source of research questions. These labels are sometimes an excuse for poorly designed studies, but when they are not, they may contain seeds of new studies. Even when they are methodologically inadequate, the student with a good knowledge of the designs can improve upon them as long as the basic idea is sound. Good exploratory studies suggest emerging trends in the field. They often suggest the topic of the future.

Descriptive studies can also be a source of new experimental investigations. Some of the original investigators of descriptive studies suggest further experimental studies on the issue. Many descriptive studies, however, do not have any hints of experimental studies. In such cases the student is alone in going beyond the descriptions provided by the investigator and thinking of experimental questions.

The student should not ignore scholarly exchanges between authors as a source of research questions. Some journals publish such exchanges, which are typically found toward the end of an issue. In the journals published by ASHA, exchanges between authors are published as Letters to the Editor, which typically are critical responses to published research followed by the author's rebuttal. Some of these exchanges can fail to illuminate the issues on hand because of a personal and subjective tone, but several of them can suggest questions for further research.

Additional sources of information can be found in books. After having reviewed the basic information and some journal articles, the student may be ready to read some specialized books. Books on recent advances are occasionally published in every field, and most contain critical reviews and summaries of recent research information. Such books can serve the student well by giving both a current overview and suggestions on potential research questions.

Books on controversies in selected clinical or theoretical issues can be helpful to students and more advanced researchers. Books on controversies are edited by an expert, and the individuals who write the chapters are also experts, who are generally known for their contrasting viewpoints. Students should not shy away from controversial issues, since, as suggested earlier, they are a good source of research problems.

Finally, there are the workshops, symposia, seminars and presentations at professional meetings and conventions that are expected to give the most recent information on a variety of topics and issues. The quality of presentations at such gatherings varies tremendously, however. With a critical approach, the student can find some research questions. A significant advantage of professional meetings is the opportunity to meet researchers who have done exceptional research in the selected area. Through these meetings, the student researcher can often get expert advice. Such advice, however, can be sought at any time during the planning and implementation of a study by contacting experts.

Identify the Classic Questions

Many graduate students and professionals find it attractive to do research on topics of recent interest. Therefore, there is often an overemphasis on finding current trends in the search for a research question. Research on current topics is generally more easily published than those that explore unknown, unappreciated, or unpopular areas and viewpoints.

There is nothing wrong in doing research on one of the currently popular topics, but a potential problem must be avoided. One cannot assume that current trends of research are necessarily the most creative or worthwhile. Research and theory also have their fashionable trends, which are called, in a more obscure way, zeitgeist. Some current trends may be nothing more than a passing fancy, though highly regarded for a while. Therefore, it is good to remember that current research trends are not the only ones that generate original research. Researchers should not be discouraged from asking old, unusual, novel, or unpopular questions. Problems are of current interest as long they need to be solved. Questions are worthy of investigation as long as they have a potential for producing new knowledge or replicating old knowledge when such a replication is deemed necessary.

A significant question that has been asked in the past may be still unanswered. Past methods may have been inadequate and unproductive. As a result, investigations on that question may have dwindled. An investigator may now be able to study the same problem with new and more productive methods. Advances in the field may make it possible to approach the problem from a new perspective. In such cases, it is appropriate to renew an old line of investigation.

The basic experimental questions of causality are timeless. In clinical research, questions relative to the effects of treatment procedures and refinement of those procedures are never out of date. In fact, new trends have a tendency to emerge in the theoretical explanation of phenomena. When one is interested in the basic experimental and empirical analysis of phenomena, most of the procedures are well established, and the questions are classic.

Concentrate Upon a Specific Area of Research

After the preliminary information-related research on a general topic, such as language acquisition or the treatment of phonological disorders, the student should think of narrowing the problem down to a more specific area of investigation. In language acquisition, for example, one might think of morphological acquisition. Even more specifically, the acquisition of the irregular morphemes, adjectives, or some specific sets of semantic or pragmatic notions may be considered. The research done so far should guide the student in this regard. Obviously, the student would not select a research question that has been overly and perhaps quite adequately researched. The initial survey of the literature should have indicated that the problem or some aspect of it still needs to be investigated.

When the student has selected a specific area, more reading is needed. The student must go back to the journals and read more papers on the major studies relative to the specific area being considered. This reading is also more intensive, critical, and analytical. The student should carefully read and critique theoretical and conceptual information. Detailed notes should be taken of the methods and procedures of the studies, because the student may decide to use some of those methods. Another reason to study the methods of the previous studies carefully is that the student may wish to avoid their deficiencies.

Formulate a Specific Research Question

A critical reading of a particular area should lead to a more specific research problem. The student should know that the journey from a general topic to a particular research problem can be long and frustrating. One may have a desire to do some research on language treatment, but a specific research question may not emerge for some time.

At this point, it may be useful to write a general description of the research problem. Once again, the student should recheck the major sources to make sure that the problem either has not been researched, has not been researched in the manner being considered, or has been researched but with room for significant methodological improvement. One of the most difficult problems faced by a majority of students at this point is to determine that the study as planned has not been done. Students often find themselves discarding their pet ideas one by one because the previous investigators were ahead of them.

Writing research questions takes some skill and practice. They should be as direct as possible and as technical as necessary. Research questions are typically about some objective phenomenon. The question can ask whether the phenomenon exists and if so what are its descriptors. Research questions can also ask whether a certain variable (such as a treatment) has an effect, and whether two or more variables interact. Purely descriptive research involves somewhat simpler questions than experimental research. For example, how many phonemes are produced by 2-year-old children is a relatively simple descriptive question. On the other hand, whether two or more phonological treatment components have certain independent and interactive effects, and if so to what extent, is a more complex experimental question.

A variety of research questions were described in Chapter 10. The kind of research questions for a particular investigation depends upon the type of research contemplated. Normative and standard-group comparison types of research mostly involve questions that ask for descriptions. Ex post facto, experimental, and correlative types of research ask questions of relation between two or more variables. Specifying the variables of a study is probably the most crucial step involved in planning a study, and therefore we shall address this question next.

Specify the Variables in Technical Language

The student will find that a serious attempt to specify the variables to be investigated will force clearer thinking about the entire research plan. The student must try to answer such questions as these: What are my dependent variables? How many dependent variables do I have? What are my independent variables? If so, how do I control them? What kind of relation is to be studied? Cause–effect relations? Correlative relations? Additive and interactive relations? Direct answers to questions such as these will help clarify the research problem and design appropriate methods.

The dependent and independent variables must be clearly separated in studies that include both of them. The typical dependent variables in communicative disorders include various kinds of speech, language, and hearing behaviors and their disorders. In a particular study, a specific aspect of these behaviors constitutes a dependent variable. In other words, although language can be described as a dependent variable, one needs to specify a particular aspect of it, for example, the production of the plural morpheme at the word level. Stuttering can be a dependent variable, but it is better to specify what exactly will be measured to document the occurrence of that variable. In essence, the dependent variable must be described in measurable terms. It must be unambiguous and specific.

An independent variable, being the manipulated or suspected cause of the dependent variable, should also be described in equally specific language, because this is the variable whose effects are determined in experimental studies. While reading the literature, the student should pay particular attention to the way the dependent and independent variables are described by different investigators. Often, students will find themselves confused about the status of the variables in their study. The student should keep in perspective the definitions of different kinds of variables (see Chapter 3).

The operational specification of variables also involves considerations of measurement. As we know from Chapter 5, variables can be measured in different ways, some more suitable than others to given problems. The student should always think in terms of more objective, more direct, and more discrete types of measures of the behaviors under study. Sometimes, it may be found that the problem is very intriguing, but the variables involved cannot be measured easily.

After specifying their variables, some investigators formulate their hypotheses. A research investigation does not require a hypothesis, but if one is preferred, it must be written clearly so that it does specify the variables to be investigated. See Chapter 3 for additional information on hypotheses.

Talk to Someone

Talking to someone about a research problem can be a great help. The person you talk to need not be an expert on the subject. In the process of talking, the student may find that he or she has not thought through some methodological aspect of the contemplated research. The student may also find out gaps in his or her understanding of some theoretical concepts involved in the study. Such deficiencies in understanding of the research topic or the procedure will force more homework or clearer thinking. This step can be taken at the very beginning and repeated at every stage of the investigation.

Talking to an expert, however, can have additional advantages. The expert can help the student avoid false starts or dead-end projects. In talking with the expert, the student may find out that a particular study has or has not been done. The expert may also pose gentle and supportive challenges so that the student attains greater clarity in thinking. The student may gain more confidence in the idea being considered, and under the best possible conditions, the exchange may inspire and motivate the student to go ahead with the project.

Evaluate the Significance of the Research Questions

In the process of selecting a research problem, the student must judge whether it will be a valuable study. The question to be researched must be of some scientific, theoretical, or applied significance. Some of the most common questions asked in evaluating the significance of research questions include the following: Is the research meaningful? Is it likely to contribute new knowledge or to expand upon the existing knowledge? Does it help solve a problem? Does it have the potential to explain an event hitherto unexplained? Does the research show a new method of studying a difficult problem? Does it improve clinical technology? Does it produce an effect unobserved so far? Does it help detect an effect that has been suspected but not observed? These are some of the many questions one can ask in evaluating the significance of research questions.

In order to judge that a given piece of research is valuable, one need not seek an affirmative answer to all the questions just posed. A single affirmative answer may be sufficient to justify a study. In other words, a study can be justified on the basis of a single evaluative criterion.

Evaluation of the significance of research problems and questions is one of the most difficult tasks, however. We shall return to this important issue in Chapter 14.

Think of the Methods

It is generally assumed that the researcher thinks of the methods only after having decided upon the problem. In practice, however, such a sequence may or may not be realized. Sometimes, methods must be considered even during the process of selecting a problem or rejecting others. If the investigator cannot think of a procedure for researching a particular question, then that question may have to be rejected or postponed for future consideration. In fact, one way to screen out poor research ideas is to realize their methodological impracticality.

Other practical considerations assume importance in the process of problem selection. The student must keep in perspective the availability of subjects, special equipment, and physical laboratory facilities. For example, if it is known that laryngectomy patients are not being served in a particular clinic, questions of the effectiveness of a certain laryngectomy treatment procedure may not be practical unless the student is willing to go elsewhere for subjects. If a particular research idea needs expensive biofeedback equipment that the department does not have, perhaps some other problem must be found. Similarly, if the research idea requires a specially constructed acoustic laboratory that simply does not exist, then that idea may have to be rejected.

When a research question is very sound, a lack of available methods (not physical instruments) should only signal a challenge to one's scientific ingenuity. The idea need not be rejected, but it may not be implemented immediately. It may take some time before an appropriate method is devised to study the problem. Meanwhile, the graduate student needs a practical problem for the thesis or some specific assignment so that he or she can graduate within a reasonable period of time. Even a seasoned researcher is likely to move on to something that can be done more easily than the project that takes extra time, effort, and thinking.

Questions that are too broad (what causes language disorders?) or too vague ("I want to know how children acquire language") do not lend themselves to methodological planning. As soon as the student begins to consider how a piece of research can be implemented, the problem itself begins to be seen in a different light. In essence, methodological considerations force problem specificity. Therefore, it is a good idea to think about the problem and the methods in an interwoven fashion. However, once a specific problem has been found, the investigator can spend more time on working out the details of methods.

One of the first methodological considerations is the subjects of a study. The student must decide upon the number of subjects and their characteristics. Clinical or nonclinical subjects and their social, personal, health, and other relevant characteristics must be considered. The age and sex of the subjects should also be decided upon. The clinical and nonclinical subjects must be described in terms of the criteria used in separating them. If "aphasic" patients are going to be used in the study, how are they going to be diagnosed? Who are not aphasic? Who will make the judgments? By what means? How and where are they going to be found? By what criteria are they finally going to be included in the study? These questions refer to subject selection procedures or criteria. There are both inclusion and exclusion criteria: They specify the characteristics that will admit individuals to the study as well as those that will exclude individuals from it.

Whether one wishes to use a large random sample or a small group of homogeneous subjects is also an important question. In most clinical studies, available subjects are used, with a few restrictions. For example, an investigation concerned with language disorders may exclude those with neurological handicaps or hearing impairment. Certain syndromes or special conditions that complicate language problems may be excluded. A relatively narrow age range may be specified as acceptable. With some such restrictions, the subjects may be selected on the basis of availability.

A difficult aspect of planning for a study is to determine the kinds of instruments that will be used in it (Curtis & Schultz, 1986). The term *instruments* includes all the kinds of equipment or apparatus that will be used in the study. The type of instruments needed for a study depends mostly upon the nature of the dependent variables and the kind of measures selected for the study (see Chapter 5 for details).

The stimulus materials that must be prepared by the clinician are also part of the instruments. Questions designed to evoke responses, modeling, and the specific target behaviors, and instructions to be given the subjects, should all be prepared beforehand.

Another important aspect of the procedure is the overall plan and the specific design of the study. The selected design may be of the single-subject or group variety. The design typically dictates the number and sequence of the conditions of the study. These conditions, such as the pretest, experiment, and posttest, must be specified. As we noted in Chapter 10, the selection of a design depends upon the nature of the research question asked.

Finally, the student must have some idea of what kind of data the study will generate and how they will be analyzed. The method of analysis is mostly determined by the design and the kinds of data. Studies of group designs generate data that are appropriately handled by statistical methods of analysis, whereas single-subject design studies generate data that can be evaluated visually and by qualitative methods.

When statistical methods of data analysis are used, the student must understand the limitations and appropriateness of the tests to be used. Each statistic is based on certain assumptions, such as the normal or non-normal distribution of the dependent variable measured and the methods of measurements used (continuous, categorical, and so on). The data for which the selected statistic is applied should not violate those assumptions. Most students need to consult an expert in statistics before selecting statistical techniques of analysis.

The foregoing is by no means an exhaustive survey of questions that must be addressed in planning a research study. It can, however, promote understanding of some major steps that must be taken in developing a research study.

PREPARATION OF THESES AND DISSERTATIONS

In a majority of graduate programs in communicative disorders, a master's thesis is optional. A few programs may require a thesis of all candidates for the master's degree. A dissertation, however, is always required of doctoral candidates.

In formulating questions for a thesis or dissertation, the student follows the same steps as described earlier. However, theses and dissertations take a more careful and thorough literature search than that needed for a class project. It is expected that a student planning a thesis or dissertation has a good background in the field, and therefore the search can be more specific and goal-directed from the beginning.

An initial step in the preparation of a thesis, however, is to find a faculty advisor who is willing to direct the research. Unlike class projects and research assignments, theses and dissertations need close supervision from the advisor. The student often works closely with the faculty member in completing an original study.

It is in the best interest of the student to find a faculty advisor who is an expert in the particular area selected for investigation. In this way, the student can be sure of getting expert advice and help in the conduct of the research study. Generally speaking, the student and the advisor will spend much time discussing potential research problems. When a problem is finally selected, it is the student's responsibility to make sure that current information on the topic has been thoroughly researched. The design and the procedures of the study are then discussed and finalized.

Most theses and dissertations are evaluated by a committee of three to five members. The advisor serves as chairman of the committee. The student, in consultation with the advisor, selects members for the committee. Depending upon the research problem being investigated, the student may select a member from outside the department. Psychologists, statisticians, linguists, and medical and other professionals may be selected by the student.

Once the committee is formed, the student must write a detailed proposal of the study and submit it for approval. Usually, an oral presentation is also made. During this oral presentation, the student briefly reviews the literature and justifies the study and its procedures. The committee's task is to ensure that the student understands all aspects of the proposed research and that the methods and procedures are appropriate. If necessary, the committee may suggest changes in particular aspects of methodology.

After obtaining the approval of the committee, the student must submit the proposal to an Institutional Review Board (IRB), which reviews the proposal from the standpoint of human or animal subject protection. An IRB's task is to determine whether the study poses any risks to the subjects, and if so, what steps are taken to minimize them. Chapter 15 offers discussion of the ethical issues involved in the conduct of research, along with human and animal subject protection procedures.

The student can begin the actual investigation only after the study has been approved by the thesis or dissertation committee and the IRB. When the study is completed, it is written according to the guidelines established by the student's department and the graduate school of the university. Most departments of communicative disorders use the guidelines established by the American Psychological Association (APA). The student must consult the third edition of the APA Manual, published in 1983.

Once again, the student works very closely with the advisor (the committee chairman) in writing the thesis or dissertation. Most students revise the thesis or dissertation several times before the advisor accepts it tentatively. Finally, when the advisor considers it appropriate, an oral examination is scheduled. The entire committee once again meets to judge the appropriateness of the thesis or dissertation for the degree being sought.

During the oral examination, the student describes the study and its results and conclusions, and also relates the findings to previous research and theories. In essence, the student defends his or her work during this oral examination. Approval is granted when the committee is satisfied with the thesis or dissertation and its defense. Following this approval, any changes and corrections suggested by the committee are incorporated, and the final copy of the thesis or dissertation is submitted to the graduate school. If it is deemed appropriate, the graduate school then accepts the document on behalf of the university.

Completing a thesis or dissertation can be extremely time-consuming. It takes hard work and typically involves extra expense. However, it is a worthwhile aspect of graduate education in any field. It is the only opportunity for students to do a piece of original research evaluated and approved by a team of experts in the field. There is no better way of learning about research than completing a thesis or dissertation. Well-planned and well-conducted theses or dissertations meet standards of publication. Therefore, they can be rewarding as well. ■

S T U D Y G U I D E

1 What are research questions? Where do you find them?

2 What are the nine steps you should take to formulate research questions?

3 Describe how the process of formulating a research question proceeds from a review of a broad area of research to a narrowly specified research question.

4 Describe the usefulness of a published review article in your search for an investigation.

5 What are the main sources of information on the current trends?

6 What do you mean by "classic research questions"? Why are they important?

7 Why is it necessary to specify the variables of a research question in technical language? Give an illustration by writing a research question that specifies its variables in technical language.

8 What are the advantages and disadvantages of talking to experts and lay persons?

9 What are some of the questions you would ask in determining the significance of research questions? Are the answers to those questions always clear and objective? Why or why not?

10 Specify why methodological impracticality is one of the early considerations in the selection of research problems.

(continued next page)

Study Guide *(continued)*

11 Formulate a research question that would be considered "classic" in its import. Specify the variables in technical language. Write a brief justification of the research the question would lead to.

12 Formulate a research question that would reflect a recent trend in your subject matter. What makes it recent? What are your variables? Justify your study.

■ CHAPTER 13

How To
Write
Research
Reports

■ Format of scientific reports, 364

■ Writing without bias, 373

■ Good writing: Some principles, 374

■ Structural principles, 374

■ Conceptual considerations, 384

■ Writing style, 394

■ Write and rewrite, 395

■ Study guide, 396

W riting is an integral part of research activity. The completion of an investigation leads the investigator to think about writing the report and having it published. Researchers and professionals are also interested in other kinds of writing. Integrative articles, critical reviews, philosophical essays, books, manuals, and a variety of reports, are also of interest to scientists and professionals.

Most universities require adequate writing skills of their graduate as well as undergraduate students. Students who wish to complete a thesis as part of the requirement for graduate degrees are especially concerned with writing skills.

In this chapter, we shall be concerned with writing in general and writing research reports in particular. I shall describe five aspects of scientific and professional writing: (1) the format of organizing a research article, (2) writing without bias, (3) some principles of good writing, (4) conceptual considerations, and (5) style.

FORMAT OF SCIENTIFIC REPORTS

Each professional and scientific community has an accepted format for reporting scientific studies. These formats encourage a relatively uniform way of writing scientific articles. Such uniformities are imposed by editors of journals and books and also by professional organizations. Uniform writing formats are helpful for several reasons. First, they make the job of editorial evaluation manageable. If different authors were to report their studies in vastly different formats, the editorial evaluation would be distracted by the problems inherent to the organization of data. Second, the mechanical aspect of printing differently reported material in a single publication such as a journal can be unnecessarily complicated. Third, a uniform reporting format is desirable for readers as well. Readers of particular journals find it easy to understand and evaluate reports written in a uniform format.

The prescriptive formats are especially required of articles submitted for publication in scientific and professional journals. Books, manuals, and other kinds of written materials are not as strictly controlled by such formats. Therefore, we shall be mostly concerned with journal article formats in this section.

A widely used format for journal articles is that of the American Psychological Association (APA). Concern for a standard format of reporting scientific studies was expressed as early as 1929 by a group of anthropological and psychological journal editors. The first publication guide was published in 1944 and became known as the *Publication Manual*. This guide was expanded in 1952 and revised in 1957 and 1967. The second edition of the *Manual* was published in 1974. The *Manual* gained wide acceptance by several editorial boards. Many nonpsychological journals also began to use the APA format. The third edition of the *Manual* was published in 1983.

The American Speech-Language-Hearing Association (ASHA) publishes four journals: *Asha, Journal of Speech and Hearing Disorders, Journal of Speech and Hearing Research*, and *Language, Speech, and Hearing Services in Schools. Asha* is published monthly; the others are published quarterly. On a periodic basis, ASHA also publishes several technical *Reports* and *Monographs*. Reports are typically a collection of papers presented in a special symposium sponsored by ASHA, whereas monographs are small books dealing with a particular clinical or research topic.

The ASHA publications had their own format until 1980. Brief guidelines on how to prepare manuscripts to be submitted were printed on the inside back cover of most of the journals. The authors were also encouraged to use the *Chicago Manual of Style* published by the University of Chicago. In 1980, the ASHA Publications Board adopted the APA format for all its journals and other publications.

Most graduate programs require their students to write papers, theses, and dissertations according the an accepted format. In many behavioral and related disciplines, the APA format is probably the most frequently used.

Journal articles can be either reports, review articles, or theoretical articles. An original research study is typically written in the form of a *report*. Reports have a fairly rigid format: Introduction, Method, Results, and Discussion. A *review article* makes a critical assessment of published research in a given area of investigation. Review articles point out the advances made in a particular area of research and summarize the state of the art. They highlight methodological and conceptual problems of past investigations and suggest questions for future research. A review article is both integrative and evaluative. The format of a review article is more flexible than that of a report. The article is organized in terms of the issues raised and data evaluated. A *theoretical article* either presents a new theory or critically examines existing theories in a particular area of investigation. Theoretical articles, too, have flexible formats dictated by the nature and number of issues and theories.

Many journals also publish scholarly exchanges between authors. As noted in Chapter 12, the ASHA journals publish such exchanges in the form of *letters to the editor*. The letters are often critical evaluations of an article published in one of the recent issues of the same journal. The author of the original article usually writes a rebuttal. These exchanges do not have a fixed format, and they generally do not have subheadings.

Theses, projects, and dissertations have a fixed format, but academic departments and universities may have their own variations of a general format. The formats of these documents contain certain unique aspects, such as an approval page, a table of contents, and a copyright authorization page. However, the body of the text, references, figures, tables, and appendixes may be prepared according to one of the widely accepted formats, such as that of the APA. Similar formats are used in case of projects and dissertations as well.

A *research proposal* is typically not published. Research proposals are made to various government and private agencies that support research. Each agency has its own guidelines and formats within which the proposals must be prepared. Those who seek funds must strictly follow these formats and guidelines.

Generally speaking, writing a technical report on a piece of empirical research can be considered the prototype of scientific writing. An investigator who is able to write a report is generally able to write other kinds of articles and proposals, with necessary modifications. Sections such as *introduction*, *review of literature*, and *discussion* are common to most types of scientific writing. Therefore, we shall focus on writing a technical report of an empirical investigation according to the APA format. The topics to be discussed will follow the order in which a report is eventually presented.

Title Page

The title page contains the title of the article, the author's name and affiliation, and a running head.

The title of an article must be brief and to the point. Long, wordy titles may not easily signal the essence of a paper and thus may fail to draw reader attention. It is better for the title to specify the experimental variables that were investigated. For example, the title "The Effect of Timeout on Stuttering" specifies both the dependent and the independent variable studied. The title is also direct, brief, and self-explanatory. The APA recommends 12 to 15 words for a title.

The author's name is written on a separate line, starting with the first name, the middle initial, and last name. Words such as *by* or *from* are not added to the author's name. Titles and degrees are also omitted.

The name of the institution where the study was conducted is written on a separate line below the author's name. Typically, the name of the department in which the study was done is omitted. When the author is not affiliated with an institution, the city and the state are specified below the name.

When the author has moved since the completion of the study, the new affiliation and the mailing address are written on a separate page under "author notes," and placed after the references. A journal, however, may print this information as a footnote on the first page.

An abbreviated version of the title is the running head, which is printed at the top of each page. An author places it at the bottom of the title page preceded by the phrase *running head*. The APA Manual limits the running head to 50 characters, including spaces between words.

Abstract

Almost all kinds of scientific articles require an abstract, which is written on a separate page. A good abstract will attract the reader to the whole article, whereas a bad one may turn the reader away. Therefore, it is important to write an abstract with an attractive style. The abstract must be accurate. It should highlight the problem, the methods, the procedures, and the results. It should also be self-contained. An abstract does not contain abbreviations. It should be written in direct and nonevaluative language. The APA Manual limits the abstract of a report to 100 to 150 words and that of a review article to 75 to 100 words. Theses and dissertations generally have longer abstracts.

Introduction

The text of the paper starts with an introductory section without a heading. This initial section of a paper introduces the reader to (1) the general area of investigation, (2) the general findings of past investigations, (3) the specific topic of the current investigation, (4) selected studies that have dealt with the topic in the past, (5) the problems and limitations of the past studies, (6) some of the questions that remain to be answered, and (7) the specific problem or research questions investigated in the present study.

The opening sentence introduces the reader to the broad area of which the present investigation is a part. In most cases, the problem of the study is not stated at the outset. The reader is prepared for the problem by an initial description of the general area and the findings of the past studies. For example, if the investigation to be reported is about a particular language treatment procedure designed to teach specific morphological features, the introductory section may first make a few statements about research on language treatment in general. Then, some of the relevant studies and their results may be summarized or cited. The writer then introduces the specific topic that helps focus on the investigation. In our example, the research on teaching morphological features would be highlighted. Past studies that are especially relevant to the topic investigated may then be reviewed in some detail. Methods and procedures of selected studies on teaching morphological features would be reviewed. This review would be concerned mostly with the conceptual and methodological limitations of the past studies. The review would also point out the questions that are still in need of further research. Finally, the author brings the problem investigated into sharper focus. The introduction may end with a formal statement of the research problem or problems.

A well-written introduction moves from the general to the particular. The initial general framework helps the reader place the investigation in a proper theoretical, conceptual, and methodological perspective. With each additional paragraph, the writer takes the reader closer to the particular research question investigated. Meanwhile, the author also reviews the past studies in such a way as to justify the present investigation. A smoothly written introduction does not need a separate section called "rationale" or "justification" of the investigation. The entire introductory section should make clear to the reader the need for the study and the reasoning behind it.

A critical part of the introduction is the review of the past studies. A well-written review justifies the study and sets the stage for it. The review is necessarily critical, because in many cases, a study is undertaken because of the limitations of past studies. In some cases the same question may have been researched, but inadequately. In other cases, a new method the author has used may be expected to prove more effective than previous methods in studying a phenomenon. In still other instances, the problem may not have been conceptualized at all in the manner of the investigation to be reported. Therefore, a critical analysis of the past research is often the best justification of an investigation.

The critical review must be fair and objective. Its tone should not be judgmental, emotional, or polemical. Nevertheless, it should be direct. The limitations of the past studies must be stated honestly and unambiguously. Therefore, the literature review should not be an exercise in diplomacy. Some can write critical reviews more tactfully than others, but tact should never be so successful as to cover up valid criticisms that help advance the cause of knowledge.

The introduction written to a direct or systematic replicative study does not involve much critical assessment of past studies and their methodologies. Direct replication studies need very brief introductions, which mainly justify the need for replication. Systematic replication studies do this and also describe in what specific ways the present study is different from the original study.

The review of literature should point out the logical or empirical relation between the past studies and the present research. It should show how the study is built upon the past evidence and methodology. It is good to remember that a vast majority of research questions are hinted at or directly suggested by past studies. Knowledge is both continuous and evolving; utterly original studies are often the stuff the junior scientist's dreams are made of. Therefore, the past studies are not criticized to show that the present study is so original that it bears no relation to other studies or present knowledge. Instead, it should show how the present study is conceptually and methodologically related to the past research while also pointing out its innovative aspects.

Toward the end of the introduction, the research question is formally stated. Hypotheses, if proposed, may be stated at this point. The research questions and hypotheses must be written in direct, clear, and terse language.

Method

The second section of a research article describes the method of the study. The method is described in detail so that a reader can evaluate its appropriateness to investigate the research questions. The description should be specific enough to permit a replication of the study by other investigators.

The method section of an empirical study has at least three subsections: the *subjects*, the *apparatus* or *materials*, and the *procedure*. Additional headings may be used when necessary. For example, clinical treatment studies may describe the *pretreatment measures* or *baselines, treatment procedures*, and *probe* or other *posttreatment* procedures under separate headings. Reports of multiple experiments are also likely to have additional subsections.

SUBJECTS. The subject characteristics, number, and selection procedures are described in this subsection. Studies in communicative disorders describe the subjects' age, sex, health, geographical location, family background, and communicative behaviors. In most cases, studies provide detailed information on the subjects' speech, language, voice, fluency, and hearing. Other relevant characteristics may be described.

The number of subjects who were initially selected and who eventually completed the study must be specified. In a group design, the number of subjects assigned to different groups must be also be described.

The subject selection procedure must be described in detail. Was it a random sample? Were the subjects selected simply because they happened to be available? Was the investigator trying to achieve a sample representative of the population? Were they clinical subjects who were seeking professional services? Were there criteria by which potential subjects were excluded from the study? How were the subjects screened? These are some of the questions that are answered in describing the subject selection procedure.

APPARATUS. In this section, the physical setting in which the study was carried out and the equipment and materials used are described. Instruments and materials that are commonly used in the discipline need not be described in detail. Their name, model number, and the manufacturer must be specified, however. Custom-made or rarely used instruments must be described in detail. If needed, drawings, photographs, and additional descriptions may be given in an appendix.

PROCEDURE. Details on how the study was implemented are given in this subsection. A commonly used experimental design is simply mentioned by name, but an uncommon design may be described in greater detail. Instructions given to the subjects, how the variables were measured and manipulated, and the time schedules followed in completing the study are also described. How different groups of subjects were treated differently or how the separate conditions of an experiment differed from each other must be specified. Finally, how the reliability of the data was established is described in this section.

It is not possible to specify everything that must be included in the subsection on procedure. It is the author's responsibility to report *everything relevant that he or she did* in completing a study. There should be a valid reason for not reporting something done by the author. The author can use the criterion of replicability in determining whether procedures were described in full. If by reading the article, another investigator can replicate the study, then the descriptions are adequate.

RESULTS

This section opens with a brief statement of the problem investigated and the general findings of the study. An overview of the results is followed by a detailed presentation of quantitative, qualitative, graphic, and tabular presentation of the findings.

In the results section, the findings are simply reported without interpretations and evaluations. Quantitative data may be presented concisely in tables. The changes noted in the dependent variables across experimental conditions are better represented graphically. Group design studies do not report individual data, but single-subject designs do. Tables and graphs should supplement, not duplicate the text. Statistical tests are always reported in terms of their value, the probability level (significance level), and degrees of freedom when appropriate. The meaning of the obtained statistical value is also briefly stated.

The results section can have headings when they are considered appropriate. It may also have subsections in which different kinds of data are reported. In organizing the results of a study, the student must consult the APA Manual and several exemplary articles published in the professional journal to which the author plans to submit the paper for publication.

Discussion

In the discussion section, the author points out the meaning and significance of the results. The section opens with a brief statement of the problem and the results of the study, and proceeds to discuss the theoretical and applied implications of the findings. The results of the study are related to the findings of previous investigations. In this section, the problems and limitations of the study may also be pointed out, along with suggestions for further research.

A well-written discussion places the results of the study in the larger context of past research on the issue at hand. Ideally, a discussion is an integrative essay on the topic investigated, but it is written in the light of the data generated by the study. The similarities between present and past findings are highlighted, as are the differences. When the results are consistent with past findings, the discussion will give a coherent but possibly advanced picture of the phenomenon investigated. When the results contradict previous findings, the author may discuss possible reasons. Methodological problems and differences typically explain such contradictions.

The discussion should answer the research questions posed in the introductory section. The author should try to answer them as directly as possible. The answer may be positive or negative, but they must be stated clearly. Possibly, the author may say that the results failed to answer the questions. In any case, vagueness and hedging should be avoided. It is possible, though, that the results of a study do not support a strong and direct answer. In such cases, some authors prefer to be vague and tentative. Even then, a direct statement that the results were ambiguous is preferable to vagueness that leaves the reader confused.

Hypotheses, when proposed by the author, are supported or refuted in the discussion section. Clarity and directness are important here, too. Some authors may be reluctant to admit that their hypotheses were not supported by data, and the discussion may therefore be vague or distorted. There may be reasons to suspect the results, however. If so, the reasons may be clearly stated, along with better tests of the hypotheses. Even then, the author should state unambiguously that the results themselves did not support the hypotheses.

A common problem in many discussions is a labored effort to explain the results, especially when the results are unexpected from a particular viewpoint. Excessive speculation is the result. Such speculations are typically so far removed from the results that the discussion and the results seem almost independent. Why the results were the way they were is an interesting question, but it should not lead to unnecessary speculation. The best approach is to describe implications that are close to data. Obviously, data that cannot be explained need further study. Speculation will not explain them unless verified by additional experiments.

SINGLE-SUBJECT STUDIES AND MULTIPLE EXPERIMENTS. Discussion of single-subject studies and those of multiple experiments is handled differently. In a single-subject study, a common discussion section is appropriate as long as the research questions and methods were common across the subjects. However, sometimes a single-subject study may involve more than one experiment, each with a single or multiple subjects. The questions researched may be different though closely related. Such may be the case within a group study as well. Then it is better to write the discussion separately for the experiments. In this case, brief discussion follows the results of each experiment. However, at the end, a general discussion of the experiments is also needed. Different experiments are a part of a single study mainly because they are related in some conceptual and methodological manner. Therefore, a common discussion is needed to suggest the significance of the results and their interrelations.

References

Within the body of a paper, references support statements made by the author about past investigations and the viewpoints of other authors. The authors and their works cited in the text are listed under the references. The reference list is placed after the discussion section.

The citations in the text and the reference list should match perfectly. There should be no citation in the text that is omitted from the reference list, and there should be no reference that is not cited.

A reference list should not be confused with a *bibliography*. A reference list contains only those studies that are cited in an article. Studies not mentioned in the text, no matter how relevant, are not included in a reference list. A bibliography, on the other hand, is a comprehensive list of published studies on a particular topic or area of investigation. One can prepare a bibliography without writing an article, but a reference list is always a part of an article.

The APA Manual (1983) specifies the rules for citing references and arranging a reference list. The reader must consult the *Manual* for details.

Appendix

The use of appendixes has declined in recent years. They increase the production cost of journals and books. When necessary, appendixes are prepared to provide information that cannot be integrated with the text. For example, a new test protocol, detailed description of a new equipment, and drawings of certain stimulus materials may be provided in an appendix.

Appendixes are used more frequently in dissertations, theses and projects. Raw data on individuals or groups of subjects, instructions, papers relative to human subject protection, and details of statistical analyses may be placed in appendixes.

Following the APA Format

Authors in communicative disorders, including student writers in most educational and clinical programs, are expected to follow the APA format. The APA *Manual* must be studied carefully in preparing manuscripts. To begin with, the *Manual* gives a brief description of the content and organization of manuscripts. In subsequent chapters, it gives comprehensive guidelines on the format of research articles. There are guidelines on punctuation, spelling, capitalization, use of italics, abbreviations, arranging headings and subheadings, quotations, the use of numbers, the metric system, preparation of tables and figures, reporting statistical and mathematical formulas, footnotes and notes, reference citations, and reference lists. In addition, the *Manual* also gives detailed instructions on how to type a manuscript.

The APA *Manual* will not be summarized here. Every author should have a copy for constant reference. In their preparation of reports, projects, and scientific articles, students need to refer repeatedly to the *Manual*. Once the paper is written, the student must make sure that it conforms to the format. It is the author's responsibility to prepare the manuscript according to the *Manual*.

Prescriptive formats are not intended to discourage interesting and unique writing styles. When a scientific article is boring, it is not because of the rigidity of the format, but because of a lack of style on the part of the author. Within an acceptable format, one can write with an interesting individual style. A mistaken assumption is that scientific writing must be devoid of individual style and that research reports must be necessarily monotonous and uninteresting. This misconception is due to a confusion between lack of style and objectivity in scientific reporting. Scientific writing can have an attractive style while retaining objectivity. However, scientific writing style does have certain characteristics that may not be found in literary writings. We shall discuss some of these differences in later sections.

WRITING WITHOUT BIAS

Scientific writing is objective in that it is free from bias. It avoids words and expressions that unfavorably reflect upon individuals and groups. Stereotypic and prejudicial expressions about sexes, individuals, and ethnic groups are often found in everyday language. They may be used by persons who do not necessarily share the implied sexism or racism. Nevertheless, such expressions are offensive and inappropriate in everyday usage as well as in scientific writing. In their pursuit of knowledge, scientists are committed to fair treatment of individuals and groups of persons.

Among the biases that can creep into writing, racism and sexism are probably most common. Racist expressions in describing subjects and exploring the meaning of research findings must be avoided. If it is necessary to identify subjects belonging to particular ethnic or cultural groups, terms that are nonevaluative must be used. The best practice is to select the terms the groups themselves use to refer to themselves in formal writings and discussions. Such expressions as *culturally deprived* or *disadvantaged* have a pseudoscientific connotation, but they are also biased. They imply that one culture is the standard against which other cultures are evaluated. In communicative disorders, the expression *standard English* is often contrasted with black English. This expression implies that the language spoken by one group is the standard by which the language spoken by the other group is judged. Another mistake made by many writers is to describe foreign languages they know very little about as *dialects*.

Many expressions that imply sexism are a part of long-established traditions of language usage, and therefore, they may not be easily recognized as sexist. One of the most inappropriately used personal pronouns is *he*. It is often used to refer to any child, student, customer, or client. Indiscriminate use of male personal pronouns may imply that all executives, doctors, nurses, firefighters, engineers, supervisors, department heads, garbage collectors, or professors are male. A frequently misused noun that implies sexism is *man*. It is the *man* who searches for knowledge, achieves great things, provides the work force. It is *mankind* that experiences great problems or solves those problems. In cases such as these, other terms, including human beings, people, persons, humanity, and humankind, are appropriate.

Since 1977, the American Psychological Association has required authors submitting articles to APA journals to use language without racial, sexual, or other kinds of biases. The APA *Manual* (1983) contains guidelines on writing without bias. In 1979, the Asha Committee on Equality of Sexes, formed by the American Speech-Language-Hearing Association, adopted the APA guidelines. With minor modifications, the Committee published the guidelines in *Asha* (1979).

Besides implying bias, indiscriminate use of certain words may create ambiguity. The word *men* in a given context may refer to people of both sexes or only to male persons. The APA/Asha guidelines give specific suggestions for avoiding both biased and ambiguous references. The guidelines give many examples of common expressions that are unacceptable and show how they can be rewritten to avoid ambiguity and bias. The student must consult the Asha (1979) publication and the APA *Manual* (1983) for the details.

GOOD WRITING: SOME PRINCIPLES

A format of research articles, such as the one discussed earlier, may not necessarily assure good writing. Scientific writing must be good writing, and it should also adhere to an accepted format. Good writing involves an understanding of both structural principles and conceptual considerations.

Structural Principles

Grammar specifies the structural principles of language. The term *grammar* includes the morphological as well as the syntactical aspects of language. In addition, one should also consider punctuation. Minimally, good writing is grammatically correct. It is not possible to specify all the rules of grammar here; the student must consult a good source on grammar. Many books on writing include basic information on grammar and correct usage. The student must have one or two such books for permanent reference (Baker, 1981; Barrass, 1978; Bates, 1980; Hargis, 1977; Kirszner & Mandell, 1986; Streng, 1972; Turabian, 1973; Zinsser, 1980). *The Holt Handbook* by Kirszner and Mandell is a useful reference book. It has good chapters on all aspects of writing, including grammar. The APA *Manual* (1983) also has a brief section on grammar.

Grammar and usage are two closely related but separate matters. Grammar is a collection of finite and fixed rules, whereas usage is a matter of change and diversity. Grammatical rules are not empirical, but usage always is. How people are talking and writing and what kinds of changes they are thus forcing in their language are a matter of usage. Scholars are concerned with usage for several reasons. In some cases, popular usage may violate the rules of grammar. In other cases, popular usage may be grammatically correct but not effective, direct, clear, or concise. Generally speaking, popular usage forces changes in language mostly at the level of vocabulary, syntax, idiom, and expression. These changes may promote or hinder direct communication in writing or speaking. Therefore, the writer should be aware of the usage of language at any given time.

There are excellent books on the contemporary usage of the English language. *Modern American Usage* by Follett (1966), the *Harper Dictionary of Contemporary Usage* by Morris and Morris (1975), and *The Elements of Style* by Strunk and White (1979) are among the best sources. Written with a great sense of humor, *A Civil Tongue* by Newman (1976) is a delightful book on the contemporary misuse of American English.

Though it will not be possible to review rules of grammar here, it is necessary to point out a few common problems that must be avoided in writing research papers. There are also some guidelines that are not a matter of correct or incorrect grammar but rather of preference.

Sentence Structure

By definition, a sentence is grammatical: it is correct and complete. Therefore, the writer should avoid sentence fragments that result from a lack of certain grammatical features or inappropriate punctuation.

Missing grammatical features create sentence fragments of the following kind:

> The group was scheduled to come to the laboratory on Monday. *But got there on Tuesday.* (Subject missing.)
> The author finally found the subjects. *In the psychology 10 class.* (Finite verb missing.)

Many problems arise when punctuation marks are used to break strings of words at inappropriate junctures. For example, a subordinate clause, which needs an independent clause, should not be punctuated as a sentence:

> The testing was completed in two sessions. *Because the instrument broke down.* (Subordinate clause punctuated as a sentence. *Revised*: The testing was completed in two sessions because the instrument broke down.)

Similar problems arise when a prepositional phrase, a verbal phrase, an absolute phrase, an appositive, a compound sentence, or an incomplete clause is punctuated as a "sentence." None of these can stand alone as sentences. An example of each illustrates these problems:

The stutterer's dysfluency rate decreased dramatically. *In the final two sessions.* (The prepositional phrase punctuated as a sentence. *Revised:* The stutterer's dysfluency rate decreased dramatically in the final two sessions.)
The experiment had 50 subjects. *Divided into two groups.* (Participial phrase, a type of verbal phrase, punctuated as a sentence. *Revised:* The experiment had 50 subjects. They were divided into two groups.)
The subjects were eight men. *Their speech characterizing severe stuttering.* (An absolute phrase punctuated as a sentence. *Revised:* The subjects were eight men. Their speech was characterized by severe stuttering.)
The subjects were tested in a sound-treated room. *A room that was especially built for the experiment.* (An appositive, punctuated as a sentence. *Revised:* The subjects were tested in a sound-treated room, a room that was especially built for the experiment.)
Many aphasic patients have word-finding problems. *And may also find it difficult to remember names.* (Part of a compound sentence punctuated as a separate sentence. *Revised:* Many aphasic patients have word-finding problems and may also find it difficult to remember names.)
Regulated breathing, a highly researched technique and known for its effectiveness with young stuttering children, which is developed by Azrin and associates. [The subject *Regulated breathing* has no predicate. *Revised:* Regulated breathing, a highly researched technique known for its effectiveness with young stuttering children, was developed by Azrin and associates. (Relative pronoun *which* deleted; the predicate *was developed* added.)]

It must be apparent to the reader that many grammatically incorrect sentences can be rewritten in different ways because the same idea can be expressed in different forms. Therefore, the revised versions of incorrect sentences must be considered only illustrative.

Generally speaking, the longer the sentence, the easier it is to make a mistake in its structure and the harder it is to find the missing element or confusing feature. Shorter, simpler sentences are preferable because they reveal their problems relatively easily. Such sentences are also easy to understand.

Verbs

It is preferable to use verbs in their *active voice.* Active voice is more direct and emphatic. Active voice is also brief.

The children were brought to the clinic by their mothers. (*Revised:* The mothers brought their children to the clinic.)

However, *passive voice* may be preferable when the agent of an action is unimportant or unknown:

An increased prevalence of stuttering in the female population *was reported* in the literature.

Most scientific papers are written in the *past tense*. Reports of empirical studies review past studies and describe a completed study. Therefore, the review, the methods, and the results are reported in the past tense.

Smith (1985) reported similar findings. Ten adult stutterers were selected. The scores of male and female subjects were the same.

When reporting something that started at an unspecified time in the past and has been continuous since then, the present perfect tense is used:

Many clinicians have used the same treatment procedure.
Over the years, many scientists have used the same instruments.

It would be incorrect to use "many clinicians used" or "many scientists used" in the above constructions.

It is preferable to write the discussion section in the present tense, however:

The data suggest a need for further research.
The result shows that it is better to use both the treatment procedures.
One of the conclusions of the study is that reduced rate of speech affects the frequency of dysfluencies.

A common mistake is to change tense abruptly. The author must be consistent in using a given tense in particular portions of a manuscript.

Agreement

Agreement between various elements of a sentence is one of the critical tests of grammatically correct sentences. Mistakes are often made in this case. Subjects and verbs must agree in number and person, whereas pronouns and their antecedents must agree in number, person, and gender.

SUBJECTS AND VERBS. Singular subjects take singular verbs and plural subjects take plural verbs:

The *result is* questionable.
The *results are* reliable.

In most simple and direct sentences, it is easy to see a mistake in subject and verb disagreement. On the other hand, disagreement may be less conspicuous in complex sentences. Mistakes are likely when intervening phrases are included in a sentence. For example:

This *result*, also reported by many past investigators, *are* not consistent with the theory. (Incorrect.)

This *result*, also reported by many past investigators, *is* not consistent with the theory. (Correct.)
These *techniques*, when used appropriately by a competent clinician, *is* known to be effective. (Incorrect.)
These *techniques*, when used appropriately by a competent clinician, *are* known to be effective. (Correct.)

Intervening phrases such as *as well as, along with, in addition to, including, and together with* do not change the number of the subject:

The *accuracy* of phoneme productions as well as the rate of correct responses *increase* during treatment. (Incorrect.)
The *accuracy* of phoneme productions as well as the rate of correct responses *increases* during treatment. (Correct.)
Error *scores*, along with the correct score, *was* used in the analysis. (Incorrect.)
Error *scores*, along with the correct score, *were* used in the analysis. (Correct.)

Generally, compound subjects joined by *and* have plural verbs (Mother *and* child *were* interviewed together). Exceptions are when an expression, though containing *and*, suggests a single concept or individual:

Who says country *and* western *is* dead?
The president *and* chief executive officer *is* Mr. Smith.

Additionally, a singular verb is used when *each* or *every* precedes a compound subject joined by *and*:

Each test and measurement procedure *was* pilot-tested.
Every *child* and adult *goes* through the same procedure.

When two subjects are linked by *or, either/or*, or *neither/nor*, the verb must be plural if both the subjects are plural and singular if both the subjects are singular:

Either verbal praise or informative feedback *is* combined with modeling.
Either verbal reinforcers or tokens *are* combined with modeling.

However, when a singular and a plural subject are linked by *neither/nor, either/or*, or *not only/but also*, the verb form is determined by the subject that is nearer to it:

Neither the treatments nor the *result are* replicable. (Incorrect.)
Neither the treatments nor the *result is* replicable. (Correct.)
Neither the treatment nor the *results are* replicable. (Correct.)
Not only the instruments, but also the *procedure are* described. (Incorrect.)
Not only the instruments, but also the *procedure, is* described. (Correct.)
Not only the instrument, but also the *procedures, are* described. (Correct.)

A few indefinite pronouns (*both, many, several, few, others*) are always plural and therefore take plural verbs. Most others (*another, anyone, everyone, each, either, neither, anything, everything, something*, and *somebody*) are singular and therefore take a singular verb:

> Anyone is acceptable, providing the subject selection criteria are met.
> Something was missing in that procedure.
> Everything is fine.
> Either of them is acceptable.

However, some indefinite pronouns such as *some, all, none, any, more,* and *most* can be singular or plural. The verb form is singular or plural depending upon the noun the pronoun refers to:

> None of the *subjects were* pretested.
> None of the *technique was* correct.
> Some of this *effect is* understandable.
> Some of the *techniques are* useless.

Collective nouns also take singular or plural verbs. A collective noun that refers to a single unit takes a singular verb; one that refers to individuals or elements of that unit takes a plural verb:

> The *group* was tested in a single session. (Singular.)
> The number of subjects was small. (Singular.)
> The *members* of the control group were tested separately. (Plural.)
> A number of subjects were absent. (Plural.)

As a general rule, *the number* is singular, *a number* is plural. But phrases that refer to fixed quantities (*majority, three quarters*) are considered collective nouns:

> The majority was against the idea. (Singular.)
> A majority of people were against the idea. (Plural.)
> Three quarters of the amount is withheld. (Singular.)
> Three quarters of those completing the treatment improve significantly. (Plural.)

Some subjects that are typically in the plural form still take singular verbs:

> The *news* is bad.
> *Statistics is* but one method of data analysis.
> *Economics is* not an exact science.
> *Politics does* not thrill me.

However, when words like *statistics* refer not to a *set* of techniques but to certain *data*, a plural verb is appropriate:

> The *statistics show* that the treatment of aphasia is successful.

Certain nouns have unusual plural forms and should not be used with singular verbs:

The baseline *data were* recorded on a separate sheet. (Plural.)
The *datum is* as solid as it can be. (Singular.)
Similar *phenomena were* observed by several scientists. (Plural.)
The same *phenomenon was* reported by other scientists. (Singular.)
The *loci* of stuttering *were* studied by Brown. (Plural.)
The locus of response control *was* shifted. (Singular.)
The *thesis was* completed on time. (Singular.)
The *theses were* too long. (Plural.)

In popular writing, *data* may be treated as singular. The singular form, *datum*, is rarely used for this reason. In scientific writing, however, *data* is always plural. A few other words have dual plural forms, though one of them may be preferred. For example, *appendices* and *appendixes* are the two plural forms of *appendix*, but *appendixes* is the preferred form. Similarly, both *indices* and *indexes* are acceptable plural forms of *index*, but *indexes* is preferred.

In using a linking verb, it is important to make sure that the verb agrees with its subject. A typical mistake is to make the verbs agree with the subject complement.

The *problem were* instruments. (Incorrect; *instruments* is the subject complement.)
The *problem was* instruments.

Correct Use of Modifiers

Modifiers connect ideas while adding information. In a sentence, the word or phrase to which a modifier refers must be clear. A *misplaced* modifier (an adjective or an adverb) refers to a wrong word or phrase in a sentence. A *dangling* modifier does not modify any word or phrase in a sentence.

Misplaced modifiers confuse the reader by not specifying which word or group of words is being modified. This is more likely to happen when the words that are modified and the modifiers are too far apart.

The author and her assistants tested the hearing of all subjects using the procedure described earlier. [(In this sentence, whether the author and her assistants or the subjects used the procedure is not clear. *Revised:* The author and her assistants, using the procedure described earlier, tested the hearing of all subjects. (Correct.)

Or,

Revised: Using the procedure described earlier, the author and her assistants tested the hearing of all subjects. (Correct.)]
Distant and mysterious, he stared at the sky. [(Who or what is distant and mysterious is not clear in this sentence). *Revised:* He stared at the sky, distant and mysterious. (It is the sky that is distant and mysterious.)]

Generally speaking, it is better to place modifiers immediately before or after the words or phrases that are modified. Certain modifiers (only, hardly, simply) must be placed before the words they modify. Different placements will change the meaning of sentences:

The past studies only offer limited solutions to this problem. (Incorrect.)
The past studies offer only limited solutions to this problem. (Correct.)
The male subjects scored a mean of 23.9 but the female subjects scored only a mean of 14.6. (Incorrect.)
The male subjects scored a mean of 23.9 but the female subjects scored a mean of only 14.6. (Correct.)

The implications are simply not clear. (Incorrect.)
The implications simply are not clear. (Correct.)

The results hardly are impressive. (Incorrect.)
The results are hardly impressive. (Correct.)

Sentences with *dangling modifiers* must be rewritten to include words or phrases that are indeed modified:

Several additional effects are observed *using this technique.* (Incorrect because the modifier has no reference in the sentence.)
Several additional effects are observed in *clients* using this technique. (Correct.)

Or,

Several additional effects are observed when *therapists* use this technique. (Correct.)

Using the standard procedure, the subjects were screened for hearing problems by the experimenter. (Incorrect.)
Using the standard procedure, the experimenter screened the subjects for hearing problems. (Correct, because the experimenter, not the subjects, used the standard procedure.)

Consistent with past studies, Johnson and Williams (1985) found that their female subjects performed better than the male subjects. (Incorrect.)
Johnson and Williams (1985) found that their female subjects performed better than the male subjects. This result is consistent with that of past studies. (Correct, because the result, not Johnson and Williams, is consistent with past studies.)

Parallel Forms

Sentences expressing parallel ideas can be especially troublesome. Parallel ideas must be expressed in the same grammatical form: words, phrases, clauses, or sentences. Parallel forms are used for emphasis, clarity, and variety. Such forms help maintain continuity of ideas. When used judiciously, parallel forms add force to writing. They also facilitate conciseness. Many parallel forms require a careful use of coordinating conjunctions: *and, but, or,* and *nor.*

The author studied books, charts, and tables.
The clients found the procedure complex but useful.

The experimental subjects were either adults or children.
The responses were neither correct nor adequate.

Parallel forms are necessary in expressing paired ideas:

His comment was brief but forceful.
Stuttering is aversive, but silence is painful.
The research was concerned with immediate generalization and subsequent maintenance.
The more patients you treat, the more you learn.
The treatment phase was over; the maintenance phase was beginning.

Parallel forms can also help highlight contrast or opposition between paired elements in a sentence:

It is better to treat stuttering children than to merely counsel the parents.
Establishing target behaviors is easier than making them last.

Several mistakes result in faulty parallelism. A common mistake is to write the different terms of a parallel construction in different terms:

Many stutterers have suffered in the past because the therapists lacked adequate training, supervised experience, and the therapists' knowledge of stuttering has been limited. (Incorrect because of an interjected nonparallel final clause of the sentence.)
Many stutterers have suffered in the past because the therapists lacked training, supervised experience, and scientific knowledge of stuttering. (Correct because the revision restores parallelism.)

Another mistake is a failure to repeat a parallel element in a series that signals parallelism. The result is a broken pattern. Such sentences must be revised to restore parallelism:

Communicatively handicapped persons have difficulty talking, reading, and self-confidence. (Incorrect because of a failure to repeat the parallel element.)
Communicatively handicapped persons have difficulty talking, reading, and maintaining self-confidence. (Correct because all three elements are parallel.)

Some of the side effects of punishment are aggression, emotionality, and the client may also learn to punish others. (Incorrect because of mixed constructions.)

Some of the side effects of punishment are aggression, emotionality, and imitative punishment. (Correct because of restored parallelism.)

Differential reinforcement helps maintenance by not allowing a rapid extinction, increasing the response strength, and improving the chances for generalization. (Incorrect because *not* does not apply to all the elements in the series.)
Differential reinforcement helps maintenance by not allowing a rapid extinction, by increasing the response strength, and by improving the chances of generalization. (Correct because the preposition *by* is repeated to prevent confusion between the elements in the series.)

Regulated breathing, developed by Azrin and associates (1975), which was researched by many other investigators, is known to be effective. (Incorrect because of a failure to start the second clause with *which*.)
Regulated breathing, *which* was developed by Azrin and associates (1975), and *which was* researched by many other investigators, is known to be effective. (Correct because *which* is used before *which was*.)

Shifts Within and Between Sentences

Sentences and paragraphs must be consistent in tense, voice, mood, person, and number. Wrong or unnecessary shifts in them confuse the reader:

The therapist *told* the client that she would not take him to outside situations unless he *maintains* fluency in the clinic. (Incorrect because of a shift in the tense.)
The therapist *told* the client that she would not take him to outside situations unless he *maintained* fluency in the clinic. (Correct because of the same tense.)

The clinician *was* well *trained*. She *knows* how to treat a variety of communicative disorders. Nevertheless, she *had* difficulty treating this particular client. (Incorrect because of a shift in tense between the sentences.)
The clinician *was* well *trained*. She *knew* how to treat a variety of communicative disorders. Nevertheless, she *had* difficulty in treating this particular client. (Correct because the same tense is maintained.)

Van Riper first *developed* "cancellation" and later "pull-outs" *were also* developed. (Inconsistent because of a shift from the active to the passive voice; who developed "pull-outs" is not clear.)
Van Riper first *developed* "cancellation" and later developed "pull-outs." (Consistent because the same voice is maintained.)

It is important that a client *possess* a tape recorder and *uses* it regularly to record his speech. (Inconsistent because of a shift from subjunctive to indicative mood.)
It is important that a client *possess* a tape recorder and *use* it regularly to record speech. (Consistent because the same mood is maintained.)

When *one* is reviewing the literature, *you* find that not many studies have been done on the issue. (Inconsistent because of a shift from second to third person.)
When *one* is reviewing the literature, *one* finds that not many studies have been done on the issue. (Consistent because the same pronoun form is maintained.) ("A review of the literature shows that not many studies have been done on the issue" is probably preferable to either of those sentences.)

If a *client* does not attend at least 90 percent of the treatment sessions, *they* will not show significant improvement. (Inconsistent because of a shift in number.)
If a *client* does not attend at least 90 percent of the treatment sessions, *he* or *she* will not show significant improvement. (Consistent because the same number is maintained.)

Punctuation

The student writer must consult a good source such as *The Holt Handbook* (Kirszner & Mandell, 1986) for a complete discussion of punctuation and mechanics. The APA *Manual* (1983) has a section on punctuation. It specifies the correct use of the period, the comma, the semicolon, the colon, the dash, quotation marks, parentheses, and brackets. The student must be able to use these elements of punctuation according to the recommendations given in the *Manual*.

Other Structural Matters

The APA *Manual* (1983) also refers to several other structural matters the student should be familiar with. It has sections on capitalization, italics, abbreviations, headings and series within a manuscript, quotations, numbers, metrication, tables, figures, reference citation, reference lists, and so on. In writing scientific papers, the student must adhere to the recommendations made in the *Manual*.

Conceptual Considerations

A mastery of the principles of grammar, punctuation, and related matters will help the writer organize a piece of writing. Those principles are matters of structure necessary for correct and acceptable expressions. However, a mastery of those principles may not necessarily assure concise, adequate, clear, and coherent writing. In spite of a good command of the structural principles, a writer may find it difficult to write well. Such a difficulty is typically a result of conceptual, rather than structural, problems.

While matters of structure are governed by relatively fixed principles, matters of conceptual considerations can be discussed only in general terms. There are no finite and explicit rules that dictate conciseness, comprehensiveness, clarity, and coherence. These parameters of writing are often judged by readers' response to a piece of writing. If readers are distracted by unnecessary words and expressions, then the writing is not concise. If readers think that some information is missing, then the writing is not adequate. If readers are not sure what is said, then the writing is not clear. Finally, if readers become confused, then the writing is not coherent. Good writing is effective. Therefore, good writing is often judged by its effects on the reader.

Knowledge of the Readership

A knowledge of the readership can help writing to be effective. One of the main difficulties of writing is that the author knows what he or she wishes to say even without writing it out, but the reader does not know. Therefore, though his or her writing is deficient, the author will have no difficulty "understanding" it. Unfortunately, what is perfectly clear to the author may be ambiguous to the reader.

The writer should try to read what is written from the viewpoint of the reader. The writer should be able to read his or her own writing and determine whether a reader without the same knowledge of what is being said can understand the material. This skill in reading one's own writing from the viewpoint of a naive reader is important for a writer.

The author should know the educational level of the readership. The extent of a readership's technical sophistication will determine the overall writing style, the number of examples given, and the amount of elaboration. Successful writers always know who their audience is and adjust their writing styles accordingly.

Concise Writing

Many first drafts are too long. Therefore, conciseness should be a major concern in preparing the second draft. If new sentences must be added, the writer must see whether a comparable number of sentences can be deleted to make the paper concise. Long papers tend to be wordy, clumsy, redundant, and indirect. The writer can usually cut the number of words, phrases, and sentences to make it more readable. It is best to read what you have written with the assumption that the length as well as the number of sentences can be cut.

You must examine every sentence and judge whether it is necessary and whether it can be shortened. The meaning of a sentence must be understood by the reader at the first reading. A sentence that must be reread in order to be understood is probably too long, clumsy, or ambiguous. Shortening it may help achieve effective as well as concise communication. Some experts suggest that the average sentence length should be 20 words or less (Bates, 1982). Most readers prefer shorter to longer sentences. Therefore, other factors being equal, the author is more likely to hold the reader attention with shorter sentences than with longer ones.

Neither the sentence length nor the type should be monotonously uniform, however. There should be a balance between shorter and longer sentences. Also, not all long sentences are necessarily difficult to understand. Some longer sentences can be made more readable by breaking them up with chunking devices such as semicolons and dashes. Other longer sentences can be clear and direct without such devices. Longer sentences are sometimes necessary to express a complex concept. When longer sentences are used sparingly and mixed with shorter ones, the reading becomes less monotonous.

Simple, active, declarative sentences are typically short and direct, but they can be dull, too. Therefore, an interesting piece of writing usually has a mixture of different types of sentences. Some sentence types, such as the passive, generally tend to be longer than other types. A shorter sentence type must be preferred as long as it is just as effective as the longer type.

Writing is not concise when it is redundant and wordy. Saying the same thing in different ways is sometimes necessary in teaching a difficult concept. However, when it seems necessary, the writer should check whether the clarity of the first statement can be improved. If a statement can be tightened up, a subsequent redundant statement can be avoided.

A typical redundancy is a result of saying the same thing in both positive and negative ways:

> The female subjects generally performed better on the experimental task. The male subjects' performance was inferior to that of the female subjects.

The second sentence says in negative terms what the first sentence says in positive terms. One of them is unnecessary, and most experts prefer the positive sentence forms.

Some of the warning signs of potentially redundant statements are phrases such as *in other words, to put it differently, to repeat, to reiterate.* What follows such phrases or clauses can be redundant.

Some redundancy in talking and writing is necessary to facilitate a proper understanding of complex materials. In scientific articles and books, summaries and abstracts repeat what has been elaborated in the body of the text. Readers are better able to focus on the text when they are given the gist of the material at the very beginning. A summary at the end may help readers remember the main points of the text. Such devices that reinforce a reader's understanding are not considered redundant.

Wordiness results when words that do not add any meaning at all are used in a sentence. Needless words and phrases and circumlocution cause wordiness. The result is an unnecessarily long sentence:

> It seemed to the author that it is important to consider many factors in selecting a specific design for the study. (*Revised*: Many factors were considered in selecting a design for the study.)

In many cases, phrases such as *who were (are), which were (are), that is,* and *there were (are)* can be eliminated:

> Eighteen persons *who were* living in rural areas were subjects. (*Revised*: Eighteen persons living in rural areas were subjects.)

> Two instruments, *which were* in good calibration, were used in the study. (*Revised*: Two instruments in good calibration were used in the study.)

> The study *that is* well known was done by Smith (1980). (*Revised*: The Smith (1980) study is well known. Or, Smith's 1980 study is well known.)

> *There were* several factors that prompted the selection of only the male subjects. (*Revised*: Several factors prompted the selection of only the male subjects.)

A number of standard phrases often used to initiate sentences can also be eliminated:

As far as the results are concerned, they appear reliable. (*Revised*: The results appear reliable.)

For all intents and purposes, the two treatment techniques are similar. (*Revised*: The two treatment techniques are similar.)

With reference to the Smith (1980) study, the methods were appropriate. (*Revised*: The methods of the Smith (1980) study were appropriate. *Or*, Smith's (1980) methods were appropriate.)

In terms of its effects, the treatment was good. (*Revised*: The treatment was effective.)

Many words used as fillers are known as *utility* words (Kirszner & Mandell, 1986). They are also often unnecessary:

It was *actually* a good study, but it did not produce worthwhile data. (*Revised*: It was a good study, but it did not produce worthwhile data.)

The deteriorating response *situation* was a problem. (*Revised*: Response deterioration was a problem.)

Certain needlessly wordy, though popular, phrases must be replaced with single words or shorter phrases:

due to the fact that	because
in spite of the fact that	though
on account of the fact that	because
at the present time	now
at this point in time	now
until such time as	until
used for the purposes of	used to (for)
the question as to whether	whether
have the ability to	be able to
hands on experience	experience
in the event that	if
by means of	by

Certain other, longer, phrases include words with overlapping meanings. Such phrases can be reduced to single words or shorter phrases:

future prospects	prospects
advance planning	planning
absolutely incomplete	incomplete
exactly identical	identical
repeat again	repeat
each and every	each *or* every
totally unique	unique

uniquely one of a kind	one of a kind (*or* unique)
reality as it is	reality
solid (*or* actual *or* true) facts	facts
famous and well-known	*either* famous *or* well-known
goals and objectives	goals *or* objectives
three different kinds	three kinds

Although concise writing is a virtue, writing that is too concise can pose problems for the reader. Depending upon the readership, some elaboration is necessary. Sometimes the same thing needs to be said differently. Examples duplicate what is said otherwise, but they are considered essential in any kind of writing. Therefore, conciseness should still serve the purpose of effective communication. The final criterion is economical as well as effective communication.

Journal articles are written for specialists with technical knowledge and therefore are more concise. Books are written for readers with different levels of formal and informal education, and therefore have a greater range of style than journal articles.

Theses, dissertations, term papers, and other pieces of writing that are expected to demonstrate a writer's knowledge of an area are more comprehensive than concise. Details are expected in these writings so that the knowledge of the writer can be evaluated. Though the instructor who evaluates the writing "knows what the student is talking about," the student must still furnish the details necessary for an evaluation.

Adequate Writing

Most books on writing do not emphasize adequacy in writing. The typical mistake made by an established writer is to write too much rather than too little. Therefore, books on writing tend to emphasize concise writing. On the other hand, beginning writers, especially student writers, tend to write too little rather than too much. Essay answers at the undergraduate and graduate levels are more often overly restricted. Important information is often missing in such restricted writings. The first drafts of theses and projects tend to omit necessary details. Most graduate students are asked to expand their first drafts to include various details.

Inadequate writing is as problematic as excessive writing. In scientific reports, theses, and essay examinations, the writing must be adequate. These pieces of writing are evaluated by other individuals. Those who read essay answers must judge whether the student knows the information requested. Inadequate answers are taken to represent inadequate knowledge. Students often complain that "they knew the material" but just did not write all they knew; but it is the students' writing, not their knowledge, that the instructor has access to. Therefore, answers must be adequate.

Scientific reports, including theses and dissertations, are also evaluated by other individuals. This evaluation is done to find out, among other things, if the procedures used were appropriate to answer the research questions and whether the results were reliable. In order to make this evaluation, the reader must have sufficient details about the procedures, results, and methods of analysis. The reader should also have enough background information. An adequate overview of past research must be available in a report. Omission of significant details makes it difficult to evaluate the significance of a study.

Inadequate writing is one of the main reasons why certain scientific reports cannot be replicated. Insufficient information on the types of subjects used, experimental manipulations, independent and dependent variables, and control procedures can make it difficult for other investigators to replicate a study.

Clear Writing

Clear writing is important in both science and everyday life. When there is no clarity, there is no communication. Much worse, there may be serious misunderstanding or even tragedy, as eloquently expressed by Strunk and White (1979, pp. 79–80):

> Muddiness is not merely a disturber of prose, it is also a destroyer of life, of hope: death on the highway caused by a badly worded road sign, heartbreak among lovers caused by a misplaced phrase in a well-intentioned letter, anguish of a traveler expecting to be met at a railroad station and not being met because of a slipshod telegram. Usually we think only of the ludicrous aspect of ambiguity; . . . But think of the tragedies that are rooted in ambiguity; think of that side, and be clear!

Clear writing cannot be achieved by doing just one thing right. Several factors contribute to clarity. Writing is clear when all or most of those factors are present. To write clearly, the author should avoid ambiguity, euphemism, jargon, cliches, colloquial expressions, and dead metaphors and similes. At the same time, the author should use the right words, and exercise care in the use of abstract words, concrete words, and figures of speech.

Ambiguity results from many structural problems of the kind discussed in some of the previous sections. For example, misplaced and dangling modifiers, faulty parallelism, inappropriate shifts within and between sentences, and wrong punctuation can make the meaning of sentences unclear. Structural accuracy, combined with directness and simplicity, will reduce ambiguity.

Unclear writing may also result from words and phrases that, for a variety of reasons, do not convey the precise meaning to the reader. Euphemisms, cliches, colloquial expressions, and ineffective figures of speech are some of the reasons for this lack of precision.

AVOID EUPHEMISMS. Euphemisms are neutral or positive-sounding words and phrases that replace negative-sounding words or phrases. Several euphemistic expressions have become a part of everyday language. Retarded children are *exceptional children*, poor people are *disadvantaged*, and the older persons are *senior citizens*. Failing students are not dismissed out but *counseled out*, and a student is not asked to retake an examination but is *given another opportunity to demonstrate knowledge*. Such euphemistic expressions hamper clarity.

Technical-sounding euphemisms can distort meaning in scientific reports. Instead of saying that some speech clinicians do not like to treat stutterers because of lack of training, one may say that the treatment of stuttering is negatively affected by some clinicians' unfavorable attitude toward stutterers. It is difficult to determine the meaning of this sentence, but it could possibly be that *the negatively affected treatment* is ineffective treatment, and *the clinicians' unfavorable attitude* may be a euphemistic reference to clinicians' inadequate training or incompetence. Intellectual honesty is an important aspect of scientific writing. Euphemism is anything but intellectual honesty and therefore has no place in scientific writing.

AVOID JARGON. Jargon is defined as the technical or specialized terms of a particular discipline as well as useless and incomprehensible vocabulary (See *The Random House Thesaurus*, 1984; and Follett's *Modern American Usage*, 1966). Scientific reports cannot be written without technical terms. Technical terms are often preferable to lay terms because of the latter's imprecise and varied connotations. Therefore, jargon, in the sense of technical and specialized terms, cannot be altogether avoided in scientific writing.

Technical words must be used only when necessary, however. A nontechnical word may be preferred to the technical if it conveys the same meaning with the same precision. For example, if the word *language* will do, there is no sense in using *linguistic competence*. Of course, thee may be a reason to prefer *linguistic competence* over *language*. In essence, the use of every technical word must be justified.

When a scientist or a professional writes for the general public, extra care must be taken in the selection of words. Technical words must be used most sparingly and with enough explanations in everyday language.

The most debilitating form of jargon is pseudotechnical gibberish. Its sole purpose is to obscure the message and presumably impress the naive audience. Careful writers avoid this kind of jargon. Sometimes, acceptable jargon in one field may be befuddling nonsense that gives an air of pseudotechnicality in a different field. Speech–language pathology is full of this kind of borrowed and grafted jargon: input, output, end gate, information processing, governor, filter, comparator, and so on. Most of it is borrowed from engineering and computer science. The relevance of such jargon for speech–language pathology is mostly presumed and theoretical.

Unless there is a scientific justification, jargon borrowed from other disciplines should not be used. It makes very little technical sense to say that *the child seems to have processed the linguistic input as a single unit* when all that the child did was to point to the right picture when requested to do so.

AVOID CLICHES. Some standard phrases give brevity and clarity to writing. Minimal use of standard phrases such as *wear and tear* and *at its best* is acceptable. However, overuse of cliches, which are standard expressions that have become dull and meaningless because of overuse, obscures writing. A writer who uses too many standard phrases betrays a lack of creativity in his or her use of language. Besides, many overused standard phrases have lost their precise definition. As a result, the writing becomes vague.

A clinician who writes that *this technique is not my cup of tea* is not saying anything clearly. The statement may mean, among other things, that the technique is ineffective or that the clinician simply does not know how to use it. Or, when a clinician writes about the *dashed hopes and aspirations of parents of language handicapped children*, we do not know whom to blame.

AVOID COLLOQUIAL EXPRESSIONS. With few exceptions, technical writing should not contain colloquial expressions. In fact, colloquial expressions are not appropriate in formal writing of any kind. In a scientific report, *the author feels that* is too loose and colloquial. The author's feelings are probably irrelevant in the context. *Feels that* should be replaced by *thinks that* or *believes that*. Similarly, *language* must be preferred to *tongue*, and *stomach* to *tummy*.

Other kinds of colloquialism to be avoided includes contractions (*isn't, won't*), abbreviations such as *TV, phone*, and *exam*, and phrases such as *sort of, you know, get across*, and *come up with*.

An extreme form of colloquialism is called *slang* (*spaced out, uptight, for sure, rad*). Such expressions have no place in scientific writing unless this form of speech is itself the matter of investigation.

AVOID DEAD METAPHORS AND SIMILES. These are expressions that were once colorful and effective but now cliche. Expressions such as *dead as a door nail, a shot in the arm, off the beaten path, sit on the fence*, and *beyond a shadow of doubt* are better avoided in scientific writing. They are probably not useful in any kind of writing. In exploring the meaning and implications of scientific data, direct and nonmetaphorical use of language is essential.

USE THE RIGHT WORDS. Words with exact meaning must be selected over those that are too broad in their meaning. In scientific writing, technical words offer more precise meaning than their counterparts in everyday language. For example, in the behavioral science literature, *reinforcer* is a technical term, which should not be confused with *reward* or *award*.

Sometimes, when none of the everyday words serve the scientific purpose, new words may be created by a scientist to suggest a specific event or process. Such neologism is acceptable in scientific writing. However, neologisms of bureaucracy (including education and science), the advertising industry, and business can only obscure the meaning of a message. Many neologisms have been created by adding *-wise* and *-ize* to words that do not take those suffixes. Consequently, words such as *prioritize, sanitize,* and *finalize*; and *gradewise, economywise,* and *timewise* have become a part of everyday language. Another set of words has been created by adding the prefix *de-* to certain words resulting in such creations as *decriminalize* and *dehumanize.* Neologisms of this kind should be left out of scientific writing.

The careful writer must be aware of subtle distinctions in meaning of words. Many pairs of words are mistakenly used interchangeably. For example, in the following pairs of words, the meaning of each word is different: disinterested and uninterested, alternate and alternative, anticipate and expect, continual and continuous, farther and further, imply and infer, stationary and stationery, economic and economical, historic and historical, affect and effect. A dictionary or a thesaurus can help distinguish the meanings of these and other commonly confused words.

USE OF ABSTRACT AND CONCRETE WORDS. Abstract words refer to concepts and relations between concepts. Abstract words do not stimulate senses because they do not always refer to sensory experiences. Concrete words refer to things and events that stimulate the senses. Such words help recall sensory images of all kinds. Therefore, concrete words are more direct. They are easy to understand. To be understood, abstract words require a certain level of conceptual understanding of the subject matter.

A general rule is that concrete words are preferable to abstract words. By generating sensory consequences, concrete words help the reader understand experiences the author has written about. Concrete words are especially useful in literary essays, journalistic reports, stories, and novels. These kinds of writings conjure up vivid images and sensations. Poetry, on the other hand, consists of many abstract words. That is why a serious poem is harder to understand than a novel or a short story. Undefined abstract words lead to different interpretations. By not defining the abstract words used, the poet creates multiple meanings, which make a small poem a complex piece of writing.

Abstract words are useful in scientific writing. Scientific reports are typically about events and their relations, and many of these relations are abstract. However, unlike the poet, the scientist defines the abstract words precisely so that multiple meanings are not suggested. Many abstract words are found in the literature review and discussion sections of a scientific report.

Even in scientific reports, concrete words must be used in describing persons, things, and events. Subjects must be described in specific terms

(12-year-old male children) rather than in general terms (young people). Similarly, instruments, procedure, and results must be described in concrete terms.

SPARING USE OF FIGURES OF SPEECH. Figures of speech, including similes and metaphors, also help make the writing vivid to the reader. Similes suggest a similarity between two essentially unlike items (a new house is *like* a black hole; it sucks in all your money). Metaphors equate two dissimilar things (all the world's a stage). Analogies describe a new concept in terms of a familiar concept (the nervous system is like a telephone network). Personification attributes human qualities to inanimate entities (the dark clouds were looking mean and ferocious).

Overuse of figures of speech can hinder direct and technical communication. Once again, they are more appropriately used in literary writings than in scientific reports. An exception is scientific writing meant for the general public, which can use figures of speech to help the reader understand complex ideas.

Some forms of figures of speech are not limited to sentences. For example, *analogical reasoning* can be considered a figurative approach to thinking about a subject matter in terms of another subject matter. Descriptions of the nervous system and its functioning in computer language and the language of the industry illustrate this approach.

Coherent Writing

One writing problem shown by student writers is incoherent writing. An essay or a review paper may lack a structure, an orderly progression of ideas and concepts, and a smooth transition from sentence to sentence, paragraph to paragraph, and section to section.

Some planning and thinking can improve the coherence of writing. The different sections of a paper and the contents of each section or topic must be determined first. Next, the sequence of these sections must be determined. Sections and contents of most scientific reports are relatively fixed. Even so, subheadings under these major sections vary. Therefore, some planning is needed to make scientific reports coherent and easy to understand. The sequences of sections, headings, and subheadings of articles with more flexible formats must be carefully thought out.

When sections and their contents are planned, an orderly progression of ideas can be achieved by smooth transitions between units of writing. The paragraph is the most important of these units. Each section or topic contains several paragraphs, and therefore writing effective paragraphs with smooth transitions between them is important in good writing.

A single concept or a brief topic gives a paragraph its unity. For example, the age, socioeconomic status, and the occupational level of the subjects used in a study may be described in a single paragraph. How the subjects were selected may be described in a different paragraph, because of a change in the idea or topic. If the selection criterion can be expressed in a single sentence, it may be a part of another paragraph. The basic rule is that a paragraph should have conceptual unity. Therefore, the beginning of a new paragraph suggests a transition to a new idea, topic, or subtopic.

Paragraphs should not be too long, nor should they typically consist of single sentences. Readers find lengthy paragraphs formidable. But a succession of brief paragraphs can make the writing fragmented. A single-sentence paragraph is generally inappropriate, but it is acceptable on occasion. Single-sentence paragraphs can make a point emphatically or can highlight a transition to a new topic.

The first sentence in a paragraph may suggest the topic or concept to be described in it. If the paragraph continues with the same idea described in the previous paragraph, then a transitory sentence, which makes a reference to the previous paragraph, is needed. To achieve a smooth transition, a paragraph should begin as well as end appropriately. If the same general idea is to be discussed in several paragraphs, the end of each paragraph should be linked to the beginning of the next paragraph. Such linking can often be achieved by a common word or a phrase that is repeated in the final sentence of the previous paragraph and the first sentence of the new paragraph.

There are also many kinds of paragraphs; perhaps the most important are those that introduce and conclude a section or topic. Some topics should be introduced slowly, preparing the reader with a few sentences; other topics can be introduced without much background information. Each section or topic should begin with an introductory paragraph. The need for paragraphs that suggest conclusion is somewhat varied. They are needed at the end of major sections and topics but may not be needed at the end of subtopics. Complex and lengthy discussions almost always need paragraphs that give a summary.

So far we have discussed concise, adequate, clear, and coherent writing. These qualities of writing require a competent conceptual handling of the subject of writing. The final point we need to discuss briefly is the matter of *style*.

WRITING STYLE

In this chapter, the term *style* is not used in the same sense as a format of writing. Format refers more to the organization and mechanics of writing than to style. A format (such as that of APA), grammar (structural matters), and conceptual considerations are all necessary to write well. But a style of writing is a different matter; it is the most individualistic of the aspects of writing. It is the style, not the knowledge of grammar and other writing principles, that distinguishes one great writer from another. It is the style, among other qualities, that separates Walt Whitman from Robert Frost and James Joyce from Saul Bellow. There are good styles and bad styles, but more importantly, each outstanding writer has his or her own unique style.

Grammatical correctness does not necessarily assure a unique style. A piece of writing may be structurally flawless but boring because of a lack of style. A style is a writer's creative use of language. It is the distinguishing pattern of words that a writer creates to produce a unique effect upon the reader. Literary writers pay close attention to style. How a story is told is at least as important as what that story is. Scientific writers, on the other hand, generally tend to pay less attention to style. They concentrate more on technical, correct, clear, concise, and adequate writing. The meaning of a poem can be intentionally obscure, but the poem may still be hailed as important; obscure scientific articles generally remain obscure. Writers of scientific subjects restrict the reader response to particular meanings of words, whereas a poet or a novelist, as noted earlier, intentionally broadens the reader response by using words with multiple meanings and then by not defining them. Nevertheless, style is important in scientific writing. There is nothing wrong with the creative use of language in scientific writing as long as the principles of effective communication are not violated. In fact, a creative writing style can enhance scientific communication.

Some unreadable scientific writing may be so because of the authors' dull style. Bold and novel use of language within the limits of scientific communication can improve the readability of most research papers. An excessive concern with the structure and format make scientific papers extremely formal, and boring to read. Surely, a breezy and informal style is not appropriate for scientific discussions, but within the limits of seriousness, one can write with lucidity, style, and beauty.

Writing with a creative style that conforms to the rules of scientific and technical communication is one of the most difficult challenges faced by writers in sciences and professions. A lack of serious interest in good literature among many scientists and professionals may be one of the reasons why most scientific writings lack unique styles. A study of good literature, ideally started early in life, should help scientists improve their writing style. Such a study should focus upon great writers of contrasting styles.

WRITE AND REWRITE

Writing correctly and with a good style is a matter of writing frequently and rewriting as often as necessary. Like any other skill, writing will not improve unless one writes. Good writing needs practice. Very few writers manage to write very little yet extremely well. Most writers have to write, write, and write before they achieve a certain ease and style of writing.

The art of revising one's writing is very important for a writer. The writer is the first reader and therefore the first critic of a piece of writing. The writer also begins as a mild critic of his or her own writing, but must learn to be a strong critic of that writing, at least privately and in the process of rewriting.

It is rewriting that eventually refines the writing. Rewriting requires a critical reading of one's own writing. Most writers, especially student writers, make the mistake of not having enough time to revise what they write before it is submitted for publication or evaluation. Therefore, many problems of writing can be avoided simply by allowing enough time to make revisions of the first draft.

Even the most established writers revise their manuscripts several times. Often, the final manuscript is vastly different from the original draft. It is better to revise a paper a few days after the original writing. A few good books on writing and comments from friends and colleagues can usually help in this process. The readability and clarity of technical papers can be improved by using suggestions made by persons not familiar with the subject matter. Scientific accuracy can be improved by taking suggestions from colleagues and experts. ■

S T U D Y G U I D E

1. Go to your department or university library and select a thesis prepared in your subject matter. Make a complete outline of the format of that thesis. Note the differences between the format of a research article published in a journal and the thesis.

2. Surveying a few journals in your subject matter, select (1) an article, (2) a report of an empirical study, and (3) a set of exchanges between two or more authors. Make an outline of these publications, retaining only the major headings. Note the similarities and differences in the formats of those three types of publications.

3. What are the characteristics of a good abstract? What is its usefulness in published papers?

4. Select a report of an empirical study from one of the journals you normally read. After having read the article, write an abstract of that report. Do not use the author's abstract. Later, compare your abstract with that of the author. Can you improve yours or the author's? If so, rewrite one or both.

5 Describe the seven factors that a well written *introduction* addresses. Find a published article whose introduction is well written because it includes those seven factors. Also, find an introduction that you think is not as well written. Justify your selection.

6 What are the standard subheadings of the section on *the method* of a published empirical report prepared according to the APA Manual?

7 What is a *discussion* of a technical paper? What are its contents?

8 Select (a) two journal articles, one written by a single author and the other written by three or more authors, (b) one book edited by a single author, (c) one book written by a single author, (d) one book written by three authors, (e) a chapter published in an edited book, and (f) a thesis. Following the APA guidelines, prepare a *reference* list of these publications.

9 Distinguish between a *reference* list and a *bibliography*.

10 Select a paper you have written and critically evaluate the writing in terms of the common structural mistakes. Make sure the paper selected was not edited by someone else. Can you find faults with your own writing? Rewrite your paper to make it more effective and readable.

11 What are the conceptual considerations of good writing? What aspect of good writing seems to give you the most difficulty? How can you gain control over that aspect of your writing?

12 What six factors should a writer avoid to write clearly?

13 Give an example of (a) euphemism, (b) jargon, (c) cliche, (d) colloquial expression, and (e) dead metaphors and similes.

14 What are figures of speech? Give examples. What is their place in scientific writing?

15 What is meant by the "style" of writing? Should scientific writings have a style? Justify your answer.

16 Select a literary essay written by a famous writer and an article published in one of the *ASHA* journals. Compare and contrast them in terms of the use of metaphors and similes, the writing style, the use of language, and the general format.

17 Write a two-page essay on your professional objectives. Put it aside for 1 week. Then, reread it and critically evaluate your writing. Rewrite your essay to make it more attractive. Have someone read and criticize it for you.

(continued next page)

Study Guide *(continued)*

18 Find a well-written scientific article published in one of the scientific/ professional journals. Why is it such a good article? What aspects of that article would you like to emulate in your own writing?

19 Identify two or three outstanding contemporary American writers of fiction, poetry, or essays. Select those known to have received critical acclaim (not necessarily those on the best-seller list). Read at least one book by each of the selected authors.

How to Evaluate Research Reports

■ Professionals as consumers of research, 400

■ Understanding and evaluating research, 400

■ Evaluation of research, 401

■ Internal consistency evaluation, 402

■ External relevance evaluation, 405

■ Evaluation of research reports: an outline, 407

■ Evaluation and appreciation of research, 411

■ Study guide, 412

E valuation of research is an important task of scientists and professionals. Sometimes it is assumed that professionals who do not do research need not be concerned with its evaluation. This is a mistake, because professionals are consumers of research. Professionals who wish to integrate research information into their clinical practice must be able to determine the usefulness of that information. Because not all research studies are equally valid or reliable, a critical clinician is a better consumer of research.

PROFESSIONALS AS CONSUMERS OF RESEARCH

Clinical practice and research can influence each other when clinicians can understand and evaluate research and researchers can understand and address clinical issues. It is the duty of clinicians to understand and evaluate clinically relevant research. Clinicians who can do this have a better chance of influencing the course of research that will generate clinically useful data.

Clinicians who are not in touch with research are likely to perpetuate the use of old, less effective assessment and treatment procedures. Such clinicians may also be the permanent victims of faddish changes in theory and practice. Acceptance of new research and theories regardless of their merit can lead to an abandonment of proven procedures. A questionable promise of a "new and revolutionary" approach may discourage attempts at refining existing techniques that may prove satisfactory. Such efforts are more economical than those needed to develop new techniques.

Uncritical clinicians are more likely to perceive only the dramatic, the popular, and the forcefully promoted techniques. Those clinicians may not be able to perceive the subtle, significant, and cumulative scientific progress made by their subject matter. Clinicians who are not able to appreciate research may not be able to contribute to their body of knowledge.

UNDERSTANDING AND EVALUATING RESEARCH

The first step in evaluating research is to understand it. Many students who read research reports find it difficult to understand them. There are many sources of this difficulty, and different students may find certain sources especially debilitating.

The first source of difficulty is lack of knowledge of the subject matter or of the particular issue of a report. A grasp of the technical vocabulary and the necessary theoretical concepts is essential for understanding research. A piece of research can be evaluated only in the broader conceptual and empirical context in which it was done. Therefore, scientists capable in one field cannot necessarily evaluate fully research in another field.

The second source of difficulty is lack of knowledge of the methods of investigation. The student needs to be familiar with the basic concepts of science, such as control, causality, and causal and other kinds of analysis. The student must understand the logic and the conditions of experimental manipulations. Knowledge of the methods of analysis, especially those of statistics, is essential in understanding many research reports.

The third source of difficulty may be lack of technical understanding of various aspects of research. Journal articles are typically written for technically competent audiences. Because of space limitations and production costs, journal articles are rarely self-explanatory. Many concepts, procedures, design aspects, and theoretical backgrounds are mentioned only briefly. If the student is not already familiar with them, other sources must be consulted.

The fourth source of difficulty is lack of experience in reading research articles. Like doing research, evaluating research is also a matter of experience. Students find that as they read more and more reports, they are able to understand more and more of them.

Students who understand research reports are not necessarily able to evaluate them, however. Students may be able to make satisfactory reports on journal articles, summarize the studies adequately, and understand the rationale, methods, results, and conclusions of particular studies. Nevertheless, students may not be able to evaluate the reliability and validity of the studies they seem to understand.

Students may uncritically accept the conclusions of methodologically defective studies. Students may not perceive logical inconsistencies, faulty designs, questionable methods of analysis, and conclusions that are not warranted by the data. Many instructors find that students need instruction and practice in evaluating research reports. Students seem to benefit from instructors' modeled evaluations. Some clinicians who try to read, understand, and evaluate research studies may also experience these problems.

EVALUATION OF RESEARCH

As pointed out by Sidman (1960), research studies are evaluated for the scientific importance of the data, their reliability, and their generality. These three objectives of evaluation can be accomplished by a critical analysis of the conceptual background of a study, the research questions asked, the methods used, the procedures of analysis, and the manner in which the conclusions were drawn. This critical analysis also tries to place the study in the overall context of the subject matter of which it is a part.

Scientific studies can be subjected to two kinds of evaluation. I call the first *the internal consistency evaluation*, and the second, *the external relevance evaluation*. I shall first describe these two types of evaluations and then, in the form of an outline, offer specific suggestions for evaluating research studies.

Internal Consistency Evaluation

The internal consistency evaluation is done within the confines of the study itself. The external relevance evaluation, on the other hand, is done to judge a study's importance in enhancing the knowledge within the subject matter. Before a study's relevance to the subject matter is determined, an internal consistency evaluation must be completed.

The internal consistency evaluation judges the study on its own terms. This evaluation is concerned with the integrity of the structure of the study. It is concerned with consistency in its purpose, methods, results, and conclusions. An important task in this evaluation is to determine whether the effects produced in a study were indeed due to the experimental manipulations (internal validity). Reliability of the results is also considered in the internal consistency evaluation.

The purpose of an investigation is an important criterion of internal consistency evaluation. A study is internally consistent only in relation to its purpose. In judging the adequacy of the methods used, one cannot use absolute criteria. The methods of a study are adequate or inadequate to answer the particular questions of that study. As we have noted elsewhere, a design may be adequate to answer one type of question but inadequate to answer another type. A method of analysis may be appropriate for one kind of data but inappropriate for another kind. Therefore, what the experimenter was trying to accomplish in the study is an important basis for judging its internal consistency.

The type of question asked determines the experimental design. If the question is one of interaction between two or more variables, a factorial group or a single-subject interactional design must be used. A simple two-group design or an *ABA* design will not answer that question. When the purpose is to find a causal relation between two variables, a correlational method is not appropriate; but when the purpose is to find out if two variables co-vary, that correlational method is appropriate.

In most cases, methodological errors threaten the internal consistency of a study. In addition to selecting a wrong design to answer the research questions, the investigator can make other mistakes. The subject selection procedure may be inappropriate. When a heterogeneous set of subjects is needed or intended, the investigator may select a small number of mostly available subjects. When homogeneous subjects are needed, the selected subjects may be heterogeneous. Subjects may be matched only on some of the relevant variables. The selection criteria may be too stringent or too lenient. As a result, subjects who are appropriate for the study may be rejected, and those that are not may be selected.

Mistakes in measuring the dependent variables, instrumentation, arranging the experimental conditions, manipulation of the independent variables, and, most importantly, building effective control procedures into the experiment can also hamper internal consistency. The pretest measures or the baselines of the dependent variables may not be reliable. The method of measurement may not be accurate. When a direct measure (frequency) of the response is required to answer the questions, only indirect measures (questionnaire responses) may have been obtained. The reliability of the instruments used in measurement may have been questionable or unknown.

Experimental conditions are a part of the design. Once the right design is selected, the required conditions must be arranged accordingly. Unfortunately, even after the right design has been selected, mistakes may be made in arranging the experimental conditions. For example, in a single-subject interactional design, more than one treatment variable may be changed across experimental conditions. The results then cannot be interpreted because of the confounding effects of multiple treatments.

Effective manipulation of the independent variables is necessary to achieve the goals of most experimental studies. Weak manipulation of the selected independent variable may fail to produce an appreciable effect. For example, a treatment variable applied only briefly may not answer the question when it is concerned with long-term effects. When an everyday experimental schedule is required, a twice-weekly schedule may be ineffective. The intensity of the independent variable may also be weak. The verbal "wrong," for example, may be delivered in a weak, unsure, soft, voice. An investigation on the effects of masking noise on stuttering may use only a 30-dB masking noise, which may be less than what is required to produce an effect.

The reader can recall from Chapter 6 that appropriate controls are necessary to establish the internal validity of an experiment. Internal validity assures that the changes observed in the dependent variable are indeed due to the manipulations of the independent variables. Internal validity can be achieved by various means, including a no-treatment control group, multiple baselines, reversal, and withdrawal of treatment. In the group design studies, mistakes in achieving equivalent groups are common. Was a population accessible for sampling? Were there both random selection and random assignment of subjects? Was the matching done on all relevant variables? When answers to questions such as these are negative, control procedures of a study are not adequate.

In single-subject designs, the baselines may be too brief, unstable, or improving. Some of the baselines in a multiple baseline design may show changes without treatment. When the treatment is withdrawn, the effects observed earlier may not dissipate. These and other problems question the adequacy of control procedures and hence the internal consistency of a single-subject study.

Faulty analysis of results is another problem that thwarts the internal consistency of research studies. In group design studies, inappropriate statistics may be used in data analysis. For example, parametric statistical techniques may be used when the data warrant nonparametric statistics. In case of a pretest–posttest control group design, the pretest and posttest means of the experimental group may be compared with a *t* test and the corresponding means of the control group may be tested with another *t* test. It was pointed out in Chapter 7 that this is an incorrect method of analysis.

In single-subject design studies, comparisons of nonadjacent experimental conditions may be made to demonstrate experimental effects. For example, an investigator who administers reinforcement for a desirable behavior in one condition may compare reinforcement and punishment for an undesirable behavior administered in another condition when these two conditions are separated by a baseline. This is a wrong procedure, because in the evaluation of multiple treatment effects, only adjacent conditions can be compared.

Finally, mistakes are made in drawing conclusions from research studies. When faulty methods of analysis are used, wrong conclusions are inevitable. The most common of these mistakes is to draw conclusions that are not consistent with the results. The results may show weak experimental effects, but the conclusions may suggest strong effects. Experimental effects may be inferred when there were none. In the statistical approach, this mistake is known as a Type I error (a null hypothesis is rejected when it should have been retained). On the other hand, an effect may be denied when there was one. In statistical analysis, this is known as Type II error (the null is retained when it should have been rejected).

Many other mistakes are possible in the interpretation of data. Subtle distortions in data are thought to result from author's convictions that are not supported by the data. Some investigators have greater faith in their own convictions than in demonstrated empirical relations. In such cases, authors may try too hard to explain the results away.

The effects of wrong statistical analyses and misinterpretations of results need not totally invalidate a study, however. As long as the report describes the results separately and completely, the methods of analyses and the author's conclusions can be separated from those results. The evaluator can come to his or her own independent conclusions. A clear separation between the results and the author's conclusions is an important aspect of internal consistency evaluation. Beginning students often cannot make this distinction. They tend to equate "the study showed that" with "the author concluded that." Obviously, those who cannot distinguish the results from the wrong conclusions of a study will be misled by the author.

The reliability of the results of a study is often judged on the basis of the internal consistency evaluation. Though the author has reported acceptable inter- and intra-subject reliability measures, serious mistakes in the implementation of a study are grounds for questioning the reliability of the results. There is no assurance that if the procedures are properly implemented, the same results would be observed.

When internal consistency questions have been satisfactorily answered, external relevance evaluation becomes important. However, should the internal consistency evaluation reveal serious problems with the study, the external relevance evaluation is a moot issue. Unreliable results of invalid experimental operations do not have external relevance to the subject matter.

External Relevance Evaluation

The object of external relevance evaluation is to determine the importance of scientific data to their subject matter. The experimental data of a given study may be reliable and internally consistent, but their significance to the subject matter may still be limited. Do the data advance the cause of understanding the phenomenon? This is the question of external relevance evaluation.

Compared with the internal consistency evaluation, the external relevance evaluation is more global. This global evaluation is done at different levels or within different contexts. The importance of data is evaluated by placing them in the larger context of research on the phenomenon addressed by the study. In turn, the particular phenomenon is also placed in the context of the larger subject matter of which it is a part. In fact, the contexts in which the data are placed for evaluation may be multiple and ever-increasing in scope. In other words, data are placed first in the smaller context of the research questions asked by the study, then in the larger context of the topic of investigation, then in the still larger context of the subject, and finally in the context of the total subject matter. The number of contexts in which the data are evaluated depends upon the scope of the questions investigated and that of the subject matter.

The multiple contexts of ever-increasing scope that are used in evaluating the importance of a research study can be illustrated with an example. Suppose that a study asks the question whether the known normative sequence of morphological acquisition can be altered by experimental teaching. Taking young children, the investigator teaches selected grammatical morphemes ahead of the developmental schedule and in a reversed order. The author concludes that it is possible to teach morphemes ahead of, and in a sequence other than, the normative sequence.

In making the external relevance evaluation of this study, the student first places the data in the context of studies on language acquisition. What kinds of studies have been done in the past? What is the significance of this study? Does this study use an approach that is different from the approaches of the past studies? Does it say anything new about the language acquisition process?

The significance of the study is evaluated next in the larger context of the analysis of language, not just language development. Does it offer a way of analyzing language behavior? Does the experimental method contribute anything new toward an understanding of language behavior in general? What kinds of theoretical statements do the results support?

In the third and still larger context, the significance of the data can be evaluated in terms of their relevance to the treatment of language disorders. Are the data related to the clinical treatment of language disorders? Do they shed light on the selection of target behaviors? Do the results have implications for sequencing target behaviors in clinical treatment?

Finally, the study may be placed in the context of communicative behaviors and disorders in general. Does it have implications for studying normal communicative behaviors? Does it suggest that similar methods of analysis can be used in studying phonological or other norm-based behaviors? Possibly, the study can be placed in the still broader context of analysis of developmentally based behaviors of all kinds.

Another concern of external relevance evaluation is the generality of data. An internally consistent study may or may not have external generality. However, as noted in Chapter 6, no single study can assure all kinds of generality. Generality is a function of replication. Therefore, an evaluation of generality attempts to determine the potential for replication. The main question to be answered is whether the study is described in sufficient detail to make replications possible. The research questions, procedures, designs, and experimental variables must be described operationally. The study then can be replicated by other investigators in other settings using different subjects. A report that does not describe its procedures (including the dependent and independent variables) in sufficient detail is evaluated negatively from the standpoint of generality.

The external relevance evaluation is the more difficult of the two evaluations because it involves a value judgment. This evaluation asks simple but difficult-to-answer questions: Is this study important, valuable, and relevant to the field of investigation? Does it make a significant contribution to the subject matter? These questions are difficult to answer, for several reasons. First, students need to have broad scholarship in the subject matter to judge the overall significance of a study. Second, individual evaluators almost always judge the importance of scientific data from the standpoint of their personal perspectives. This is necessarily so because scientists who evaluate the scientific significance of their colleagues' data do not have a common set of criteria. What is considered an important criterion by one evaluator may be considered trivial by another evaluator. After a thorough discussion of the evaluation of scientific importance of data, Sidman (1960, p. 41) said this: "If science is to use the importance of data as a criterion for accepting or rejecting an experiment, it must have a set of rules within which the scientist can operate when he has to make his evaluation. Do such rules actually exist? The answer is no."

Lack of objective rules and the subjective nature of evaluation of the external relevance of data suggest that we should be careful in rejecting any experimental data as unimportant. Negative evaluation of external relevance of a study is often made on the basis of one's own theoretical biases and convictions arising from personal experiences. If the results are not consistent with such biases and convictions, a negative judgment may be rendered. However, this can be a bad practice, because the value of certain experimental data can be independent of theoretical viewpoints and personal biases. This is true of the biases and convictions of both the evaluator and the original investigator. If it appears that the methods and procedures of a study were appropriate, the data whose significance is not clear must be afforded the benefit of doubt. Such data may have been rejected by the original investigator because they did not support his or her preconceived ideas. An evaluator may think that the data are trivial because of his or her own limited perspective. In such cases, the best course of action is to reserve judgment. Sound experimental data survive negative judgments rendered by fellow scientists.

The difficulties involved in making external evaluation should not discourage us from trying, however. For both scientific and professional reasons, it is important that we judge the importance of the studies we read. One must try to make the best possible judgment and remain open to a different judgment. An uncritical acceptance of everything, perhaps desirable for personal reasons, is not helpful in advancing the science of a subject matter. Uncritical acceptance of scientific literature can be detrimental to the professional's integrity and to the progress of clients under treatment.

What follows is an integrated outline for making a summative evaluation of research studies. It includes questions of both internal consistency evaluation and external relevance evaluation.

EVALUATION OF RESEARCH REPORTS: AN OUTLINE

Before using this outline, the student must make sure that he or she is familiar with the subject matter and understands the concepts, methods, and procedures of the study to be evaluated. Only after achieving a thorough understanding of the study and its background can a student make an evaluation of it.

The student must ask and try to answer the following questions as well as possible:

Significance of the Problem Investigated

Was the problem investigated significant?
Does it concern with an important area of investigation?
Does it advance our understanding of the issues involved?
Does it have basic implications, applied implications, or both?

Introduction and Literature Review

Was the introduction section clear and complete?
Did it help focus on the problem investigated?
Did it review the literature in sufficient detail to justify the study?
Was the review objective, impartial, and appropriately critical?
Did it give a historical perspective if one was required to understand the
     investigation?
Did it point out the strengths and limitations of previous studies?
Did the introduction place the research questions in the context of
     previous investigations?
Overall, did this section tell you why the study was made?

Statement of the Problem

Was the problem stated clearly?
Did the problem statement specify the variables in operational terms?
Was the problem statement clear enough to permit a replication?
If hypotheses were made, were they stated clearly?
If there were no hypotheses, did the author specify the research questions?

Methods

Were the methods described clearly and adequately?
Could you replicate the methods?
Did the author tell you who the subjects were?
Did you understand how many subjects were selected?
Was the selection procedure adequate for the purpose and design of the
     study?
How were the subjects divided into experimental and control groups?
Were they matched, and if so, on what variables?
In a group design study, did the author use both random selection and
     random assignment?
In a single-subject or small group study, were the subjects homogeneous
     or heterogeneous? In either case, were the individual subjects described
     in sufficient detail?
In a clinical study, did the author tell you enough about the disorder,
     its history, and measured severity?
Did the author describe the instruments and give their make and model
     numbers?
Was there information on reliability of the instruments used?
Were there sufficient descriptions of the functioning of complex and new
     instruments used in the study?
Were the instruments selected appropriate for the purposes of the study?

Were the procedures described adequately?

Did you understand what the author did and how it was done in the study?

What was the design of the study?

Was it appropriate for answering the research questions?

Was the selected design used correctly?

Were the experimental conditions arranged logically?

Did the design include adequate controls?

Did the control procedures rule out the sources of internal invalidity to a satisfactory degree?

What were the dependent and independent variables?

How were the variables measured?

How were the subjects instructed?

What were the stimulus materials?

How were the pretests and baselines established?

Were the pretreatment measures reliable?

How were the independent variables manipulated?

Were the manipulations strong and unambiguous?

Did the experimenter establish reliability and validity of the dependent variable measures? By what procedures?

Were the reliability indexes satisfactory?

Results

What were the results of the study? Were they described objectively and without evaluations and interpretations?

In a single-subject design study, did the author describe the results of individual subjects separately?

Were the single-subject results visually represented?

In a group design study, were the group performances clearly distinguished?

In small group studies, did the author summarize individual differences in results?

Did the author describe data qualitatively?

Did the author describe data quantitatively?

What were the methods of analysis?

Were they appropriate?

Did the author use statistical procedures correctly?

Did you find descriptive statistics in sufficient detail?

Did the author report the value of inferential statistical tests and their probability levels?

Were the figures, tables, and appendixes used effectively?

Was the overall data presentation orderly and logical?

Discussion

> Did the author discuss the results adequately? Did the discussion section examine the meaning and implications of the results?
>
> Did the author try to answer the research questions in light of the data?
>
> Did the author clearly state whether the hypotheses were supported or not supported by the data?
>
> Did the author relate the observations to previous findings?
>
> Did the discussion examine the theoretical implications of the results? Did it suggest applied implications? Were the applied implications specific enough? Can you implement these suggestions in your clinical practice?
>
> Did the discussion suggest additional research questions?
>
> Did the discussion summarize the problems and limitations of the study?
>
> Did the author avoid excessive speculation, fruitless debates, and questionable attempts to explain the results?
>
> Did the author accept negative findings?

Reference List

> Did the author follow the selected format in arranging the references? Was the reference list accurate?
>
> Did the author list all of the works cited in the text?
>
> Did the author not include works not cited in the text?

Appendix

> Did the author provide needed additional materials in the appendix?
>
> Was the appendix section used prudently?
>
> Was it necessary and sufficient?

The outline just given is not meant to be comprehensive, but to alert the student to some of the important questions that must be answered in evaluating a research study.

It must be evident to the student that some evaluative questions, such as those concerned with the scientific importance of an investigation, are harder than others to answer. Also, it is better to do this evaluation after all other questions have been answered. Evaluation of the introduction and literature review and procedures requires conceptual as well as technical knowledge. Evaluating the discussion section also needs broad scholarship in the subject matter. Evaluation of data presentation, reference, and appendixes needs knowledge of the accepted format, such as that of the APA.

As noted before, evaluation is a judgmental process. Though it may be difficult, the student should not hesitate in making judgments and checking them with those of others who are more knowledgeable.

EVALUATION AND APPRECIATION OF RESEARCH

Clearly, the theme of this chapter is critical evaluation of research reports. Without counteracting that theme, I should also like to state that we must learn to appreciate research. A critical consumer of research is not necessarily the one who is always looking for the perfect study. Students working on research project assignments often think that their studies must be perfect in all respects. It is good to remember that a perfect study is more easily designed than conducted. It is also good to remember that a perfect study has not been conducted yet. Studies designed by even the best researchers are not likely to be perfect.

Since all studies tend to have some limitations, it is important to be able to weigh those limitations against the strengths of a given study. In some cases, the conceptual or methodological limitations of a study can be so serious as to render the data worthless. A student must be able to recognize such limitations. On the other hand, the limitations of other studies may be such that the results are still meaningful within those limitations. A student must be able to recognize this as well.

The results of scientific studies on given issues can be arranged on a hierarchy of broad patterns and rough stages of progression. Some studies are uncontrolled, some have a certain degree of control, and others are more tightly controlled. The results of each of those studies must be evaluated in light of their limitations. For example, the results of a one-group pretest–posttest study or an *AB* single-subject study may indicate that a given treatment was followed by notable changes in certain client behaviors. That there was no control in the study is certainly a serious limitation, but the results may still be considered worthwhile. An evaluation that the treatment is worthy of further experimental manipulation is favorable as well as acceptable. On the other hand, an evaluation that the treatment and the changes in the client behaviors were causally related is favorable but not acceptable. The judgment that the results do not mean anything is unfavorable as well as questionable.

It may be helpful to distinguish serious *errors* in the design and implementation of a study from *limitations* that are a part of any research design and acceptable *compromises* that are often made in the execution of a study. Only serious errors in the design of a study invalidate the results. Design limitations, on the other hand, set limits within which meaningfulness of results can be interpreted.

It is possible to retain a critical outlook on research while maintaining a certain degree of enthusiasm for research. A critical outlook is not the same as a cynical outlook. After all, one who reads and evaluates research regularly must find some research interesting and stimulating. If not, there is no guarantee that that person will continue to read and evaluate research reports. ■

S T U D Y **G U I D E**

1 What is the difference between *understanding* and *evaluating* scientific reports?

2 Why should clinicians who are not expected to do research understand the research methods and concepts of science?

3 What kinds of difficulties do you, as a graduate student, face in understanding research articles? What can you do to overcome those difficulties?

4 What are Sidman's three criteria by which scientific studies are evaluated?

5 What is internal consistency evaluation? How is it done?

6 What is external relevance evaluation? How is it done?

7 Are there objective rules by which scientists can determine the scientific importance of data?

8 Select a journal report that you understand well. Make sure the report is of an empirical investigation (not a review or theoretical article). Using the outline of evaluation given in this chapter, evaluate the report. Have your instructor or someone knowledgeable take a look at your evaluation.

■ C H A P T E R   **15**

Ethics of Research

■ Honesty and integrity of scientists, 414

■ Effects of science on society, 416

■ The ethics of treatment evaluation, 417

■ Protection of human subjects, 420

■ Ethical issues relative to animal subjects, 427

■ Dissemination of research findings, 428

■ Study guide, 429

H istorically, the practice of science has raised many ethical issues because science is both a personal and a social activity. Science is powerful. It can change lives and living conditions. Its effect can be desirable or undesirable. The products of science can be beneficial when used by responsible individuals and agencies. But science can be dangerous in the hands of wrong people. Therefore, it is no surprise that such a powerful enterprise should be under ethical constraints. Such constraints are welcomed by both scientists and nonscientists so that the practice of science does not adversely affect individuals and society.

Scientists consider research to be an ethical activity. Scientists seek knowledge, try to solve practical problems, design new methods of treating diseases and disorders, and try to develop new technologies that benefit humankind. But they also have the responsibility of doing all of this in an honest, responsible, open, and ethically justifiable manner.

Clinical research in medicine and human service professions raises some additional ethical issues. Treatment-related research can sometimes pose a dilemma concerning the client's right to receive prompt and appropriate treatment and the profession's need to evaluate treatment procedures. Our discussion of ethical issues will consider the problems involved in clinical as well as nonclinical research.

In this chapter, I shall address six fundamental ethical issues that affect research: (1) the honesty and integrity of research scientists, (2) the effects of science on society, (3) the ethics of treatment evaluation, (4) the protection of individuals who serve as subjects in research studies, (5) ethical issues relative to animal subjects, and (6) the dissemination of research findings.

HONESTY AND INTEGRITY OF SCIENTISTS

Scientists produce data and evidence about the behavior of natural phenomena. These data and evidence constitute our knowledge of those phenomena. Normally, the reliability and validity of this knowledge are judged on methodological grounds. The results of scientific observation and experimentation are tentatively accepted when it is determined that the methods and procedures were appropriate and used correctly. Typically, in other words, faulty methods and procedures of research studies are considered to be the main source of questionable data.

There is another source of questionable data, which is more global and more difficult to determine: the personal conduct of scientists themselves. Both the scientific and the general community believe, most appropriately, that scientists are people with integrity. The observations they report are normally not suspected on personal grounds because it is believed that (1) the data and evidence scientists report are a product of honest work, (2) the methods and procedures were indeed implemented the way they were described in the report, and (3) the reported quantitative values were actually observed and recorded during the study.

A majority of scientists report only the findings of work actually done by them. Studies may have methodological problems, but scientists try to implement the selected procedures in the best possible manner. They record the quantitative value of the studied variables as truthfully as they can. Nonetheless, the history of science has occasionally documented instances of fraudulent conduct of certain scientists. Cases of fraudulent data have been uncovered in many disciplines. It is known that in 1912, an archaeologist reported the discovery of a human skull and jaw bone so different from the known forms of historic and prehistoric skulls that it forced scientists to think of a different evolutionary sequence. The skull came to be known as the "Piltdown man" because it was discovered in Piltdown Common, England (Campbell, 1976). However, during the 1950s, it became clear that a human skull and an ape jaw were used to construct the new find. Obviously, such a combination was puzzling to scientists.

In more recent years, one of the better-known cases of possible fraud is that of the famous British psychologist Cyril Burt, who claimed that intelligence is mostly inherited. His evidence was that identical twins reared in different environments are still very similar in their intelligence as measured by standardized tests (Burt, 1972). His work had a significant impact on the practice of education and on the study of intelligence and inheritance of behavioral traits. Because of what was considered to be a significant contribution to science, Burt was widely recognized as an international authority on the genetics of intelligence. He received numerous prestigious awards and was knighted by the British government.

To the surprise of the scientific community, it was reported in 1976 that Burt may have falsified much of his data on identical twins. The number of identical twin pairs he actually studied became questionable. The existence of several sets of identical twins Burt is supposed to have studied could not be documented. Whether he indeed had some of the research assistants mentioned in his publications was also questioned (Kamin, 1974; "Taint of," 1976).

Although outright fraud in terms of cooked-up data is not discovered frequently, subtle distortions in the results and their interpretations are more commonly found. There may be actual or perceived pressure to produce certain kinds of data. Some scientists who are well known for their theories may be especially under this kind of pressure. It is not uncommon that a particular laboratory typically produces data that are consistent with one viewpoint, whereas another laboratory equally typically produces contradictory data on the same issue. It is believed that some hired research assistants are prone to distort the data they collect on behalf of professors and scientists whose theories are widely accepted (Diener & Crandall, 1978; Shaughnessy & Zechmeister, 1985).

As we discussed in Chapter 3, a public position taken by a scientist in the form of theories and hypotheses can create pressure to uphold those positions regardless of the actual data. Instead of contradicting his or her previously stated positions, the scientist may resort to distortions in observations and interpretations of data. One way of avoiding the personally troublesome situation of having to contradict oneself is to refrain from prematurely committing oneself to a particular viewpoint.

It must be recognized that many scientists will not hesitate to reverse themselves or modify their positions in light of new data. Scientists are expected to say only what their data suggest, and those who practice this are the exemplary ones whom students and other scientists should emulate.

It must also be recognized that a commitment to a viewpoint or a philosophy cannot be avoided forever. Accumulated experimental data have theoretical as well as philosophical implications, and they cannot and should not be ignored. Commitment to a viewpoint at a time when replicated experimental data have accumulated can reduce the chances of having to contradict oneself too soon.

It should be clear, too, that particular viewpoints and experimental data can be questioned inappropriately. In such cases, defense of those viewpoints and data is appropriate. A scientist has every right to defend his or her position and point out the inappropriateness of apparently contradictory positions.

As we noted in Chapter 3, the tendency to value data and evidence more than a particular point of view is characteristic of all good scientists. Within the best traditions of science, scientists do not try to "prove" or "disprove" any particular viewpoint. Instead, they seek truth. It is only as a byproduct of this search that a particular viewpoint is either supported or rejected.

EFFECTS OF SCIENCE ON SOCIETY

The effects of science and research on society are also an ethical issue. Generally speaking, scientific research is for the good of society, but like all desirable ventures, it can produce some bad side effects. Such bad effects have become increasingly clear in the natural sciences.

Atomic research has vastly increased our knowledge of the physical world and has produced various kinds of benefits, including improved medical treatment procedures, but it has also increased the chances of the annihilation of humankind. Genetic research has helped us better understand the mysteries of life, with many desirable effects on society, but it has also raised the prospects of new and dangerous forms of life being inadvertently created. The chemical sciences have formulated new chemicals that are effective in treating various diseases, killing pests, and destroying crop-threatening weeds, but they have also adversely affected life in a chemically polluted world. Ethical issues such as these are complex, since the risk/benefit ratio must be weighed carefully and objectively. Unfortunately, objectivity in this case is more easily preached than practiced.

Scientists face a tremendous challenge in this case. On one hand, they are asked to solve a variety of problems so that life can be prolonged and its quality improved. On the other hand, they are asked to accomplish it in such a manner that no undesirable side effects emerge. Regardless of such societal demands, scientists are committed to increasing their knowledge and improving the quality of life with the least amount of risk to the society. They have an obligation to assess the amount of both the long-term and the short-term risks of their research efforts and devise methods to eliminate or reduce those risks. Conducting atomic explosions in underground sites and developing chemicals that eat up other kinds of deadly chemical wastes illustrate this kind of effort on the part of scientists.

THE ETHICS OF TREATMENT EVALUATION

A special concern of clinical researchers is the effects of experimentation on clients who seek professional services. The concern is serious in the evaluation of treatment. An apparent ethical dilemma is whether to experiment or not experiment with different treatment procedures. It is sometimes suggested that clients should be treated and not experimented upon. This suggestion implies that experimental treatments are somehow more detrimental to clients than nonexperimental treatments.

A closer examination of the issue reveals that the distinction between experimental and nonexperimental treatments may be less meaningful than that between effective and ineffective (or dangerous) treatments. It is the ineffective or dangerous treatment that is detrimental to clients regardless of whether it is considered experimental or routine. Therefore, what is unethical is the practice of ineffective or dangerous treatment procedures.

When is a treatment experimental? This question is easily answered when a clinician calls a treatment experimental. The clinician then systematically collects data, uses certain control procedures, and thus tries to evaluate the effects of a particular treatment procedure. The effects may be positive, and the clients may have benefited just as much as those under an equally effective but routine treatment procedure. However, what about the use of a treatment procedure whose effects have never been experimentally evaluated? Is this an experiment? Most people tend to think that as long as a procedure is more or less routine, and it is not called experimental by the clinicians who use it, it is not experimental. This assumption has created a false issue of ethics in treatment research.

As pointed out by Barlow, Hayes, and Nelson (1984), a treatment may be considered research or experimental when the clinician systematically collects data during the course of the treatment. Experimental treatment always involves operational definitions of the procedures, objective goals and criteria, and systematic collection of data to evaluate the effects of treatment. On the other hand, when the clinician uses a certain procedure routinely, does not collect data, and assumes that it is effective, it is more likely to be considered treatment. Even more importantly, when the treatment procedure is not clearly defined, the goals are subjectively stated, and the improvement criteria are not specified, most people may not consider that treatment experimental.

In speech–language pathology, the practice of many treatment procedures is not based on experimental evaluations. Apparently, the practice of those procedures is based on clinical traditions and experiences. In many cases it is much worse, as pointed out by Minifie (1983): "our clinical strategies . . . are based upon trial-and-error empiricism and clinical hunch, rather than upon a strong scientific data base" (p. 31). The trial-and-error approach may constitute an endless series of errors. When a clinical hunch is wrong, nothing better may be available, and therefore the same ineffective practice may be perpetuated. Presumably, ineffective procedures continue to be used because the clinician either does not know that the technique does not help clients or cannot implement a better procedure. Oddly enough, not many ethical concerns are raised about this kind of clinical practice.

Another kind of clinical practice is also oblivious of ethical concerns: that based on complex, impressive, but nevertheless speculative theories. These theories are a collection of unverified hypotheses but are not recognized as such. Theories of this kind are sometimes so prestigious that in the judgment of many clinicians, a treatment procedure that works well but is not a part of an accepted theory must be discarded. This is what Perkins (1986) has called the "malfunctions" of a theory. The converse may also be practiced. If a procedure does not seem to work, but a theory suggests that it should, then the technique and the theory may both be kept. Unfortunately, this practice puts both service and knowledge in jeopardy.

It is when clinicians wish to determine the effects of treatment objectively that ethical concerns seem to be pressing. Addressing this issue, Barlow et al. (1984) stated that "indeed, our current societal posture at times seems to assume that if the intervention is poorly specified; goals are unclear; and if measures are weak, infrequent, or nonexistent, then there is *less* of an ethical worry. Our own cultural ambivalence about science has turned vice into virtue, sloppiness into safety" (p. 285).

The ethics of treatment evaluation involves at least three related issues. The first is whether treatment evaluation is necessary. The second is whether treatment evaluation is ethically justified. The third is whether treatment and treatment research are different kinds of activities. I shall briefly address these three issues.

The question whether treatment evaluation is necessary may not sound like an ethical issue, but it is at the heart of the ethical controversy. Those who question the ethics of treatment evaluation imply that it is not necessary.

When the necessity of treatment research with regard to a particular disorder is questioned, two assumptions may be implied. The first assumption is that an effective procedure to treat that disorder already exists and that the effects are objectively documented. The second assumption is that there is no room to improve the efficacy of that procedure. In many cases, one or both of these assumptions may be mistaken. Many diseases and disorders do not have effective treatments. Also, the efficacy of effective treatments can perhaps be improved by controlled research. In case of communicative disorders, no one asserts that we have perfectly effective treatment procedures that cannot be improved upon. When we need effective procedures, and we need to know that we are using effective procedures, then there is no choice but to experiment.

If it is concluded that treatment evaluation is necessary and that it is no more harmful to clients than are unverified procedures that might actually be ineffective or dangerous, then the second issue, whether treatment evaluation is ethically justified, appears in a different light. Obviously, treatment evaluation is justified. Indeed, it has been argued that systematic and objective evaluation of treatment procedures is one of the ethical responsibilities of clinical professions (Barlow et al., 1984; Perkins, 1985). Continued practice of treatment procedures whose effects are not objectively documented must be considered ethically objectionable. Whether a treatment is old or new is not of consequence. Procedures that have been used widely and for a long time may still be ineffective and hence detrimental to clients. When seen from this standpoint, whether clinicians should experiment with their treatment procedures is a false question.

It may be sometimes assumed that experiments that produce no effects or negative effects are of greater ethical concern than those that produce positive effects. Therefore, when treatments are evaluated and the results are nonexistent or negative, the clients may be said to have been used as "guinea pigs." This logic is also faulty in that the same procedure, used routinely, may not raise the same ethical question. Experiments showing that certain procedures are not useful or even harmful may prevent the widespread use of such procedures. Therefore, the outcome of an experimental treatment is hardly a basis on which to judge the ethics of clinical experimentation. Efforts at empirical determination of the positive, neutral, or negative effects of treatment procedures is a necessary and ethical activity of clinicians. We know only when we evaluate a technique. As pointed out by Barlow et al. (1984, p. 287), systematic "evaluation [of a treatment] is not what makes it experimental. It just keeps us from fooling ourselves when it is."

The third issue, whether routine treatment and controlled treatment evaluation are different kinds of activities, has been discussed occasionally (Siegel and Spradlin, 1985). When it is concluded that they are different, ethical concerns emerge. If treatment evaluation is inherently different from treatment, then is there a justification for subjecting clients who need treatment to something other than treatment? There is no question that in some specific respects, controlled evaluation of treatment can differ from routine treatment. However, the difference does not lead to the conclusion that treatment evaluation is unjustified. Before a procedure is used as routine treatment, it must undergo treatment evaluation. Therefore, treatment and treatment evaluation ought to be different, and both are necessary.

The discussion so far is not intended to suggest that there are no ethical problems in conducting treatment research. There are such problems, but they arise only because of the necessity of experimental treatment evaluations. In other words, whether clinicians should experimentally evaluate their procedures is not an ethical or otherwise valid question. The answer to that question is yes, and therefore we have ethical concerns.

In evaluating treatment effects, the researcher must take precautions to reduce the risk, if any, to the clients who serve as subjects. In fact, steps to reduce the risks to human subjects must be taken in all kinds of research, not just clinical treatment research. We shall now turn to this important ethical issue.

PROTECTION OF HUMAN SUBJECTS

In this section, I shall address the issue of protection of human subjects in general and, when appropriate, point out special ethical considerations relative to clinical treatment research.

Responsible scientists have always been concerned with the welfare of individuals who serve as subjects in various medical, biological, behavioral, and other kinds of experiments. Scientists have known that the need to produce knowledge that will benefit humankind must be balanced with the risks that such an enterprise might pose to the human subjects. Nonetheless, abuses of human subjects have occurred, especially in such institutional settings as mental hospitals, prisons, and military research installations (Metz & Folkins, 1985). Fortunately, the National Research Act, signed into law in 1974, has been a significant instrument in promoting the welfare of human subjects in research studies. Revised and expanded federal regulations have been published in 1981 (Federal Register, January 16, 1981).

Professional organizations such as the American Psychological Association (APA) have also been concerned with the protection of human subjects in research. In 1973, the APA published its own ethical guidelines on the use of human subjects. The guidelines were revised in 1982. Metz and Folkins (1985) have provided a brief historical account of the federal government's role in the protection of human subjects along with a discussion of the issues in speech and hearing research.

The federal regulations to protect human subjects apply only to investigations funded by the United States Department of Health and Human

Services (HHS). However, all branches and agencies of the federal government that support research may adopt the HHS guidelines in the near future (Metz & Folkins, 1985). Under the current regulations, research involving common educational techniques, educational tests, surveys and interviews, observation of public behaviors, and the use of existing data may be exempt from the human subject protection procedures (Federal Register, January 16, 1981).

Although human subject protection procedures are not required by law, most research institutions, including universities and hospitals, have established them even for those research studies that are not supported by government funds. The federal regulations were designed to protect research subjects as well as the investigators and their institutions. Therefore, most institutions and agencies that support research require that some form of human subject protection procedures be followed in conducting research studies.

The most salient feature of the human subject protection procedures is the review of research proposals by an Institutional Review Board (IRB). Most colleges and universities have multiple IRBs functioning at the level of a department and the school in which the department is housed. Usually, there is also a university-wide IRB, which receives reports from IRBs at the lower levels.

It is now standard practice to submit all research procedures to one of these IRBs, which are also known as Human Subjects Committees. These committees or boards review the proposal to determine whether the study poses any risk to the subjects and if it does, what steps must be taken to reduce it. The human subjects committee may also deny approval to carry out a study on the basis of unacceptable risks to the participants, but this is rare.

Since human subject protection procedures apply only to individuals who participate in research and not to routine clinical or educational procedures, a clear understanding of the legal concept of research is necessary. According to the regulations, any systematic investigation designed to develop or contribute to generalizable knowledge is research. If the purpose is to treat a client but no attempt to produce knowledge is contemplated, then it is not research. In such cases, new treatment procedures may be used without institutional review of the procedures. However, if the clinician plans to determine the effects under controlled conditions and publish the results in order to make a scientific contribution, then it is research and the proposal must be reviewed by an IRB.

All theses and dissertation proposals are routinely submitted to an IRB. A clinician who is not sure whether an undertaking contains an element of research or is simply a routine clinical procedure should submit a written description of the activities to an IRB for review and advice.

Institutional Review Boards must have at least five individuals. The HHS regulations also stipulate that IRBs should contain at least one person who is not a scientist, and one person who is not affiliated with the institution where the research will be conducted. The person without a scientific background may also be the one not affiliated with the institution. Most college and university IRBs that review in-house proposals that do not receive funds from HHS do not recruit members from outside the university. Proposals that do not involve risks to subjects may also be reviewed by one or two members of a university department's review committee, and a report of this action made to a higher, fully constituted IRB. When risks are involved, such expeditious reviews are not allowed. Studies that pose risks may be reviewed by multiple IRBs within an institution. The author of a research proposal may be asked to speak to the committee but does not take part in the review process.

The major concerns of an IRB in reviewing research proposals include the risk/benefit ratio, informed consent, and the privacy of the participants.

Risk/Benefit Ratio

It is assumed that participation in any kind of research may involve risk to the subjects. Some of the risks may be psychological. For example, research involving the experimental evaluation of the effects of shock or white noise on stuttering may create emotional stress or anxiety in stutterers. The procedures may also create physical harm or injury. Certain other procedures may cause social embarrassment. For example, a study may be designed to evaluate the maintenance of target behaviors in natural settings. A stutterer's treated fluency may be monitored in a supermarket, where the client may be forced into speaking in difficult situations. In medical research, new medical or surgical treatment procedures may pose significant risks to the lives of the patients.

In this case, the IRB's task is to determine whether the study poses risks to subjects, and if so, whether it is minimal, and if not, how to handle the unacceptable level of risk. It is judged that the risk is minimal when the expected level of risk does not exceed the level experienced in daily life situations. As a rough guideline, the amount of risk (stress) experienced while taking ordinary psychological or physical tests is considered minimal. In such cases, an IRB may give quick approval to the study.

When the risk is judged to be more than minimal, the IRB does not necessarily deny permission to conduct the study. Instead, it reviews the procedures set forth by the investigator to handle that risk. The IRB may suggest modifications in the procedure. The intensity of potentially damaging experimental stimuli such as shock and noise may be limited. The subjects may be allowed to determine the intensity levels presented to them. Stutterers may not be taken to social situations to test their fluency until after they have demonstrated fluency in more controlled, less embarrassing situations.

Potential risks to certain populations, such as children, may be viewed more conservatively. Whether the subjects are children or adults, an IRB may suggest less stressful methods of data collection or, when this is not possible, require constant and professional monitoring of the subjects' reactions to the experimental procedures. For example, the IRB may require the presence of a physician or a clinical psychologist when the experimental procedures are thought to cause physical or psychological stress. The IRB may also require that the experiment be terminated when unacceptable levels of emotional reactions are shown by subjects.

The IRBs evaluate not only the potential risks but also the potential scientific benefits. It is important to realize that the scientific benefit, not the benefit to the participant, is what is evaluated. Other factors being equal, a research study that provides no benefits to the subjects may be approved as long as the study is expected to generate scientific information. However, in this context, IRBs face a difficult task because they are generally not expected to evaluate the methodological or theoretical soundness of the studies they review. When it is considered appropriate, an IRB may seek an independent evaluation of the proposal's scientific merits from qualified scientists.

The federal regulations and the guidelines of professional organizations and universities are not designed to prevent all research studies that pose risks to human participants. Rather, they are intended to make sure that adequate protective measures are taken when there is risk. Many research studies that do pose various levels of risk to the participants are considered valuable from the standpoint of scientific knowledge and eventual benefit to people. It may be noted that many people volunteer for risky experiments that may eventually benefit society. Those who volunteer for experimental medical or surgical treatments such as new drug evaluations, organ transplants, and artificial heart surgeries are a case in point.

Most research studies in speech–language pathology and audiology involve only a minimal risk to subjects, and many clinical treatment studies actually improve the client's clinical conditions.

Informed Consent

A person's informed consent to participate voluntarily in research is one of the most important ethical principles of research. Informed consent involves three components. First, the subjects must fully understand the procedures of the study as far as their participation is concerned. Second, they must freely and voluntarily consent to participate in the study. Third, the subjects must be free to withdraw from the study at any time with no consequence.

It must be noted that potential subjects should not be contacted until after the approval of the IRB. This is because the method of subject contact itself may involve some coercion. For example, an instructor may ask his students to participate in an experiment in such a way as to imply that a lack of participation may have punitive consequences. A clinician may ask clients to participate in an experimental treatment while giving the impression that no other treatment is available. Therefore, an IRB must screen the method by which the potential subjects are initially contacted.

In obtaining informed consent from potential subjects, the researcher must fully describe the procedures and purposes of the study. The individuals must know what is expected of them, what kinds of stimulus conditions they will be exposed to, what kinds of responses they will be asked to make, and how long they need to participate in the study. They must understand the risks and benefits of participation. In clinical treatment research, the availability of alternative treatment procedures must be specified. When the risk is more than minimal, the possibilities of compensation must also be described. The potential subjects must be informed of the names of persons (other than the author) they may contact about the research. The potential subjects must understand that participation is entirely voluntary and that they are free to withdraw from the study at any stage with no penalty or prejudice. Finally, the individuals contacted must be told whether and to what extent their anonymity will be protected during and after the study.

The potential subjects must have all the information in writing. They usually sign their name on the same document, called the informed consent form, to indicate their willingness to participate in the study. The writing must be simple and nontechnical so that the individuals can understand the full implications of their participation. When the subjects are children, parents give informed consent. Children 7 to 18 years old may also sign the informed consent form along with their parents. The children must be informed at a level appropriate for them to understand the procedures. Special efforts are needed to make sure that communicatively handicapped individuals understand the procedures of a study before deciding to participate.

The Problem of Full Disclosure

Some of the requirements of informed consent can create potential problems for many research studies. The most important of these problems is the scientific consequence of informing the subjects about certain procedures and their expected effects.

When the subjects are given the full details of the purposes and procedures of certain treatment techniques, a biasing effect may be created. This effect may then confound the effects of the treatment itself. For example, if stutterers are told that the purpose of the experiment is to decrease their stuttering by saying "no" every time they stutter, some subjects may be able to monitor their stuttering more carefully. Such monitoring may produce its own effect on the frequency of stuttering.

A verbal conditioning study has documented the effects of disclosing the purpose of an experiment to the subjects (Resnick & Schwartz, 1973). In this study, one group of subjects was told that the purpose was to increase a certain class of verbal behaviors by verbal reinforcers, which was the actual purpose of the study. Another group was simply told that the purpose was to study certain aspects of communication. The group that was informed of the actual purpose of the experiment did not show an increase in behaviors that were followed by the experimenter's verbal stimuli, whereas the group that was not informed showed the typical increase.

There are also research questions that cannot be answered unless the purposes of a study are concealed. For example, if a psychologist studies anger in a contrived laboratory situation, telling the potential subjects about the purpose and the procedure of the study may make it impossible to subsequently evoke anger. Similarly, if a psychologist studies the conditions under which people express surprise, full disclosure of the stimuli to be used in evoking surprise will leave nothing to study. In clinical studies of covert measurement (see Chapter 5), the clients are not supposed to know that their behavior is being measured. However, telling a stutterer that his or her stuttering will be measured in a particular situation negates covert measurement.

Many researchers in the past have not fully disclosed the purpose and the procedures of their studies to the subjects. This has raised the ethical question of deception (Kelman, 1972; Milgram, 1977). Deception may be mild or extreme. A general description of the purpose and procedure may be provided while some crucial information is withheld from the subjects. Deception may also involve total misrepresentation of the purposes of the study. A certain degree of deception or misrepresentation that does not create additional risks to the subjects and that is considered absolutely essential to the study may be acceptable. As in the case of all adverse procedures, the judgment will be based on the risk/benefit ratio. The potential harm from lack of full disclosure must be weighed against the scientific benefits of the study.

Subjects who are not informed of some aspects of the study must be *debriefed* as soon as their participation is over. In debriefing, the subjects are given a full description of the actual purposes and procedures of the study with an explanation as to why the information was withheld from them until the end of their participation. This is done to avoid any potential negative effects of the experimental procedures and the deception. For example, individuals who were made to experience anxiety, anger, or some other strong emotion in front of an audience may feel better when they find out the true nature of the experiment.

The Privacy of the Subjects

The privacy of the subjects of research studies is another important ethical issue. Clinicians know that the privacy or confidentiality of clients is an important professional issue regardless of research concerns. Like clinicians, research investigators must take every possible step to protect the privacy of their subjects.

Most research studies are published in one form or another. Publication will include descriptions of subjects. Therefore, the subjects must give informed consent to such publication. The typical procedure is to inform the subjects that their confidentiality will be protected when the studies are published. In most cases, the subjects' name and other identifying data will not be published.

In some situations, subject identity will be revealed in certain kinds of publications. For example, the picture of a client may be a part of a research article showing various physical characteristics of certain genetic syndromes. In such cases, explicit written permission to publish pictures must be obtained from the clients, their guardians, or both. Similar permission must be obtained when audiotaped or videotaped materials are expected to be published in some form. Most speech and hearing centers routinely obtain such permission from the clients, their guardians, or both. This procedure facilitates the future research use of client information.

Throughout the study, information obtained about individuals, their families, institutions, and organizations must be kept strictly confidential. The subjects must be informed of the procedures by which the confidentiality of the subjects and institutions will be maintained. An investigator may propose, for example, that the individuals will be coded and the names of the subjects will not be used in any stage of data analysis. Access to confidential information about individuals may be restricted. Only the principal investigator may know the names of the subjects. An IRB may find that the safeguards need improvement and make suggestions to that effect. Eventually, the potential subjects or their guardians judge for themselves whether the proposed methods of protecting confidentiality are acceptable.

The ethical issues discussed in this chapter are not always amenable to objective and unambiguous resolution. The regulations and guidelines do recognize the difficulty involved in assessing the risk/benefit ratio, the need for deception, and the possibilities of the invasion of privacy of research subjects. The investigator and the IRB make the best possible judgments, taking all of the important factors into consideration.

As we have noted, IRBs are responsible for making sure that individuals who serve as subjects in research studies are treated fairly and honestly. However, the presence of such boards and committees does not reduce the responsibility of the investigator. It is the investigator who is ultimately responsible for his or her conduct in the course of research investigations. Most authors propose research studies with adequate safeguards already built into them. The IRBs have to trust the authors in following the approved procedures. When a violation occurs, the IRB does not have the power to take punitive steps against the investigator. The authorities of the institution where violations occurred must handle them.

ETHICAL ISSUES RELATIVE TO ANIMAL SUBJECTS

We have concentrated on the ethical treatment of human subjects in this chapter because of the preponderance of research involving human subjects in speech and hearing. However, ethical guidelines must also be followed when animal subjects are used in research.

Animals are frequently used in many laboratory and field experiments. Research studies in medicine, biology, ethology, psychology, and pharmaceutics involve animals. Most new drugs are first used with animal subjects. New surgical procedures are often experimentally performed on animals. When the effects of new chemicals (other than drugs) are studied, once again animals are the primary subjects. In behavioral and psychological research, animals have been subjected to various stimuli under both normal and altered neurophysiological structures. Any new research on the brain that involves an invasive procedure is first tried out on animals. Monkeys, rats, mice, cats, dogs, and fish are often used in these experiments.

In communicative disorders, the use of animal subjects is limited. However, there are special problems that are studied with animals. In the study of the evolution and functioning of phonation, various species of animals are studied. Some of these studies may involve surgical procedures to analyze the structures of phonatory mechanisms. Animals are probably more frequently used in the study of audition. Chinchillas, for example, have been used frequently in the study of hearing because their auditory mechanism is similar to that of humans.

The appropriateness of using animals in potentially dangerous experiments has been an issue in recent years (Larsen, 1982; Rosenfeld, 1981; Wade, 1976). Advocates of animal rights have argued that many scientific experiments in which animals are subjected to painful procedures are unethical and should be banned. Those who justify the use of animal experiments remind us that many life-saving drugs, vaccines, and surgical procedures would not have been developed without animal experimentation.

It is quite possible that animals will continue to be used as subjects in scientific experiments. Therefore, the need to follow ethical guidelines in the care of laboratory animals is clear. There are various local, state, and federal laws pertaining to the use of animals in scientific research. The American Psychological Association (1981) has published guidelines on the care and use of animals in research laboratories. These guidelines suggest that the acquisition, care, use, and disposal of animals must follow federal, state, and local laws. The guidelines specify that those who engage in animal experimentation receive special training in the care of animal subjects. The experimenters are expected to minimize discomfort, illness, deprivation, stress, and pain due to the experimental procedures. Scientists must make sure that before animals are subjected to such procedures, alternative methods are considered. Painful or stressful procedures must be justified in terms of the scientific, educational, or applied benefit. While in the custody of scientists, animals must receive humane care.

DISSEMINATION OF RESEARCH FINDINGS

In the final analysis, research is justified when it is worthwhile in some empirical sense. The worth of a piece of research is judged by other scientists, and when possible, by the society at large. However, people, including scientists, can make this judgment only when research findings are disseminated. In this sense, dissemination of research findings is an ethical responsibility of researchers.

One can argue that if research findings are never going to be published, any amount of risk that the subjects experience is unacceptable. Even when no risk is involved, efforts are involved. As subjects, individuals give their time for research. Many experience inconvenience because of their participation in research. Individuals are expected to volunteer for research on the assumption that they contribute to the advancement of scientific knowledge. Unpublished results, unfortunately, do not advance scientific knowledge.

The information generated by scientific studies must receive the widest possible dissemination and the most appropriate dissemination. A majority of scientific studies are appropriately first published in scientific journals. When certain findings are technical and subject to misunderstanding by the general public, it may not be desirable to publish those findings in popular media. When it is judged that the findings of a treatment study are highly tentative, it may not be appropriate to disseminate them to potential clients who may be candidates for that or similar treatment. Most scientists prefer that the initial findings be published in a scientific or professional journal so that other experts can evaluate those findings and, if possible, replicate them. Scientists typically react negatively to publications of "new" and "revolutionary" scientific findings and clinical treatment procedures in popular media. Scientifically well-established findings, of course, must receive the widest possible dissemination. Such findings may be published in popular sources as well.

In conclusion, it may be stated that when scientists pay due attention to the ethical principles that govern research and publication, a responsible practice of science emerges. Ethical principles are meant to reduce the undesirable side effects of scientific research and thereby increase the potential of benefit to humankind. Every researcher must be fully knowledgeable in ethical principles so that the practice of science will be as responsible as its products are enlightening. ■

S T U D Y **G U I D E**

1 What are the sources of questionable data?

2 How are theories and hypotheses related to the questions of reliability and validity of data?

3 Describe some of the undesirable side effects of science and technology. What steps do you suggest to counteract them?

4 What is an apparent ethical dilemma of clinical experimentation?

5 When is a treatment experimental?

6 What are some of the false questions relative to the ethics of clinical experimentation?

7 Is the question "Should we experiment with treatment procedures or not?" ethically or otherwise valid? Justify your answer.

8 Can you experiment with an untested treatment procedure that has been used widely over a number of years? Why or why not?

9 Does the practice of a treatment procedure, when it is not called experimental, raise questions of ethics? Under what conditions are such questions likely to be raised?

10 What is "research" according to the National Research Act?

11 What is an Institutional Review Board?

12 How is the membership of an Institutional Review Board constituted?

13 What are the major concerns of an Institutional Review Board?

14 What is a risk–benefit ratio? How is it determined? In this process, whose risk and whose benefits are evaluated?

15 Does the presence of risk to the subjects automatically mean that a study cannot be conducted? Justify your answer.

16 What are the three components of informed consent?

17 Can you contact potential subjects before obtaining permission from an Institutional Review Board? Justify your answer.

18 You wish to evaluate a stuttering treatment program using one of the group designs. Describe the procedures for obtaining informed consent from your subjects.

(continued next page)

Study Guide *(continued)*

19 What are the problems of full disclosure? How would you handle them?

20 What procedures would you use in protecting the privacy of your clients who participate in research studies?

REFERENCES

Altman, J. (1974). Observational study of behavior: sampling methods. *Behavior, 7,* 227–267.

American Psychological Association. (1981). Ethical principles of psychologists. *American Psychologist, 36,* 633–638.

American Psychological Association. (1982). *Ethical principles in the conduct of research with human participants.* Washington, DC: Author.

American Psychological Association. (1983). *Publication manual of the American Psychological Association* (3rd ed.). Washington, DC: Author.

Bachrach, A. J. (1969). *Psychological research: An introduction.* New York: Random House.

Baer, D. M., Wolf, M. M., & Risley, T. R. (1968). Some current dimensions of applied behavior analysis. *Journal of Applied Behavior Analysis, 10,* 117, 119.

Baker, S. (1981). *The practical stylist* (2nd ed.). New York: Harper & Row.

Bannister, D. (1966). Psychology as an exercise in paradox. *Bulletin of British Psychological Society, 19,* 21–26.

Barlow, D. H. & Hayes, S. C. (1979). Alternating treatments design: One strategy for comparing the effects of two treatments in a single subject. *Journal of Applied Behavior Analysis, 12,* 199–210.

Barlow, D. H., Hayes, S. C., & Nelson, R. O. (1984). *The scientist practitioner: Research and accountability in clinical and educational settings.* New York: Pergamon.

Barlow, D. H. & Hersen, M. (1984). *Single case experimental designs* (2nd ed.). New York: Pergamon.

Barrass, R. (1978). *Scientists must write.* New York: Wiley.

Bates, J. D. (1980). *Writing with precision.* Washington, DC: Acropolis.

Batten, M. (1968). *Discovery by chance: Science and the unexpected.* New York: Funk & Wagnalls.

Bauer, H. (1985). Single-subject research designs in communicative interaction and disorders. In R. D. Kent (Ed.), Application of research to assessment and therapy. *Seminars in Speech and Language, 6,* 67–102.

Bloodstein, O. (1980). *Handbook on stuttering.* Chicago: National Easter Seal Society.

Bracht, G. H. & Glass, G. V. (1968). The external validity of experiments. *American Educational Research Journal, 5,* 437–474.

Brinton, B. & Fujiki, M. (1984). Development of topic manipulation skills in discourse. *Journal of Speech and Hearing Research, 27,* 350–358.

Brown, R. (1973). *A first language: The early stages.* Cambridge, MA: Harvard University Press.

Browning, R. M. (1967). A same-subject design for simultaneous comparison of three reinforcement contingencies. *Behavior Research and Therapy, 5,* 237–243.

Burt, C. (1972). Inheritance of general intelligence. *American Psychologist, 27,* 175–190.

Campbell, B. G. (1976). *Humankind emerging.* Boston: Little, Brown.

Campbell, D. T., & Stanley, J. C. (1966). *Experimental and quasi-experimental designs for research.* Chicago: Rand McNally.

Campbell, N. (1952). *What is science?* New York: Dover.

Cannon, W. (1945). *The way of an investigator.* New York: W. W. Norton.

Capelli, R. (1985). An experimental analysis of morphologic acquisition. Unpublished master's thesis, California State University, Fresno.

Chomsky, N. (1957). *Syntactic structures.* The Hague: Mouton.

Christensen, L. B. (1980). *Experimental methodology* (2nd ed.). Boston: Allyn & Bacon.

Cohen, L. H. (1979). The research readership and information source reliance of clinical psychologists. *Professional Psychology, 10,* 780–786.

Connell, P. J. & Thompson, C. K. (1986). Flexibility of single-subject experimental designs. Part III: Using flexibility to design or modify experiments. *Journal of Speech and Hearing Disorders, 51,* 214–225.

Cook, T. D. & Campbell, D. T. (1979). *Quasi-experimental design: Design and analysis issues for field settings.* Chicago: Rand McNally.

Costello, J. M. (1979). Clinician and researcher: A necessary dichotomy? *Journal of National Student Speech and Hearing Association, 7,* 6–26.

Costello, J. M., Punch, J., Schery, T., & Schriberg, L. (1984). Asha interviews. *Asha, 26,* 27–36.

Curtis, J. F. & Schultz, M. C. (1986). *Basic laboratory instrumentation for speech and hearing.* Boston: Little, Brown.

De Cesari, R. (1985). Experimental training of grammatic morphemes: Effects on the order of acquisition. Unpublished master's thesis, California State University, Fresno.

Diener, E. & Crandall, R. (1978). *Ethics in social and behavioral research.* Chicago: University of Chicago.

Eddington, E. S. (1967). Statistical inference from N=1 experiments. *Journal of Psychology, 65,* 195–199.

Edwards, A. L. (1960). *Experimental design in psychological research* (rev. ed.). New York: Rinehart.

Feldman, A. S. (1981). The challenge of autonomy. *Asha, 23,* 941–946.

Feldman, A. S. (1984). In support of the professional doctorate. *Asha, 26,* 25–33.

Ferster, C. B., & Skinner, B. F. (1957). *Schedules of reinforcement.* New York: Appleton-Century-Crofts.

Fisher, R. A. (1925). *Statistical methods for research workers.* London: Oliver & Boyd.

Fisher, R. A. (1942). *Design of experiments.* London: Oliver & Boyd.

Fisher, R. A. (1956). *Statistical methods and scientific inference.* London: Oliver & Boyd.

Flower, R. M. (1983). Keynote address: Looking backwards and looking forward: Some views through a four-decade window. In N. S. Rees & T. L. Snope, (Eds.), *Proceedings of the 1983 national conference on undergraduate, graduate, and continuing education.* (pp. 9–15). Washington, DC: ASHA Reports no.13.

Follet, W. (1966). *Modern American usage.* New York: Hill & Wang.

Freeman, H. E. (1977). The present status of evaluation research. In M. Guttentag (Ed.). *Evaluation studies annual review.* Beverly Hills: Sage Publications.

Gadlin, H. & Ingle, G. (1975). Through the one-way mirror: The limits of experimental self-reflection. *American Psychologist, 30,* 1003–1009.

Gittleman-Foster, N. (1983). Observer reliability in the measurement of dysfluencies with trained and untrained observers. Unpublished master's thesis, California State university, Fresno.

Glass, G. V., Wilson, V. L., & Gottman, J. M. (1974). *Design and analysis of time-series experiments.* Boulder: Colorado Associated University Press.

Goldstein, H. (1984). Effects of modeling and corrected practice on generative language learning of preschool children. *Journal of Speech and Hearing Disorders, 49,* 389–398.

Goodman, N. (1967). The epistemological argument. *Synthese, 17,* 23–28.

Grmek, M. D. (1981). A plea for freeing the history of scientific discoveries from myth. In M. D. Grmek, R. S. Cohen, & G. Cymino (Eds.), *On scientific discovery* (pp. 9–42). London: D. Reidel.

Hargis, C. H. (1977). *English syntax.* Springfield, IL: Charles C Thomas.

Hartman, D. P. & Hall, R. V. (1976). The changing criterion design. *Journal of Applied Behavior Analysis, 9,* 537–532.

Hayes, S. C. (1981). Single-case experimental design and empirical clinical practice. *Journal of Consulting and Clinical Psychology, 49,* 193–211.

Hegde, M. N. (1980a). Issues in the study and explanation of language behavior. *Journal of Psycholinguistic Research, 9,* 1–22.

Hegde, M. N. (1980b). An experimental-clinical analysis of grammatical and behavioral distinctions between verbal auxiliary and copula. *Journal of Speech and Hearing Research, 23,* 864–877.

Hegde, M. N. (1985). *Treatment procedures in communicative disorders.* San Diego: Little, Brown/College-Hill Press.

Hegde, M. N., Noll, M. J., & Pecora, R. (1978). A study of some factors affecting generalization of language training. *Journal of Speech and Hearing Disorders, 44,* 301–320.

Horner, R. D., & Baer, D. M. (1978). Multiple probe technique: A variation of the multiple baseline. *Journal of Applied Behavior Analysis, 11,* 189–196.

Howie, P. M., Woods, C. L., & Andrews, G. (1982). Relationship between covert and overt speech measures immediately before and immediately after stuttering treatment. *Journal of Speech and Hearing Disorders, 47,* 419–422.

Huck, W. S., Cormier, W. H., & Bounds, W. G., Jr. (1974). *Reading statistics and research.* New York: Harper & Row.

Hurtig, R. (1977). Toward a functional theory of discourse. In R. O. Freedle (Ed.), *Discourse production and comprehension.* Norwood, NJ: Ablex.

Ingham, R. (1984). *Stuttering and behavior therapy: Current status and experimental foundations.* San Diego: College-Hill Press.

Johnson, W. (1955). A study of the onset and development of stuttering. In W. Johnson & R. R. Leutenegger (Eds.), *Stuttering in children and adults.* Minneapolis: University of Minnesota.

Johnson, W. & associates (1959). *The onset of stuttering.* Minneapolis: University of Minnesota.

Johnston, J. M. & Pennypacker, H. S. (1980). *Strategies and tactics of human behavioral research.* Hillsdale, NJ.: Lawrence Erlbaum.

Kamin, L. J. (1974). *The science and politics of I. Q.* Hillsdale, NJ: Lawrence Erlbaum.

Kazdin, A. E. (1982). *Single-case research designs: Methods for clinical and applied settings.* New York: Oxford University.

Kearns, K. P. (1986). Flexibility of single-subject experimental designs. Part II: Design selection and arrangement of experimental phases. *Journal of Speech and Hearing Disorders, 51,* 204–214.

Kelman, H. C. (1972). Human use of human subjects: The problem of deception in social psychological experiments. *Psychological Bulletin, 67,* 1–11.

Kent, R. D. (1983). Issue IX: Role of research: How can we improve the role of research and educate speech–language pathologists and audiologists to be competent users of research? In N. S. Rees & T. L. Snope (Eds.), *Proceedings of the 1983 national conference on undergraduate, graduate, and continuing education* (pp. 76–86). Washington, DC: ASHA Reports no.13.

Kent, R. D. (1985). Science and the clinician: The practice of science and the science of practice. In R. D. Kent (Ed.), Application of research to assessment and therapy. *Seminars in Speech and Language, 6,* 1–12.

Kent, R. D. & Fair, J. (1985). Clinical research: Who, where, and how? In R. D. Kent (Ed.), Application of research to assessment and therapy. *Seminars in Speech and Language, 6,* 23–34.

Kerlinger, F. N. (1973). *Foundations of behavioral research.* New York: Holt, Rinehart, & Winston.

Kirszner, L. G. & Mandell, S. R. (1986). *The Holt handbook.* New York: Holt, Rinehart, & Winston.

Larsen, C. C. (1982). Taub conviction revives centuries-old debate. *APA Monitor,* (January), *1,* 12–13.

Lee, B. S. (1950) Effects of delayed speech feedback. *Journal of the Acoustical Society of America, 22,* 824–826.

Lee, B. S. (1951). Artificial stutter. *Journal of Speech and Hearing Disorders, 16,* 53–55.

Martlew, M. (1980). Mothers' control of strategies in dyadic mother/child conversations. *Journal of Psycholinguistic Research, 9,* 327–347.

McCall, W. A. (1923). *How to experiment in education.* New York: Macmillan.

McReynolds, L. V. & Engmann, D. L. (1974). An experimental analysis of the relationship between subject noun and object noun phrases. In L. V. McReynolds (Ed.), *Developing systematic procedures for training children's language.* (pp. 30–46). Rockville Pike, MD: Asha Monographs no.18.

McReynolds, L. V. & Kearns, K. P. (1983). *Single-subject experimental designs in communicative disorders.* Baltimore: University Park.

McReynolds, L. V. & Thompson, C. K. (1986). Flexibility of single-subject experimental designs. Part I: Review of the basics of single-subject designs. *Journal of Speech and Hearing Disorders, 51,* 194–203.

Metz, D. E. & Folkins, J. W. (1985). Protection of human subjects in speech and hearing research. *Asha, 27,* 25–29.

Milgram, S. (1977). Subject reaction: The neglected factor in the ethics of experimentation. *Hastings Center Report,* October.

Minifie, F. (1983). Knowledge and service: Does the foundation of the profession need shoring up? *Asha, 25,* 29–32.

Moll, K. (1983). Issue II: Graduate education. In N. S. Rees & T. L. Snope (Eds.), *Proceedings of the 1983 national conference on undergraduate, graduate, and continuing education.* (pp. 25–37). Washington, DC: *ASHA* reports no. 13.

Morris, W. & Morris, M. (1975). *Harper dictionary of contemporary usage.* New York: Harper & Row.

Newman, E. (1976). *A civil tongue.* New York: Warner.

Newsom, C., Favell, J. E., & Rincover, A. (1983). Side effects of punishment. In S. Axlerod & J. Apsche (Eds.), *The effects of punishment on human behavior* (pp. 285–316). New York: Academic.

Patton, M. Q. (1978). *Utilization-focused evaluation.* Beverly Hills: Sage.

Perkins, W. H. (1985). From clinical dispenser to clinical scientist. In R. D. Kent (Ed.), Application of research to assessment and therapy. *Seminars in Speech and Language, 6,* 13–21.

Perkins, W. H. (1986). The functions and malfunctions of theories and therapies. *Asha, 28,* 31–33.

Peterson, H. A. & Marquardt, T. P. (1981). *Appraisal and diagnosis of speech and language disorders.* Englewood Cliffs, NJ: Prentice-Hall.

Random House (1984). *The Random House thesaurus.* New York: Author.

Reiner, B. J. & Ludlow, C. L. (1981). Using MEDLINE for literature retrieval in the communicative disorders. *Asha, 23,* 655–662.

Resnick, J. H. & Schwartz, T. (1973). Ethical standards as an independent variable in psychological research. *American Psychologist, 28,* 134–139.

Ringel, R. L., (1972). The clinician and the researcher: An artificial dichotomy. *Asha, 14,* 351–353.

Ringel, R. L., Trachtman, L. E., & Prutting, C. A. (1984). The science in human communication sciences. *Asha, 26,* 33–37.

Rosenfeld, A. (1981). Animal rights vs. human health. *Science, 18,* 22.

Rusch, F. R. & Kazdin, A. E. (1981). Toward a methodology of withdrawal designs for the assessment of response maintenance. *Journal of Applied Behavior Analysis, 14,* 131–140.

Scherer, N. & Olswang, L. B. (1984). Role of mothers' expansions in stimulating children's language production. *Journal of Speech and Hearing Research, 27,* 387–396.

Shaughnessy, J. J. & Zechmeister, E. B. (1985). *Research methods in psychology.* New York: Alfred A. Knopf.

Sidman, M. (1960). *Tactics of scientific research.* New York: Basic Books.

Siegel, G. M. & Spradlin, J. E. (1985). Therapy and research. *Journal of Speech and Hearing Disorders, 50,* 226–230.

Sinclair, W. J. (1901). *Semmelweis: His life and his doctrine.* Manshester, England: Manchester University Press.

Skinner, B. F. (1953). *Science and human behavior.* New York: Free Press.

Skinner, B. F. (1956). A case history in scientific method. *American Psychologist, 11,* 221–233.

Skinner, B. F. (1969). *Contingencies of reinforcement: A theoretical analysis.* New York: Appleton-Century-Crofts.

Skinner, B. F. (1972). *Cumulative record: A selection of papers* (3rd ed.). New York: Appleton-Century-Crofts.

Skinner, B. F. (1974). *About behaviorism.* New York: Alfred A. Knopf.

Snow, C. E. & Ferguson, L. A. (1977). *Talking to children: Language input and acquisition*. London: Cambridge University.

Solomon, R. L. (1949). An extension of control group design. *Psychological Bulletin, 46,* 137–150.

Stevens, S. (1951). Mathematics, measurement, and psychophysics. In S. Stevens (Ed.), *Handbook of experimental psychology*. New York: Wiley.

Streng, A. H. (1972). *Syntax, speech, & hearing*. New York: Grune & Stratton.

Strunk, W., Jr. & White, E. B. (1979). *The elements of style* (3rd ed.). New York: Macmillan.

Taint of scholarly fraud (1976). *Time,* December 6, p. 66.

Tucker, D. J. & Berry, G. (1980). Teaching severely multihandicapped students to put on their own hearing aids. *Journal of Applied Behavior Analysis, 13,* 65–75.

Turabian, K. L. (1973). *A manual for writers of term papers, theses, and dissertations* (4th ed.). Chicago: University of Chicago.

Ulman, J. D. & Sulzer-Azaroff, B. (1975). Multielement baseline design in educational research. In E. Ramp, & G. Semb (Eds.), *Behavior analysis: Areas of research and application* (pp. 377–391). Englewood Cliffs, NJ: Prentice-Hall.

Ventry, I. M. & Schiavetti, N. (1980). *Evaluating research in speech pathology and audiology*. Reading, MA: Addison-Wesley.

Vetter, D. K. (1985). Evaluation of clinical intervention: Accountability. In R. D. Kent (Ed.), Application of research to assessment and therapy. *Seminars in Speech and Language, 6,* 55–65.

Wade, N. (1976). Animal rights: NIH cat sex study brings grief to New York museum. *Science, 194,* 162–167.

Wanaska, S. K. & Bedrosian, J. L. (1985). Conversational structure and topic performance in mother-child interactions. *Journal of Speech and Hearing Research, 28,* 579–584.

Wilson, D. (1976). *In search of penicillin*. New York: Alfred A. Knopf.

Yoder, D. (1984). To market. *Asha, 26,* 23–26.

Young, M. A. (1969a). Observer agreement: Cumulative effects of rating many samples. *Journal of Speech and Hearing Research, 12,* 135–143.

Young, M. A. (1969b). Observer agreement: Cumulative effects of repeated ratings of the same samples and knowledge of results. *Journal of Speech and Hearing Research, 12,* 144–155.

Young, M. A. (1975). Observer agreement for marking moments of stuttering. *Journal of Speech and Hearing Research, 18,* 530–540.

Zimmermann, G. N. (1984). Knowledge and service: Does the foundation of our science need shoring up? *Asha, 26,* 31–34.

Zinsser, W. (1980). *On writing well: An informal guide to writing nonfiction* (2nd ed.). New York: Harper & Row.

■ A P P E N D I X

List of Journals

The following list of journals is relevant for a literature search. It is not an exhaustive list. Periodically, new journals come into existence and some old ones cease publication. Also, not every issue of every journal listed contains papers on speech, language, or hearing. However, depending on the research question, a student may find it necessary to consult several of these journals.

Journals Published by the American Speech-Language-Hearing Association

Asha. This is a monthly journal devoted mostly to scientific, professional, governmental, organizational, and public affairs relative to speech-language pathology and audiology.

Journal of Speech and Hearing Disorders. Published quarterly, this journal contains papers that are of immediate clinical relevance. It publishes experimental and review articles, reports, and letters to the editor.

Journal of Speech and Hearing Research. Published quarterly, this journal contains studies on the processes and disorders of speech, language, and hearing. It publishes experimental, theoretical, review, and tutorial articles, and letters to the editor.

Language, Speech, and Hearing Services in Schools. This journal publishes papers that are especially relevant to the clinical services offered in the public schools.

ASHA Reports. These are periodic publications of proceedings of conferences on speech, language, and hearing sponsored wholly or partly by the American Speech-Language-Hearing Association.

ASHA Monographs. These are published irregularly. Each monograph is devoted to a particular issue or topic in speech, language, or hearing.

Other Journals of Interest to a Study of Communication and its Disorders

This list includes not only journals of speech, language, and hearing, but also selected medical, educational, psychological, and behavioral journals that are relevant to a scholarly literature research on specific topics of communication, communication disorders, and treatment.

Academic Therapy
Academy of Rehabilitative Audiology
American Annals of the Deaf
American Journal of Mental Deficiency
Annals of Dyslexia
Annals of Otology, Rhinology, and Laryngology
Applied Psycholinguistics
Archives of Otolaryngology-Head and Neck Surgery
Audiology
Australian Journal of Audiology
Australian Journal of Communication Disorders
Behavior Modification
Behavior Research and Therapy
Behavior Therapy
Behavioral and Brain Sciences
Behavioral neurosciences
Behaviorism
Brain: A Journal of Neurology
Brain and Language
British Journal of Audiology
British Journal of Disorders of Communication
Cleft Palate Journal
Child Development
Cognition
Cognitive Psychology
Cognitive Therapy and Research
Contemporary Psychology
Cortex
Developmental Psychology
Ear and Hearing
Folia Phoniatrica
Geriatrics
Hearing Instruments
Journal of Applied Behavior Analysis
Journal of Applied Psychology
Journal of Auditory Research
Journal of Autism and Developmental Disorders

Journal of Behavior Therapy and Experimental Psychiatry
Journal of Child Language
Journal of Clinical Psychology
Journal of Communication Disorders
Journal of Consulting and Clinical Psychology
Journal of Experimental Child Psychology
Journal of Fluency Disorders
Journal of Gerontology
Journal of Learning Disabilities
Journal of Phonetics
Journal of Psycholinguistic Research
Journal of Rehabilitation
Journal of the Acoustical Society of America
Journal of the British Association of Teachers of the Deaf
Journal of the Experimental Analysis of Behavior
Language and Learning
Language and Speech
Laryngoscope
Mental Retardation
Neuorology
Psychological Bulletin
Psychological Review
Scandinavian Audiology
Seminars in Hearing
Seminars in Speech and Language
Topics in Language Disorders
Volta Review

INDEX

Author

Altman, J., 115, 431
Andrews, G., 121, 433

Bachrach, A. J., 21, 41, 47, 62, 63, 431,
Baer, D. M., 27, 250, 257, 431,
Baker, S. , 374, 431
Bannister, D., 91, 431
Barlow, D. H., 9, 138, 140, 154, 217, 219,
    226, 234, 215, 255, 261, 262, 264,
    265, 283, 288, 294, 417, 418, 419,
    431
Barrass, R., 374, 431
Bates, J. D., 374, 385, 431
Batten , M., 29, 431
Bauer, H., 16, 431
Bedrosian, J. L., 116, 436
Berry, G., 257, 436
Binet, A., 106
Bloodstein, O., 114, 127
Bounds, W. G., Jr., 165, 433
Bracht, G. H., 151, 431
Brinton, B., 116, 431
Brown, R., 84, 110, 130, 431
Browning, R. M., 273, 431
Burt, C., 415

Campbell, B. G., 415, 431
Campbell, D. T., 165, 166, 175, 176, 186,
    190, 191, 431
Campbell, N., 104, 431
Cannon, W., 38, 431
Capelli, R., 83, 83, 432
Cattell, R., 106
Chomsky, N., 48, 49, 330, 432
Christensen, L. B., 140, 432
Cohen, L. H., 9, 432

Connell, P. J., 16, 217, 266, 432
Cook, T. D., 190, 191, 432
Cormier, W. H., 165, 433
Costello, J. M., 5, 8, 11, 14, 16, 432
Crandall, R., 415, 432
Curtis, J. F., 125, 358, 432

De Cesari, R., 83, 432
Diener, E., 415, 432

Eddington, E. S., 154, 432
Edwards, A. L., 165, 197, 432
Engmann, D. L., 250, 434

Fair, J., 11, 434
Favell, J. E., 264, 435
Feldman, A. S., 14, 432
Ferguson, L. A., 116, 435
Ferster, C. B., 29, 432
Fisher, R. A., 64, 165, 432
Fleming, A., 29, 38
Flower, R. M., 7
Folkins, J. W., 420, 421, 434
Follet, W., 375, 390, 432
Freeman, H. E., 98, 432
Fujiki, M., 116, 431

Gadlin, H., 91, 432
Galton, F., 106
Gittleman-Foster, N., 128, 432
Glass, G. V., 151, 190
Goldstein, H., 117, 433
Goodman, N., 49, 433
Gottman, J. M., 190, 433
Grmek, M. D., 33, 433

Hall, R. V., 270, 433
Hargis, C. H., 374, 433
Hartman, D., P., 270, 433
Hayes, C. S., 9, 217, 255, 262, 264, 274, 417, 431, 433
Hegde, M. N., 16, 48, 157, 250, 253, 254, 288, 433
Hersen, M., 138, 140, 154, 217, 219, 224, 226, 234, 251, 262, 264, 265, 283, 288, 294, 431
Hochberg, 14
Horner, R. D., 257, 433
Howie, P. M., 121, 433
Huck, W. S., 165, 433
Hurtig, R., 116, 433

Ingle, G., 91, 432
Ingham, R., 121, 433

Johnson, W., 60, 76, 77, 433
Johnston, J. M., 46, 104, 105, 106, 122, 138, 140, 141, 217, 433

Kamin, L. J., 415, 433
Kazdin, A. E., 150, 217, 219, 272, 273, 433, 435
Kearns, K. P., 16, 217, 236, 270, 433, 434
Kelman, H. C., 425, 434
Kent, R. D., 5, 7, 8, 11, 14, 15, 16, 434
Kerlinger, F. N., 62, 75, 78, 91, 129, 140, 165, 434
Kirszner, L. G., 374, 384, 387, 434
Koenigsknecht, R., 14

Larsen, C. C., 427, 343
Lee, B. S., 28, 30, 434
Ludlow, C. L., 351, 435

Mandell, S. R., 374, 384, 387, 434
Marquardt, T. P., 129, 435
Martlew, M., 116, 434
McCall, W. A., 165, 197, 434
McReynolds, L. V., 16, 217, 236, 250, 270, 434
Metz, D. E., 420, 421, 434
Minifie, F., 5, 7, 14, 15, 418, 434
Milgram, S., 425, 434
Moll. K., 5, 14, 434
Morris, M., 375, 434
Morris, W., 375, 434

Nelson, R. O., 9, 217, 255, 264, 417, 431
Newman, E., 375, 435

Newsom, C., 264, 435
Noll, M. J., 253, 433

Olswang, L. B., 117, 435

Patton, M. Q., 98, 435
Pecora, R., 253, 433
Pennypacker, H. S., 46, 104, 105, 122, 138, 140, 141, 217, 433
Perkins, W. H., 8, 11, 12, 15, 16, 418, 419, 435
Peterson, H. A., 129, 435
Prutting, C. A., 5, 8, 435
Punch, J., 8, 432

Quetelet, A., 106
Reiner, B. J., 351, 435
Resnick, J. H., 424, 435
Rincover, A., 264, 435
Ringel, R. L., 5, 8, 435
Risley, T. R., 27, 250, 431,
Rosenfeld, A., 427, 435
Rusch, F. R., 272, 273, 435

Scherer, N., 117, 435
Schery, T., 8, 432
Schiavetti, N., 129, 436
Schriberg, L., 8, 432
Schultz, M. C., 125, 358, 432
Schwartz, T., 424, 435
Shaughnessy, J. J., 165, 415, 435
Sidman, M., 23, 24, 39, 40, 62, 63, 138, 140, 141, 143, 217, 265, 283, 401, 406, 435
Siegel, G. M., 419, 435
Sinclair, W. J. , 38, 435
Skinner, B. F., 27, 29, 30, 38, 39, 47, 48, 63, 64, 106, 130, 342, 435
Snow, C. E., 116, 435
Soloman, R. L., 177, 178, 211, 214, 340, 435
Spradlin, J. E., 419, 435
Stanley, J. C., 165, 166, 175, 176, 186, 431
Stevens, S., 104, 436
Streng, A. H., 374, 436
Strunk, W., Jr., 375, 389, 436
Sulzer-Azaroff, B., 264, 265, 436

Thompson, C. K., 16, 217, 266, 432, 434
Trachtman, L. E., 5, 8, 435
Tucker, D. J., 257, 436
Turabian, K. L., 374, 436

Ulman, J. D., 264, 265, 436

Ventry, I. M., 129, 436
Vetter, D. K., 16, 436

Wade, N., 427, 436
Wanaska, S. K., 116, 436
White, E. B., 357, 389, 436
Wilson, D., 29, 436
Wilson, V. L., 190, 433

Wolf, M. M., 27, 250, 431
Woods, C. L., 121, 433

Yoder, D., 5, 436
Young, M. A., 127, 128, 436

Zechmeister, E. B., 374, 435
Zimmermann, G. N., 5, 436
Zinsser, W., 374, 436

INDEX

Subject

Abstracts
 characteristics of, 367
 how to write, 367
American Psychological Association (APA),
  364–367, 372, 374, 375, 394,
 the publication manual of, 364–367,
  372, 374, 375, 394, 420, 427
American Speech-Language-Hearing
  Associations, 365, 374
 publications of, 365
Astronomy, 52
Attrition
 as a factor in internal validity, 149

Baselines, 233–237
 criteria of, 233–237
  potential for contrast, 236–237
  reliability, 234
  stability, 234
 simultaneous multibaselines, 237–239
Basic research
 and applied experimental research, 90
 and clinical practice, 10–13
 definition of, 90

Causality and functional analysis, 56–60
 instigating versus maintaining causes,
  58–60
 multiple causation, 57–58
Clinical and applied research, 10–13, 93–96
 defined, 93
 descriptive and experimental, 94
 importance of, 94
Clinical–experimental research, 11–13, 93–96
Clinical practice
 the effect of research on, 9

Clinical psychology, 9
Clinical science, 15
Clinicians
 as consumers of research, 400
 as producers of research, 15–16
 and research, 8–9
Cognition, 56
Communicative behaviors
 measures of, 109–121
  duration, 111–112
  dyadic interaction,
  frequency, 109–111
  interresponse time, 112–113
  latency, 113–114
  momentary time sampling, 114–115
  time sampling, 114
  verbal interaction sampling, 115
Communicative disorders
 description of, 3
 historical course of, 3
 starting point of, 3
Control
 as an outcome of science, 51
Control mechanisms of group designs,
  171–173
 formation of control groups, 171–173
 matching, 171–173
 randomization, 171
Control mechanisms of single-subject
  designs
 baselines, 233–237
 criterion-referenced change, 229–230
 reinstatement of treatment, 226–228
 rapid alternations, 230–233
 replication, 221–222
 reversal of treatment, 224–226

Control mechanisms *(continued)*
  simultaneous multibaselines, 237–239
  withdrawal of treatment, 222–224
Controlling relation, 61
Correlational analysis design, 206–207
Counterbalanced within-subjects designs,
    196–205
  complex counterbalanced designs,
      200–201
  crossover design, 199–200
  description of, 196–197
  limitations of
    order effects, 201–202
    carryover effects, 202–204
    ceiling and floor effects, 205
  one-group single-treatment
      counterbalanced design, 197–199
  summary and summative evaluation of,
      205–206
Current trends. *See also* Information
    retrieval systems.
  how to identify, 349–353

Data, 27
  controlled, 71
  conclusions and
  defined, 70
  evidence and, 70–71
  replicated, 71
  uncontrolled, 71
Delayed auditory feed back, 28, 30
Dependent variables. *See* Variables
Designs of research,
  as means of controlling variability,
      141–143
  confused with statistics, 165
  definitions of, 135–136
  elements of, 135–136
  group designs
    advantages and disadvantages of,
        310–312
    carryover effects in, 202–204
    ceiling and floor effects, 205
    completely randomized factorial design,
        184–185, 210, 305, 307, 318,
        319
    complex counterbalanced designs,
        200–201
    correlational analysis design, 206–207,
        211–212
    counterbalanced within-subjects
        designs, 196–206, 212

crossover design, 199–200, 211, 318
factorial designs, 181–186, 210, 305,
    306, 307, 308, 318
formation of control groups in, 171–173
in clinical research, 207–209
Latin square designs, 200–201
multigroup posttest-only design,
    180–181, 210
multigroup pretest-posttest design,
    179–180, 210, 305, 318
multiple-group time-series designs,
    194–196, 211
nonequivalent control group design,
    187–189, 304
one-group pretest-posttest design,
    168–169, 210, 302, 318
one-group single-treatment
    counterbalanced design,
    197–198, 211
one-shot case study, 167–168, 210
order effects in, 201–202
posttest-only control group design,
    176–177, 210, 304, 318
preexperimental designs, 167–170
pretest-posttest control group design,
    173–176, 210, 304, 318
quasiexperimental designs, 186–196,
    212
randomized blocks design, 182–184,
    210, 305, 306, 319
separate sample pretest-posttest design,
    189–190
single-group time-series designs,
    190–194, 211
Soloman four-group design, 177–179,
    210
static-group comparison, 169–170, 210
summary and applications of, 210–211
terminology and characteristics of, 165
time-series designs, 190–196, 212, 304,
    305, 308, 318, 319
true experimental designs, 171–186, 211
problems common to, 313–315
single-subject designs, 241–278
  AB design, 241–242, 276, 302, 318
  ABA design, 242, 276, 278, 318
  ABA reversal design, 244–246, 304,
      318
  ABA withdrawal design, 242–244, 304
  ABAB design, 247–250, 276, 278,
      304, 305, 318
  ABACA/ACABA design, 259–261, 277,

278, 305, 318
advantages and disadvantages of,
    312–313
alternating treatments design, 261–264,
    277–278, 305, 318
BAB design, 246–247, 276, 278, 304,
    318
baselines in, 233–237
basic terminology and characteristics of
carryover and contrast effects in,
    264–266
changing criterion design, 270–71,
    277–278, 305, 318
clinical research and, 275
control mechanisms in, 221–241
criterion-referenced change in, 229–230
designs to assess response maintenance,
    271–273, 238
ineffective treatments in multiple
    treatment evaluations, 265–266
interactional design, 266–270, 277–278,
    306, 307, 308, 318, 319
multiple baseline designs, 250–259,
    277–278, 304, 305, 318
multiple treatment comparisons,
    259–271
order effects and counterbalancing in,
    263–264
periodic treatments design, 274–275
preexperimental, 241–242
rapid alternations in, 230–233
reinstatement in, 226–228
replications in, 221–222
reversal of treatment in, 224–226
simultaneous multibaselines in,
    237–239
simultaneous treatments design,
    273–274, 307, 319
summary and applications of, 276–277
withdrawal of treatment in, 222–224
structure and logic of, 136–137
variability and, 137–141
Determinism, 45
Diffusion of treatment
as a factor in internal validity, 150
Dissemination of research findings, 428
Doctorate
Professional, 14
research, 14
Dyadic interaction, 116

Education and training models

of speech–language pathologists, 13–16
Effects of science on society, 416–417
Empiricism, 45–47
Ethics of research
and effects of science on society, 416–417
and honesty and integrity of scientists,
    414–416
dissemination of research findings and, 428
evaluation of established clinical practice
    and, 417–420
protecting animal subjects and, 4278
protection of human subjects and,
    420–426
    APA guidelines of, 420
    debriefing and, 425
    disclosure problem in, 424–425
    informed consent in, 423–425
    Institutional Review Boards and,
        421–426
    National Research act and, 420–421
    privacy of subjects and, 425–426
    risk/benefit ratio and, 422–423
relative to treatment evaluation, 417–420
Ethology, 50
Evaluation of design strategies, 301–322
    advantages of group designs, 310–311
    advantages of single-subject designs, 312
    disadvantages of group designs, 311–312
    disadvantages of single-subject designs,
        312–313
    philosophic considerations in, 315
    soundness of data in, 316–317
Evaluation of research reports, 16–17,
    401–411
    an outline for, 407–410
    appreciation and, 411
    external relevance, 405–407
    internal consistency, 402–405
    the need for, 400–401
    understanding and, 400–401
Evaluation research, 98–99
    defined, 98
    types of, 98–99
        comprehensive evaluation, 99
        impact evaluation, 99
        process evaluation, 98
Evidence, 70–71
Experiment
    defined, 60
    procedures of, 60–61
Experimental control, 60
Experimental research, 87–93

Experimental research *(continued)*
basic and applied, 90–91
procedures of, 87–90
strengths and weaknesses of, 91–93
Explanation, 51
Ex post facto research, 75–79
defined, 75
procedures of, 76–77
strengths and weaknesses of, 77–79
External validity. *See* Generality

Factorial designs, 181–185. *See also* Designs
of research
Format of scientific reports, 364–373
abstract, 367
according to APA, 364–373
appendix, 372
discussion, 370
introduction, 367
method, 368–370
references
results, 370
title page, 366

Generality, 27, 151–159, 283–298, 406
defined, 151
failed replications and, 291–294
generalization and, 160
Hawthorne effect and, 158
Homo- and heterogeneity of subjects and,
296–297
multiple treatment interference and, 158
of treatment variables and treatment
packages, 294–296
pretest-posttest sensitization and, 157–158
procedures of establishing, 283–291
direct replication, 283–287
homogeneous subjects and, 285–287
systematic replication, 287–291
types of,
across experimenters, 156–157
across response classes, 157
across settings, 156
across subjects, 155–156
clinical replication, 294
inferential, 152–154
logical, 154–155

History
as a factor in internal validity, 13
Human subjects protection procedures,
420–426. *See also* Ethics of research

Hypothesis
accidental discovery and, 24
defined, 24
in scientific research, 61–65
null hypothesis, 64–65
the need for, 62–65
theory and, 62
Information retrieval systems
abstracts, 350–351
Comprehensive Dissertation Index, 350
Cumulted Index Medicus, 350
Deafness, Speech, and Hearing (dsh)
abstracts, 350
Dissertation Abstracts International, 350
Eric (Educational Resources Information
Center), 351
Exceptional Child Education Resources,
351
Linguistics and Language behavior
Abstracts, 351
MEDLINE, 351
PsychINFO, 351
Psychological Abstracts, 350
Instrumentation
as a factor in internal validity, 147
Internal validity, 144–151
factors that affect
attrition, 149
diffusion of treatment, 150
history, 145
instrumentation, 147
maturation, 146
statistical regression, 148
subject selection, 149
testing, 146

Literature search, *see* Information retrieval
systems

Matching, 172–173
Maturation
as a factor in internal validity, 146
Measurement
client assisted, 117
covert measurement, 119–121
defined, 105
idemnotic, 105
indirect measures, 118–119
levels of, 107–109
interval, 108
nominal, 107
ordinal, 108

ratio, 109
observer and, 121–124
of communicative behaviors, 109–121
philosophies of, 105, 334–336
reliability of, 126–129
self report and, 118–119
vaganotic, 105
Mentalism, 56
Multiple baseline designs, 27, 28, 250–259
across behaviors, 250–254
across settings, 256–257
across subjects, 254–256
additional controls in, 258–259
problems of repeated baselines in, 257–258
Multiple treatment evaluations, 179–185,
259–270
designs for
ABACA/ACABA design, 259–261
alternating treatments design, 261–263
factorial designs, 181–185
ineffective treatments in, 265–266
multigroup posttest-only design, 180–181
multigroup pretest–posttest design,
179–180

Nativism, 330
Normative research, 79–84
age as an independent variable in, 83–84
defined, 79
norms and, 80
procedures of, 80–81
strengths and weaknesses of, 81–84

Observation, 104–105
and measurement, 104–105
as a sensory process, 104
everyday and scientific, 104
mechanical aids and, 124
observer and, 121–124
Observer, 121–124
biases of, 121–122
training of, 122–124
Outcome of scientific activity, 50–52
control, 51–52
description, 50
explanation, 51
prediction, 51
understanding, 51

Penicillin
the accidental discovery of, 29–30
Periodic treatments design, 274

Philosophy,
as methodology, 326
handling methodological problems with,
339–342
interplay between methodology and,
342–343
of the science of speech and language,
329–339
of subject matters, 327–328
Physics, 7
Physiology, 7
Population
defined, 25, 171
in group designs, 171–172
Preexperimental designs, 167–170

Quasiexperimental designs, 186–196

Random procedure, 171–172
limitations of, 207–209
Rationalism, 330
Reasoning,
and theory construction, 66–69
deductive, 66–69
deductive and inductive compared, 68–69
inductive, 66–69
Reliability
correlation and, 128
defined, 126
interobserver, 126–128
intraobserver, 126–128
of tests vs. research data, 129
Young's formula of, 127–128
Replication, 283–299
and development of treatment packages,
294
direct, 283–287
failed, 291–294
homo- and heterogeneity of subjects in,
296–298
systematic, 287–291
Research
accidental, 28–30
apparatus failure and, 39–40
definition of, 22, 75, 421
formal view of, 31–33
formative view of, 33
reasons for doing
curiosity, 23–24, 30,
explanation of events, 24–26, 30
solve practical problems, 26–28, 30
demonstration of certain effects, 28–30

Research *(continued)*
  Science and, 21–22
  Types of
    applied 19
    basic, 9–10, 13
    clinical and applied, 9–13, 93–96
    evaluation research, 98–99
    ex post facto, 75–79
    experimental, 3, 9–13, 87–93
    normative, 11, 79–84
    research questions and, 99–101
    sample surveys, 96–98
    standard-group comparisons, 84–87
Research Designs, *See* Designs of research
Research papers
  formats of, 364–373
    appendix, 372
    discussion, 370–371
    introduction, 367–368
    method, 368–370
    references, 372
    results, 370
  types of, 365–366
  unpublished, 30–31
Research questions
  and investigative strategies, 301–310
  description of, 302–310, 347–348
  how to formulate, 348–359
  methodology and, 355–359
  significance of, 356–357
  where to find, 348–359
Response maintenance
  designs to assess, 271–273

Sample, 171–172
Sample surveys, 96–98
  defined, 96
  limitations of, 97–98
Scholasticism, 45–46
Science
  as a philosophy, 45
  as a set of methods, 49–50
  as behavior, 47–49
  definition of, 45
  methodology of, 60–65
  misconceptions about, 44
  outcome of, 50–52
  predictions in, 51
Scientific laws, 69–70
Scientific method,
  the need to study, 4–6
    the legal and social considerations and, 4

  professional and scientific
    considerations and, 5
Scientists
  characteristics of, 47–49
  misconceptions about, 47–48
Serendipity in research, 37–40
Simultaneous treatments design, 273
Single subject strategy, 16, 217–281
standard-group comparisons, 84–87
  defined, 84
  procedures of, 84–86
  strengths and weaknesses of, 86–87
Statistics, 15, 16
  and experimental designs, 15, 165
Statistical regression
  as a factor in internal validity, 148–149
Statistical versus clinical significance, 208,
    219
Subject selection bias
  as a factor in internal validity, 149
Syllogisms, 67

Technology, 26, 45–46
  defined, 26
  and research, 26
Testing
  as a factor in internal validity, 146
Theories
  and hypothesis, 62, 65
  and scientific laws, 69–70
  dangers of deductive, 68–69
  defined, 65
  deductive, 25, 66–69
  inductive, 25, 66–69
  inductive and deductive compared, 67–69
  logic and, 66–69
  process of constructing, 66–69
Theses and dissertations,
  preparation of, 359–361
Time-series designs, 190–195
Treatment
  definition of, 25
  evaluation of, 27
True experimental (group) designs, 171–185

Validity, 27
  defined, 143–144
  of experimental operations, 143–159
  types of, 151–159
    external, 151–159,
    internal, 144–151, 402, 403
Variables

active and assigned, 55
defined, 52
dependent, 53, 331–334
  integrity of, 340–441
  magnitude of change in, 341–442
  problems associated with, 331–334
independent, 53–54
  kinds of, 55
  locus of, 336–339
intervening, 56
Variability, 137–143
description of, 137–138
group designs and, 141–143
intersubject
  philosophic ways of handling, 339–340
  statistical means of handling, 142–143
single-subject designs and, 141–143
types of
  error, 140
  extraneous, 140
  extrinsic, 140–141, 339
  intrinsic, 138–139, 339

random, 140
systematic, 140

Writing scientific reports
APA format of, 364–373
and rewriting, 395–396
conceptual considerations in, 384–394
  adequate writing, 388–389
  clear writing, 389–393
  coherent writing
  concise writing, 385–388
  knowledge of the readership, 384–385
structural principles of, 374–384
  agreement, 377–380
  modifiers, 380–381
  parallel forms, 381–383
  sentence structure, 375–384
  shifts within and between sentences,
    383–384
  verbs, 376–377
style of, 394–395
without bias, 373–374